LIVING WELL WITH

Autoimmune Disease

Also by Mary J. Shomon
Living Well with Hypothyroidism

LIVING WELL WITH

Autoimmune Disease

What Your Doctor

Doesn't Tell You . . .

That You Need to Know

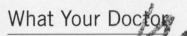
MARY J. SHOMON

HarperResource

An Imprint of HarperCollinsPublishers

HarperCollins books may be purchased for educational, business,
or sales promotional use. For information please write: Special
Markets Department, HarperCollins Publishers Inc., 10 East 53rd
Street, New York, NY 10022.

FIRST EDITION

Designed by Joy O'Meara Battista

Library of Congress Cataloging-in-Publication Data

Shomon, Mary J.
    Living well with autoimmune disease : what your doctor
doesn't tell you . . . that you need to know / Mary J. Shomon.
        p.   cm.
    Includes bibliographical references and index.
    ISBN 0-06-093819-6
    1. Autoimmune diseases—Popular works. I. Title.

RC600 .S465   2002
616.97'8—dc21
                                                        2002023305

02   03   04   05   06   WBC/RRD   10   9   8   7   6   5   4   3   2   1

This book is dedicated with love to my mother, Patricia, who has shown me that miracles do happen, and that true healing and remarkable recovery are possible.

CONTENTS

ACKNOWLEDGMENTS

I would like to acknowledge my husband, Jon Mathis, who provided tremendous support, advice, and assistance. Without his love and support, this book would not have been possible. I also want to thank my daughter, Julia, who was very patient while Mommy was "making a book."

Special thanks to family, friends, and supporters who provided love, support, assistance, patience, and encouragement along the way, including Dan Shomon, Sr.; Pat Shomon; Dan Shomon, Jr.; Barbara and Russell Mathis; Jeannie Yamine; Michele Abdow; Julia Schopick; Angela Cannon; Sandy Levy; Kate Lemmerman, MD; the Momfriends list; Ric and Diane Blake; Genevieve Piturro and Demo DeMartile; Elizabeth Mensah-Engmann; Rosario and Ana Quintanilla.

For top-notch research, writing, Internet, consulting, and technical help, I am very thankful for the assistance of Sheila Ali-Oston, Kim Conley, Willow Curry, Dale Dermott, Laura Horton, Jody La-Ferriere, Beth Weise Moeller, Louise Shapiro, Sarah Vela, and Vickie Queen.

This book would not be a reality without my agent, Carol Mann, and my editor at HarperCollins, Sarah Durand, who both helped guide its direction and were a joy to work with on this project. I also want to include special thanks to Gail Ross of the Gail Ross Literary Agency.

Special thanks go to the American Autoimmune Related Diseases Association (AARDA) and its founder, president, and executive director, Virginia T. Ladd, RT, and chairperson of AARDA's

Scientific Advisory Board, Noel R. Rose, MD, PhD, who are truly inspirational pioneers in the effort to better understand autoimmune diseases and help those who suffer with these conditions.

I offer my gratitude and appreciation to the experts, practitioners, and organizations who generously contributed time, information, and ideas, or agreed to be interviewed for the book, including Eric Berg, DC; David Brownstein, MD; Kim Carmichael-Cox; Tracee Cornforth; Phylameana lila Désy; Laura Dolson; John V. Dommisse, MD; Carol Eustice; Richard Eustice; Richard "Dr. Rich" Fogoros, MD; Gillian Ford; Paula Ford-Martin; Veronica Froman; Larrian Gillespie, MD; Rick Hall, MS, RD; Ronald Hoffman, MD; Leonard Holmes, PhD; Donna Hurlock, MD; Phyllis Jacobs; Karta Purkh Singh Khalsa; Mary Kugler, MSN, RN, C; Virginia T. Ladd, RT; Stephen Langer, MD; Lisa Lorden; John C. Lowe, DC; Gina Honeyman-Lowe, DC; Andrea Maloney Schara, LCSWA; Dr. Chuck Meece; Joseph Mercola, DO; Don Michael, MD; Viana Muller, PhD; Michael Phillips; Debra Pozen; Gary Presley; Christina Puchalski, MD; Patrick Purdue, DOM, AP; Carol Roberts, MD; Noel R. Rose, MD, PhD; Marie Savard, MD; James Scheer; Sherrill Sellman; Karilee Halo Shames, RN, PhD; Richard Shames, MD; Melissa Stöppler, MD; Alan Tillotson, PhD, AHG, DAy; and Amber Tresca. Thanks also go to the many autoimmune disease patients who generously contributed their stories and experiences.

And, finally, thanks to the millions of women and men who struggle daily with autoimmune diseases—who keep trying to get the right diagnosis and treatment, who keep getting out of bed despite the pain, who keep going to work despite the fatigue, and who keep inspiring their friends, families, and colleagues. Your sheer courage, strength, and ability to persevere have inspired me, and I can only hope to return the favor in some small way.

"Where there is great love, there are always miracles!"
—*Willa Cather*

PART I

Understanding Autoimmune Disease

1

Introduction

When I was first diagnosed with hypothyroidism, I didn't have any idea what or where the thyroid was, or what it actually did. My doctor phoned to let me know that my thyroid was a little underactive, called in a prescription to the pharmacy, and that was the extent of the diagnosis and treatment. Months after I began thyroid hormone replacement, I was still struggling with continuing symptoms. My hair was falling out and clogging the drain. I was waking up each morning with sore and achy joints and muscles. Just a few hours of typing on the computer would set off a major attack of carpal tunnel syndrome in my forearms and wrists. My eyes became scratchy and my vision blurry due to dryness. My hands and feet frequently tingled and went numb.

I decided to find out more about my condition and read a book from the 1970s explaining that the main cause of hypothyroidism was actually an autoimmune disease called Hashimoto's thyroiditis. The book offered little insight into the causes and treatment for this condition. All it suggested was that having one autoimmune disease could increase the risk of developing other autoimmune conditions. The prospect of having one poorly understood condition was frightening and was made far worse by the idea that I was also at higher risk for lupus, multiple sclerosis, diabetes, or worse.

I asked my doctor to refer me to an endocrinologist—a specialist in endocrine diseases. When I consulted with the endocrinologist, I asked her if I could be tested for Hashimoto's thyroiditis. "We could do that," she responded, "but what's the point of spending the money? Because the fact that your hypothyroidism may be caused by an autoimmune disease is not going to change anything." But the truth is, my hypothyroidism was ultimately caused by an autoimmune disease—Hashimoto's thyroiditis. And that *does* change everything.

It changes the way I should eat. The symptoms I should monitor more closely. The vitamins, minerals, herbs, and supplements I should take. The types of doctors I should visit. The ways I should manage stress. Even the water I should drink. And it changes the way I should feed my young daughter and care for her health now to protect her in the future.

That's why I wrote *Living Well with Autoimmune Disease*. Because autoimmune disease does matter . . . and because we need to know more.

Variations of my story are repeated every day when a patient with autoimmune thyroid disease wonders, as I did, if the tingling and numbness are actually signs of impending multiple sclerosis. Or when the woman with lupus asks how she got the condition and is offered nothing more than a shrug of the shoulders from a doctor. Or when a person with Sjögren's syndrome worries that the dry eyes and mouth are a harbinger of other autoimmune diseases to come but is told there's nothing that can be done to prevent them, so why worry. Or when a pregnant woman wonders whether her baby will be at greater risk of developing an autoimmune disease someday.

But for most autoimmune diseases, the best that medicine can do is keep some of the symptoms at bay. The root cause of the condition, or any potential to cure the autoimmune disease, is rarely—if at all—addressed. And that means you may ultimately feel afraid.

Afraid because once the immune system has turned on you, you may start on a seemingly downward health spiral characterized by development of other autoimmune conditions.

Afraid because multiple autoimmune conditions are frequently accompanied by dramatically worsening allergies, heightened chemical sensitivities, hormonal imbalances, and a host of other debilitating and life-changing symptoms.

Afraid because you've perhaps only just learned to deal with your diagnosed condition and now you suspect that every new symptom, every new ache or pain, might signal the onset of another new and insidious autoimmune disease.

Afraid because, for the most part, doctors throw up their hands when you ask, "What can I do about my autoimmune condition?" And afraid because your doctors just shake their heads, perplexed, when you ask, "How can I avoid getting more autoimmune-related diseases?" And afraid because most doctors don't have an answer to the critical question: "Is there anything I can do to help prevent my children from developing autoimmune diseases?"

Afraid because, over time, chronic malfunctioning of the immune system can ultimately lead to various cancers.

Afraid that there's no way to recapture your health, no way to slow or halt the inexorable march of an immune system gone haywire as it launches each new attack on another part of your body.

Afraid that there are no answers.

But there are answers.

You just aren't likely to hear them from the typical HMO (Health Maintenance Organization) doctor, who may not even recognize or easily diagnose many autoimmune conditions, much less know how to treat them—particularly given the constraints of the typical HMO-mandated 15-minute-or-less appointment.

And the answers aren't likely to be forthcoming from the average primary care doctor, or GP, or ob-gyn—the doctors most of us see for our day-to-day medical care. These doctors rush through dozens of patients a day and barely have time to keep up with key developments in the most studied conditions such as heart disease and cancer, much less time to delve into complicated and often misunderstood autoimmune diseases.

And even those doctors who consider themselves experts in treating the most common autoimmune diseases rarely venture into the uncharted territory of actually dealing with the autoimmune process itself. Most are content to focus on treating symptoms. So endocrinologists give insulin for diabetes and thyroid hormone replacement for thyroid disease. Rheumatologists prescribe pain relievers and immunosuppressives for rheumatoid arthritis. Gastroenterologists offer surgeries and drugs for Crohn's disease. But ask these doctors about the autoimmune implications of the conditions and they may draw a blank.

The term *autoimmune disease* and the concept of autoimmunity weren't even articulated or understood until the late 1950s. And although autoimmune disease has been studied by experts and researchers since that time, how and why we develop autoimmune diseases has not been widely covered by popular medicine. Most of us don't find regular newspaper reports of the latest research findings on risks and causes of autoimmune disease. We don't find pamphlets in our doctors' offices on how to avoid developing an autoimmune condition. There are no autoimmunologists—specialists who diagnose and treat the spectrum of autoimmune diseases.

This is in sharp contrast to cancer, for example. When it comes to cancer, every day new information is released about risk factors and lifestyle issues. We know that smoking can cause lung cancer, that obesity and a high-fat diet may contribute to the risk of developing breast cancer, that excessive sunbathing causes skin cancer. If you've had cancer, there are a variety of recommendations regarding diet, exercise, supplements, and lifestyle to prevent recurrence. And there are cancer hospitals, specialists, nutritionists, holistic experts, alternative clinics, and many other cancer-focused experts and resources. When you fill out a medical history form, there are questions about family history of cancer.

Why don't we have the same approach for autoimmune disease? Some people would say it's because autoimmune diseases aren't that common. But they would be wrong. The American Autoimmune Related Diseases Association (AARDA), the only national organization dedicated specifically to autoimmune diseases, states that approximately 50 million Americans, or 20 percent of the population, suffer from autoimmune diseases.

Others believe that it's because autoimmune diseases are usually chronic and because they affect primarily women. Dr. Denise Faustman, associate professor at Harvard Medical School and director of the Immunobiology Laboratory at Massachusetts General Hospital, shared her thoughts in an Associated Press interview:

Middle-aged women are not fashionable—and they are the main victims. It's fashionable to talk about young people dying, children dying. But it's not fashionable to talk about some woman who can't walk down the hallway or loses her job because of arthritis. It's slow and chronic and you don't die and get the attention.

However, autoimmune diseases are one of the ten leading causes of all deaths among U.S. women age 65 and younger. According to AARDA, separate from accidents, homicides, and suicides, autoimmune diseases are the seventh leading cause of death by disease among females ages 1 to 14 and the fifth leading cause of death by disease among females ages 15 to 44.

Finally, there's the problem that autoimmune diseases just aren't viewed collectively. Periodically, you'll hear about individual autoimmune conditions. Monaco's Princess Caroline was bald for several years due to the autoimmune disease alopecia. Former Mouseketeer Annette Funicello and talk show host Montel Williams are both publicly battling the autoimmune disease multiple sclerosis. Mary Tyler Moore is a well-known advocate for type I diabetes, having suffered from it since childhood. Radio host Rush Limbaugh suffers from autoimmune-related hearing loss. But rarely are autoimmune diseases discussed comprehensively as a category of conditions.

If autoimmune disease is overlooked at the system-wide level, it is also overlooked at the individual level. I was a fairly typical story. At age 31, I had a bad bout of Epstein-Barr virus, followed by months of slow recuperation. Then, at age 32, I started noticing slow, steady weight gain, increasing fatigue, and slight depression. When I went to the doctor three times within six months complaining about these symptoms and determined to get answers, she decided she needed to test my thyroid, and at age 33, I was diagnosed. If I date the onset of my autoimmune disease back to the viral illness, it was about 2½ years until I was formally diagnosed with Hashimoto's thyroiditis. But I was actually lucky. According to AARDA, the typical autoimmune disease patient faces years of visits to many different doctors before being correctly diagnosed.

Trusting your own instincts is really the critical first step. But some of us are our own worst enemies. We accept it as a given that after pregnancy, or during menopause, or once we hit our 60s, we're bound to lose hair, suffer appetite and weight changes, feel weak, lose our sex drive, or be unable to sleep through the night. We assume that bone-numbing fatigue is a normal by-product of a busy schedule and chronic lack of sleep. We look for quick fixes for each problem. We get depressed, so we take antidepressants. We gain weight, so we take diet drugs. We have muscle pains and aches, so we take pain relievers. We don't put the clues together ourselves and we miss the bigger picture.

Getting an expert—the right one who can make the right diagnosis—to take you seriously is another important step. Even when we haven't missed the bigger picture, doctors might. I receive hundreds of letters from patients each week, and I hear the same stories over and over again from women and men who suspect they have a health problem—some even suspect an autoimmune condition—but are told to leave the diagnosing to the experts, or whose HMOs refuse to refer them to specialists, or who are told by physicians, "Of course you're tired, depressed, and feeling sore and achy . . . you work too hard and aren't getting enough sleep." Or, most commonly, people who are being seen by doctors suffer from what I think doctors may call stressed, depressed, and PMSed syndrome, because the doctors assume that seemingly vague symptoms such as fatigue, weakness, and mild depression are signs of stress, or, in women, hormonal problems. Their doctors typically send them home with antidepressants, sleeping pills, pain relievers, or estrogen replacement, rather than looking for an underlying condition to explain the problems.

Margaret, now in her 60s, did not feel healthy most of her life. She noticed numb hands and feet in her late 20s. After having several children, the numbness returned when she was 40, along with fatigue and sleep problems. Margaret kept returning from numerous doctors with prescriptions for Valium. When she reached her 50s, the numbness worsened, and the fatigue became indescribable. Says Margaret:

> *This time, with an MRI of my brain, I was finally given a diagnosis of multiple sclerosis. I was subsequently also diagnosed with autoimmune hypothyroidism. It seems I was born a number of years too early for so complicated an autoimmune disease to be properly diagnosed and corrected.*

Another woman, Penny, was in her late 40s, with adult children, and she and her husband were finally ready to enjoy life on their own again, when, as she puts it, "my world crumbled." For two years, she suffered with shortness of breath, dizziness, and excessive fatigue. She was diagnosed as having panic attacks and was prescribed

Zoloft. After another two years, her hair was falling out in clumps, she had a large goiter on her neck, and, as she describes it, "my husband and I both thought I was having a nervous breakdown, and my twenty-five-year marriage was on the rocks." Another doctor finally diagnosed her with hyperthyroidism, and after treatment, she was able to get her health and her life back on track.

While Margaret and Penny were both diagnosed, there's not always an easy answer for every patient. Some people may have a whole host of symptoms that point to, but are not fully diagnosable as, various autoimmune diseases. These symptoms may come and go, vary in intensity, but may never be sufficient to qualify for a complete diagnosis.

After a partial hysterectomy and a bout of swollen neck glands, Joanne started experiencing facial and body spasms, difficulty walking, and reflexes that overreacted to any stimulus, such as an unexpected touch, sound, sight, or taste. Joanne was initially diagnosed with allergies. When further tests ruled out epilepsy, she was then diagnosed as having had a nervous breakdown, then tested again for epilepsy, which came up negative. Traditional doctors said she was having simple muscle spasms, and a naturopath said she had myasthenia gravis. Neurologists then ruled out the myasthenia gravis but thought perhaps it was multiple sclerosis. More time passed before doctors diagnosed a rare autoimmune disease called stiff-man syndrome. Her condition deteriorating, it was discovered that Joanne had almost no calcium, and she was hospitalized, near death. More tests revealed she had celiac disease. Subsequently, tests said that she did not have stiff-man syndrome. After months of being bedridden, a visiting nurse came to do blood work, and Joanne was also diagnosed with Hashimoto's thyroiditis and put on thyroid hormone replacement. Says Joanne:

Within four days, I was out of bed, stretching and relearning how to walk. Within two weeks, I was walking around the block. For the first time in eight years, I felt positive energy in my body and my attitude. Eventually my health improved. I am in pain, but not as much as I was. Pills have been reduced from twenty plus to around four a day. Depression and extreme fatigue are my major enemies . . . I am better. So, is it all in my mind? I know it's not. When I wake up after a night's sleep and can't move anything but my mouth, I know so. It's been a battle with doctors just to get them to understand what happens to me. Getting them to question why is even more difficult.

It is for people like Joanne, Penny, Margaret—and you—that I wrote this book. *Living Well with Autoimmune Disease* will help you trust your own instincts, pinpoint symptoms, and find the right practitioner to help you get a diagnosis.

You need this book if

- You have a variety of vague but troublesome symptoms and want to investigate your risk factors for autoimmune disease, and whether your symptoms fit any particular patterns
- You have family members with autoimmune conditions and you want to reduce your own risk wherever possible
- You have been diagnosed with an autoimmune disease and want to have a better understanding of your condition, and what autoimmunity really means
- You have been diagnosed with an autoimmune disease and are not receiving optimal treatment—conventional and/or alternative—for your condition, and are looking for more information in order to feel well
- You have an autoimmune disease and want to avoid developing related conditions
- You are an open-minded health practitioner who wants to understand patients' perspectives on autoimmune conditions,

as well as some of the cutting-edge ways other practitioners are dealing with these conditions

Living Well with Autoimmune Disease will help you go beyond treatments that merely manage symptoms, to discover cutting-edge approaches that can actually reduce and even reverse the autoimmune response, reduce or eliminate symptoms, and, in some cases, even cure autoimmune conditions entirely.

After reading *Living Well with Autoimmune Disease,* you will

- Have the knowledge and an important tool—the Autoimmune Disease Risk Factors and Symptoms Checklist, featured in Chapter 15—to help you get a proper diagnosis
- Better understand what it means to have an autoimmune disease, and the impact the autoimmune process has on current and future health
- Have far greater insight into the environmental, genetic, hereditary, nutritional, and mind–body factors that make us more or less susceptible to autoimmune disease
- Know the key symptoms, diagnostic procedures, and conventional treatments for the most common autoimmune diseases
- Learn about the most innovative and promising new and alternative treatments for key autoimmune diseases—for example, the diet that can completely cure some cases of diabetes, or the antibiotic therapy that offers hope for rheumatoid arthritis sufferers (treatments that you are not likely to hear about from your doctor)
- Find out where to go—how to find the best doctors, books, patient organizations, experts, websites, resources—for more information on conventional and alternative treatments for key autoimmune conditions
- Hear from some of our most innovative practitioners about their truly cutting-edge theories and practical approaches to

slowing, stalling, or even reversing the autoimmune disease process

Living Well with Autoimmune Disease offers practical support and advice to move beyond simply living with a condition, to actively working to balance and strengthen your own immune system. In this book, you'll find the tools you need to take a proactive role in improving your own health, and perhaps even preventing further autoimmune attacks on the body.

My hope is that you come away from this book understanding that having an autoimmune disease is like having two separate conditions: the actual condition and its obvious symptoms plus an underlying, general autoimmune dysfunction, which deserves special attention. And I also hope that you will come away from this book aware of the innovative responses to autoimmune dysfunction that may help you manage your condition, reduce symptoms, prevent future health problems, and perhaps most importantly, give you hope.

2

The Immune System and Autoimmune Disease

Your immune system is your body's defense system, its way to protect you from potentially harmful invaders such as bacteria, viruses, and other potential dangers. The immune system is an elaborate and complicated system. There's no single organ or process you can point to as your immune system. The immune system actually includes a network of cells and organs that communicate with each other to accomplish three key purposes: (1) to identify and recognize the invaders; (2) to put up barriers to prevent them from gaining access to the body's cells and organs; and (3) if bacteria or viruses do manage to attack, or cancerous cells and growths manage to proliferate, to then isolate, deactivate, and in some cases destroy those invaders or cancers, and prevent them from spreading or doing further harm to the body.

Technically, the immune system targets antigens. An antigen is a molecule—usually a protein—found on the surface of substances that can potentially harm your body. Antigens exist on living organisms such as viruses, bacteria, parasites, fungus, and molds, and on nonliving substances such as chemicals, drugs, pet dander, dust, and even components of foods.

The whole point of the immune system is to recognize and then destroy substances that have antigens. Fundamental to this process is the immune system's ability to recognize antigens versus our own cells. You, your cells, organs, tissue, blood, and so on, are all referred to as "self." The body's cells carry a marker that identifies them as self. Normally the immune system does not attack anything carrying a self marker. This process of peaceful coexistence is called *self-tolerance*.

Antigens, however, all carry markers. And the immune system has a unique ability to recognize millions of those antigens and to respond to them as "nonself." Once recognized as antigens, the immune system responds by producing antibodies, natural killer cells and other defenders that mount an appropriate defense or attack.

For example, even some of our cells have antigens called human leukocyte antigens, or HLAs. But a healthy immune system learns to recognize these HLAs as normal and won't attack them or react to them. There are as many as 10,000 different combinations of HLAs.

Another example of the immune system's unique abilities is seen during pregnancy. During a normal pregnancy, a woman's immune system changes and does not recognize the fetus as nonself. But that same immune system does not grant such special status to a transplanted organ. To avoid the body identifying such an organ as nonself and rejecting it, special antirejection drugs are given.

■ The Immune System Organs

Although there's no single organ of the immune system, there are a number we can look at as part of this system. The various ones that make up the immune system are sometimes referred to as lymphoid organs, because they have a role in the growth, development, and activities of lymphocytes, the white blood cells that are key actors in the immune system. The lymphoid organs include the tonsils, adenoids, lymph nodes, thymus, spleen, bone marrow, and intestinal surfaces, among others.

These various lymphoid organs are interconnected and linked to other organs by a network of vessels similar to blood vessels. These lymph vessels carry immune cells and foreign particles in lymph, a clear fluid that bathes the body's tissues.

The bone marrow, where all blood cells are created, plays a critical role in the immune system, because the cells destined to become immune cells are created from stem cells found in the bone marrow.

■ The Cellular Immune System

When you get into a discussion of the various cells that make up the immune system, things can get complicated.

The majority of immune system cells are lymphocytes, which are small white blood cells. The main types of lymphocytes are B cells, T cells, and killer cells. Lymphocytes move between blood and tissue, and have a long life in the body.

Some immune cells become myeloid cells, which are large white blood cells that can devour bacteria and other foreign particles. Myeloid cells include eosinophils and basophils. Eosinophils and basophils are mainly involved in allergic responses and secrete toxic chemicals to destroy cells harmful to organs and tissues.

Some myeloid cells become phagocytes, which are large white cells that can engulf and digest foreign invaders. They include monocytes, which circulate in the blood, and macrophages, which are found in tissues throughout the body. Macrophages are versatile cells; they act as scavengers, secrete a wide variety of powerful chemicals, and play an essential role in activating T cells.

Neutrophils—cells that circulate in the blood but move into tissues where they are needed—are not only phagocytes but also granulocytes; they contain granules filled with potent chemicals. These chemicals, in addition to destroying microorganisms, play a key role in acute inflammatory reactions. They prevent and treat bacteria and other antigens but die in the process. Phagocytes can also release pyrogens, which cause fever. There are specialized phagocytes found in different parts of the body. For example, synovial A cells, which are phagocytes, are found in the fluid surrounding the joints.

T Cells

Going back to lymphocytes, two major types of lymphocytes are B cells and T cells. T cells, which come from the thymus, help to destroy infected cells and coordinate the body's overall immune response. Their purpose is to remember nonself antigens, and when they encounter those substances, to protect the body in various ways.

The T cell has a molecule on its surface called the T-cell receptor. This receptor interacts with major histocompatibility complex (MHC) molecules. Think of the T-cell receptor as a lock and the MHC as a key. The MHC molecules on the surfaces of most other cells are the key that fit into the T cell's lock and allow the T cell to recognize antigens.

Some T cells are called helper cells and are identified by surface markers. These are known as special cluster determined or CD cells. CD4 T cells are known as helper cells, and they help or promote immune response. CD8 T cells are suppressor cells, and they suppress or block immune response.

The chief tools of T cells are cytokines, which are chemical messengers secreted by the T cells. Cytokines bind to specific receptors on target cells and then recruit other cells to aid in the immune response. Cytokines can encourage cell growth, promote cell activation, direct cellular traffic, and destroy target cells including cancer cells and viruses. Because they serve as a messenger between white cells, or leukocytes, many cytokines are also known as interleukins.

B Cells

B cells, the other type of lymphocyte, work by secreting antibodies. Each B cell produces one specific antibody. When a B cell meets its partner antigen, it starts to create plasma, and the plasma then generates the antibody against that antigen.

Killer Cells

There are also types of lymphocytes called killer cells, including cytotoxic T cells and natural killer (NK) cells. Cytotoxic T cells need to recognize a specific antigen in order to act. In contrast, NK cells roam and act spontaneously and don't require specific antigens in order to move into action. Both cytotoxic T cells and NK cells bind to their target and deliver chemicals that kill the invading antigens and cells. NK cells play a key role in fighting cancer, and they also release interferons, which can prevent or slow viral replication.

■ Other Immune System Components

A variety of other components are involved in the immune system.

- Interferons, released by the natural killer T cells, help prevent viral penetration.
- Interleukins are proteins that simulate white blood cell activity.
- Tumor necrosis factor (TNF) is a chemical released by macrophages and activated T cells. TNF can cause fever and even kill some kinds of cancer cells.

The complement system is another important area of the immune system. It features various proteins that work to complement the work of antibodies in destroying bacteria. These complement proteins circulate in the blood in an inactive form but are triggered when a complement molecule encounters an antibody that is bound to an antigen—that is, an antigen-antibody complex. The complement then creates a cylinder that punctures the offending cell's membrane and essentially acts as a funnel to allow fluids and molecules in and out of the target cell, eventually killing it.

Antibodies

We talked about how antibodies are made to match up with different antigens. What's interesting about antibodies is that they are shaped in a certain way so as to match up with an antigen—again, the way a key fits into a lock.

Antibodies belong to a family of large protein molecules known as immunoglobulins. Scientists have identified nine different types of classes of human immunoglobulins: four kinds of IgG and two kinds of IgA, plus IgM, IgE, and IgD.

IgG, the major immunoglobulin in the blood, can enter tissue spaces; it works efficiently to coat microorganisms, speeding their uptake by other cells in the immune system. IgD, found in the membrane of B cells, has a role in helping B cells recognize antigens. IgE is normally found in only trace amounts, but it is responsible for allergy symptoms. IgM, produced to fight antigens, functions primarily as a bacteria killer but decreases and allows IgG to take over. IgA is a major antibody in body fluids and secretions such as tears, saliva, and fluids in the the gastrointesintal system and works as a barrier to guard the entrances to the body.

Types of Immunity

How do these cells interact and act as an immune system? There are actually several key ways. One is called acquired immunity. In this case, after exposure to antigens, your immune cells that encountered the antigen develop a memory of it. That way, the next time they encounter that same antigen, they will be able to respond more quickly. An example is the acquired immunity you get after having a childhood disease such as chicken pox, which most people don't typically get twice. The next time your body encounters the chicken pox virus, the immune system is primed to destroy it quickly. This sort of immunity can be stimulated not only by exposure and infection but also by preventive vaccines such as the flu vaccine or tetanus shots.

You can also have passive or short-term immunity. That's the kind of immunity that comes from antibodies that are not your own. Mothers pass on antibodies to their newborns that help protect the infant from various illnesses, and these antibodies usually disappear in the first year of life. Some people receive gamma globulin shots, which are treatments of various antibodies that temporarily neutralize certain viruses, such as hepatitis, and boost the immune system.

■ The Immune Response

How does the immune system respond? When an organism or antigen attempts to get into the body, it must first get past the front-line barriers. The skin, skin oils, mucous membranes, cough and sneeze reflexes, and tears are some of the body's barriers designed to keep out antigens. If you think about how the tears—which are rich in IgA antibodies—flow if you get something in your eye, or how you sneeze when exposed to pollen, you're seeing the immune system's barriers in action.

Of course, antigens frequently do get through the external barriers. That's where the other aspects of the immune system step in. Invaders that get past the barriers must confront specific immune system processes and weapons tailored just for them. For example, when an antigen gets past the initial barriers, one of the most basic responses is inflammation. The inflamed tissue releases various chemicals that cause swelling and sometimes fever. The swelling then helps to isolate the antigens from the body's tissues. The chemicals released by the swelling and fever also serve as a call to action for the immune system, attracting white blood cells that come to surround, engulf, and destroy the antigens.

■ Immune Disorders

Part of understanding the immune system is recognizing some of its possible disorders. For example, allergies are an immune system malfunction. In allergies, the body perceives as a danger something that is normally harmless. Allergies to substances such as pollen or peanuts or dog dander occur when the body's first exposure to that substance triggers an inappropriately large antibody response. So, for example, after that first pollen exposure, or after an unusually heavy exposure, B cells make large amounts of pollen antibody, IgE. The IgE attaches to mast cells, which are cells found in the lungs, skin, tongue, and linings of the nose and gastrointestinal tract. The next time pollen is encountered, the IgE-primed mast cells release powerful chemicals that cause wheezing, sneezing, and other allergic symptoms.

There are also immunodeficiency disorders and immune problems such as acquired immune deficiency syndrome (AIDS). In these dysfunctions, there is a failure in all or part of the immune system. In AIDS, for example, a virus destroys helper T cells and ends up being propagated in the body by macrophages and other T cells.

Sometimes the immune system can be deliberately suppressed, such as in chemotherapy, or in giving immunosuppressive drugs to transplant patients so that they don't reject a transplanted organ.

Cancer is another disorder of the immune system. When normal cells turn into cancer cells, some of the antigens on their surface change. These new or altered antigens flag immune defenders, including cytotoxic T cells, natural killer cells, and macrophages. According to one theory, patrolling cells of the immune system provide continuing body-wide surveillance, isolating and eliminating cells that undergo malignant transformation. Tumors develop when the immune surveillance system breaks down or is overwhelmed.

■ Autoimmune Disease

Autoimmune disease is a common form of immune dysfunction. As late as the early 1960s, medical experts believed that the immune system could only be directed against foreign invaders and that the immune system could always distinguish self from nonself.

But researchers discovered that the immune system, which normally defends only against invaders, can become confused and attack self, targeting the cells, tissues, or organs of our own bodies. This concept—autoimmunity—may be taken for granted now, but it was a groundbreaking discovery at the time.

In autoimmunity, the immune system's ability to recognize what's foreign and what's part of your own body breaks down in some way. Thinking that cells or tissues or organs are foreign invaders, the immune system moves into action to be rid of the invader, starting with the manufacture of antibodies—known as autoantibodies—and the generation of T cells that have as their mission the destruction of the "invader."

Various autoimmune mechanisms cause autoimmune disease. For instance, T cells that attack and disable pancreas cells can contribute to the development of diabetes. In rheumatoid arthritis, toxic molecules are made by overproductive macrophages and neutrophils, and they invade the joints. In some autoimmune diseases, B cells mistakenly make antibodies against tissues of the body instead of foreign antigens. Occasionally, these autoantibodies either interfere with the normal function of the tissues or initiate destruction of the tissues. People with Hashimoto's thyroiditis experience hypothyroidism due to the gradual destruction of the thyroid and its hormone-producing capabilities. Myasthenia gravis patients experience muscle weakness because autoantibodies attack a part of the nerve that stimulates muscle movement. In the skin disease pemphigus, autoantibodies are misdirected against cells in the skin, causing severe blisters.

When many antibodies are bound to antigens in the bloodstream, they form a large network called an immune complex. Immune complexes can accumulate and initiate inflammation within small blood vessels that nourish tissues. Immune complexes, immune cells, and inflammatory molecules can block blood flow and ultimately destroy organs such as the kidney. A buildup of immune complexes, for example, is the reason that some cases of systemic lupus erythematosus can be extremely severe.

In some cases, damage to tissues by the immune system may be permanent, as with the destruction of insulin-producing cells of the pancreas in Type I diabetes. Whereas some conditions are progressive, some autoimmune diseases go into remission or even disappear. This happens, for example, in a small percentage of Graves' disease cases, or in multiple sclerosis, where periods of remission sometimes last for months or years. And the hair-loss condition alopecia areata frequently resolves itself after time, with no treatment.

Autoimmune diseases target different parts of the body. For example, the autoimmune reaction targets the brain in multiple sclerosis, the intestinal and bowel system in Crohn's disease and irritable bowel syndrome, and the thyroid in Hashimoto's thyroiditis and Graves' disease. In systemic autoimmune diseases such as lupus or sarcoidosis, the tissues and organs affected may vary depending on the person. One person with lupus may have affected skin and joints, for example, whereas another may have affected skin, kidneys, and lungs.

The underlying mechanism, however, is that the immune system wrongly decides that cells, tissues, or organs that are clearly self are instead nonself, and begins to put into place the attack mechanism reserved for invading antigens.

Prevalence of Autoimmune Diseases

Many of the individual autoimmune diseases are rare. But as a group, autoimmune diseases afflict millions of Americans. But exactly how many? The answer is not known with complete accuracy, because the studies have not been conducted to specifically identify the total numbers of some of these conditions. But according to Noel R. Rose, MD, PhD, chairperson of the American Autoimmune Related Diseases Association's Scientific Advisory Board and director of the Johns Hopkins Autoimmune Research Center, "taken together, the autoimmune diseases occupy the third or fourth place in the list of prevalent diseases in our country."

Dr. Rose himself has estimated that there are at least 8.5 million people with autoimmune diseases. A chart featured in his definitive textbook, *The Autoimmune Diseases,* and developed by Dr. Rose along with Drs. Jacobson and Graham, provides estimates of people with selected autoimmune diseases, identifying 17 of the estimated 80 different autoimmune diseases and indicating an estimated total of 8.5 million Americans, of which 6.7 million are women and 1.8 million are men.

The estimate, however, is a conservative one. When you look at some of the conditions that make up this estimate and compare the numbers with the estimates from patient organizations and specific population studies, it's likely that there are many more autoimmune disease sufferers.

	Estimates by Dr. Rose	Estimates by Patient Organizations
Graves' disease	3,048,636	3,500,000
Diabetes Type I	146,892	1,177,500
Multiple sclerosis	154,278	350,000
Rheumatoid arthritis	1,736,099	2,100,000
Scleroderma	8,922	55,100
Sjögren's syndrome	38,108	2,000,000
Lupus	63,052	1,400,000
Hashimoto's thyroiditis	1,490,371	5,000,000
Vitiligo	1,059,560	2,500,000
Total number of patients	7,745,918	18,082,600

And these are only 9 of the estimated 80 to 100 diseases that may be autoimmune related.

According to Dr. Rose, part of the huge difference in estimates is due to how autoimmune disease is defined and which diseases are included in the list: "Jacobson's article was a fairly conservative list. Those are diseases where we are pretty comfortable that autoimmunity plays a role. But there are many other diseases where there's evidence of an immunological abnormality but we're not sure that it's autoimmune—there are 100 diseases in that list." Dr. Rose feels that if the other conditions that are almost guaranteed to be autoimmune in nature were added in, the total would be approximately 10 million.

Dr. Rose's top estimate is only one-fifth that of the organization he advises, the American Autoimmune Related Diseases Association (AARDA), which says that approximately 50 million Americans—20 percent of the population or one in five people—suffer from autoimmune diseases.

AARDA, however, lists 58 conditions on its website, including chronic fatigue syndrome and fibromyalgia, as autoimmune-related diseases. An estimated 1 million people have chronic fatigue syndrome, and there are an estimated 7 to 10 million fibromyalgia suf-ferers, which contribute to these numbers. The following list includes all of the conditions identified by AARDA as autoimmune related:

Alopecia areata

Ankylosing spondylitis

Antiphospholipid syndrome

Autoimmune Addison's disease

Autoimmune hemolytic anemia

Autoimmune hepatitis

Behçet's disease

Bullous pemphigoid

Cardiomyopathy

Celiac sprue dermatitis

Chronic fatigue immune
    dysfunction syndrome (CFIDS)

Chronic inflammatory
    demyelinating polyneuropathy

Cicatricial pemphigoid

Cold agglutinin disease

CREST syndrome

Crohn's disease

Discoid lupus

Essential mixed
    cryoglobulinemia

Fibromyalgia/fibromyositis

Graves' disease

Guillain-Barré syndrome

Hashimoto's thyroiditis

Idiopathic pulmonary fibrosis

Idiopathic thrombocytopenia
    purpura (ITP)

IgA nephropathy

Insulin-dependent diabetes

Juvenile arthritis

Lichen planus

Lupus

Meniere's disease

Mixed connective tissue disease

Multiple sclerosis

Myasthenia gravis

Pemphigus vulgaris

Pernicious anemia

Polyarteritis nodosa

Polychondritis

Polyglandular syndromes

Polymyalgia rheumatica

Polymyositis and dermatomyositis

Primary agammaglobulinemia

Primary biliary cirrhosis

Psoriasis

Raynaud's phenomenon

Reiter's syndrome

Rheumatic fever

Rheumatoid arthritis

Sarcoidosis

Scleroderma

Sjögren's syndrome

Stiff-man syndrome

Takayasu arteritis

Temporal arteritis/giant cell arteritis	Vasculitis
Ulcerative colitis	Vitiligo
Uveitis	Wegener's granulomatosis

There are still fairly dramatic individual discrepancies in estimates. According to Dr. Rose, consistent or standardized epidemiology has not yet been applied to make particularly accurate assessments for the various autoimmune conditions.

The real message of all these discrepancies, however, is that autoimmune disease is far more prevalent than conventional medical wisdom acknowledges, and patients face a great risk of being misdiagnosed, or undiagnosed, simply because it's not medically understood how widespread these conditions really are.

Even though there is disagreement over the total number, there's definite agreement that they are far more prevalent in women than in men. This gender-based risk factor is discussed at greater length in Chapter 3, but one physician, immunologist Dr. Denise Faustman of Harvard Medical School and the Massachusetts General Hospital's Immunobiology Laboratory, estimates that between 75 and 90 percent of autoimmune disease sufferers are women. Dr. Rose's estimates find that approximately 79 percent of autoimmune disease sufferers are women. AARDA believes that an estimated 75 percent of autoimmune disease sufferers—or 30 million—are women.

Are Autoimmune Diseases on the Rise?

There's a perception that autoimmune diseases may be on the rise. The question is whether that belief is a function of increased awareness and detection or whether there is an actual increase in conditions. According to Dr. Rose:

When we started to work on autoimmune thyroid disease in the 1950s, we went to our endocrine colleagues to get serum from patients with Hashimoto's disease. Many of them told

*us it was rare, and that they "haven't seen a case in 20 years."
Now, it's very common. Does that mean there's more, or are
doctors more aware, and we have better tools for demonstrating it? I personally think it is increasing.*

AARDA's executive director, Virginia Ladd, also suspects that
the number is on the rise:

*It's a combination of things. There is more awareness of
autoimmune conditions as a group. The Internet is certainly
helpful to patients who know how to use it. And we're probably getting better at diagnosing and accepting the diagnosis.
But I still have to wonder if it's not increasing.*

We definitely know that the numbers of patients diagnosed with
fibromyalgia and certain other autoimmune conditions are on the
rise. Some research studies also reveal that there are many patients
with various autoimmune conditions who are undiagnosed. For
example, a February 2000 report in the *Archives of Internal Medicine* found that as many as 13 million Americans may have an
undiagnosed thyroid condition. This number was double the previously suspected level of undiagnosed cases in the United States.

The Costs of Treatment

The worldwide market for autoimmune therapies is currently
$7.3 billion, with treatments for rheumatoid arthritis accounting
for 48 percent of the total. However, as new therapies for psoriasis
enter the market, the total autoimmune market is expected to reach
$18.3 billion by 2006. Treatments for four of the most common
autoimmune disorders—rheumatoid arthritis, multiple sclerosis,
inflammatory bowel disease, and psoriasis—account for 75 percent
of the autoimmune drug trials worldwide. Autoimmune diseases
cost Americans $87 billion each year in total health costs.

How Are Autoimmune Diseases Diagnosed?

Autoimmune diseases can be difficult to diagnose, particularly early in the course of the disease. With a variety of symptoms, and many of them starting out with vague symptoms such as fatigue, depression, joint pain, muscle aches, and weight changes, it's very easy for autoimmune conditions to be written off as stress, depression, not enough sleep, or, in the case of women, premenstrual syndrome (PMS), postpartum fatigue, menopause, or that handy catchall, "hormonal problems."

In 1996, an AARDA survey found that patients with an autoimmune disease saw, on the average, six doctors over a six-year period before getting their diagnoses, and along the way, 60 percent of them were labeled as "chronic complainers" by doctors. According to Virginia Ladd, a new survey conducted in 2001 found that although the numbers had improved, patients were seeing an average of four doctors over five years before getting the proper diagnosis, and slightly less than half still ended up with the "chronic complainer" label. This is still a long time to wait for a diagnosis, especially when you consider that many people have symptoms of autoimmune disease for years before they even start to seek medical attention.

Diagnosing an autoimmune disease is frequently an imprecise process. Even when a doctor is looking for an autoimmune condition, there are a variety of places that the diagnosis can get derailed. In some cases, testing will allow for a specific diagnosis to be made. For example, there are clear laboratory tests and standards for diabetes, and a definite diagnosis can usually be made based on the laboratory tests. But rheumatoid arthritis presents different challenges. Higher concentrations of rheumatoid factor can suggest rheumatoid arthritis but don't guarantee it. And negative results for rheumatoid factor do not exclude the condition. In rheumatoid arthritis, a diagnosis shortly after the onset of symptoms is critical, as permanent, debilitating joint damage can occur in as little as a year, and early treatment can help slow the progress of the disease and avoid some of that damage.

Autoimmune diseases are, for the most part, considered lifelong, chronic diseases. Few are legitimately "curable," but the majority are treatable to some extent. Yet they are unpredictable. Some people have low-grade versions of conditions and never develop the full range of debilitating symptoms. Others go through periods of remission and then have periods where their condition flares. Some people go on to develop various common complications of conditions and others never do. There are no clear-cut ways to predict the course of someone's experience with a particular autoimmune disease.

How Are Autoimmune Diseases Treated?

There are a variety of ways in which autoimmune diseases are treated, and specifics are discussed in the individual chapters on the various conditions covered in this book. In some cases, treatment focuses on correcting the hormonal imbalance that results from the autoimmune condition in the first place. In Type I diabetes, for example, patients take insulin to control blood sugar and to prevent further damage to the kidneys, eyes, blood vessels, and nerves resulting from uncontrolled elevations in blood sugar. In Hashimoto's thyroiditis, thyroid hormone is frequently given because the body's attack on the thyroid impairs its ability to produce a sufficient amount.

In other cases, the objective is to slow or stop the immune system's destruction of organs or tissues. These immunosuppressive therapies—corticosteroids such as prednisone, methotrexate, cyclophosphamide, azathioprine, and cyclosporin—reduce inflammation and can sometimes help prevent the body's autoimmune reactions. A downside to these therapies, however, is that along with a host of serious side effects, in suppressing the immune system they also impair the body's ability to fight infection. For some people, immunosuppressive therapy may result in remission. Patients frequently need to remain on these therapies, as conditions often reappear when medications are withdrawn.

A whole new world of gene and cellular therapies, stem cell–based treatments, hormonally based regimens, and other options are being studied and investigated, with new announcements made every day. These treatments are discussed in Chapter 11.

3

Autoimmune Disease Causes and Risk Factors

What causes autoimmune disease and how can you know if you are at risk? These are good questions, but, unfortunately, the answers aren't clear for most autoimmune conditions.

Although there's no evidence that autoimmune diseases are contagious, we do know that some appear to be triggered—at least in part—by viruses or bacteria. But every person exposed to those offending viruses or bacteria does not go on to develop autoimmune diseases. We also know that a hereditary or genetic predisposition to autoimmune disease is a factor, but every person with a family history does not ultimately develop an autoimmune disease.

Then there are exposures to everything from sunlight, which is a factor in lupus, to occupational exposure to silica, which can increase the risk of scleroderma and other connective tissue diseases. But, again, everyone exposed to sunlight or silica does not go on to develop an autoimmune disease.

Nutritional factors can play a role as well. Celiac disease, for example, can be stopped in its tracks if a patient adopts a gluten-free diet. And over- or underconsumption of dietary iodine can trigger various autoimmune thyroid disorders. But everyone who consumes wheat gluten products or iodine does not develop these conditions.

One of the most obvious—and least understood—risk factors is gender. From 75 to 90 percent of all autoimmune disease sufferers are women. The reasons for this gender discrepancy aren't clearly understood yet.

So, risk cannot be predicted with any sort of mathematical accuracy. But taking into account the various risk factors, in particular the family history of autoimmune disease—combined with symptoms—can help to identify patterns that might be affecting you. The detailed Autoimmune Disease Risk Factors and Symptoms Checklist in Chapter 15 provides a complete listing of the various risks touched upon here, as well as a comprehensive list of symptoms. When filled out, the checklist can offer you an organized way to communicate with your practitioner.

■ Family or Personal History of Autoimmune Disease

Certainly, many, if not most, autoimmune diseases have a genetic or hereditary basis. Some diseases, such as psoriasis, may run in a family specifically. In other cases, a family with genetic tendencies toward autoimmune disease may have family members with different conditions. For example, one relative has thyroid disease, another has lupus, and another Sjögren's syndrome. According to Dr. Rose:

Most of the autoimmune diseases that have been studied show, on average, about one-third of developing an autoimmune disease is the hereditary risk. Even when family connections seem quite prevalent, genetic predisposition accounts for at most 60 percent of the absolute risk for developing an autoimmune disease. For some diseases, this genetic or hered-

itary risk is actually much lower. Genetically identical twins have less than a 40 percent chance of developing the same autoimmune diseases in most cases.

There isn't a direct cause-and-effect relationship between genetics and developing the autoimmune disease. For example, in a disease such as hemophilia, Tay-Sachs, or sickle cell anemia, there are specific and calculable risks of a child also having the disease. With autoimmune disease, a family history means that you are more likely to also have an autoimmune disease, but more than inheriting a specific condition, you inherit a higher risk of developing autoimmune diseases in general.

Genetic research now shows that autoimmune diseases have a shared genetic basis, and these findings argue for a view of autoimmune diseases as a unified group of conditions. Much like it's now known that cancers have similar mechanisms, even though different organs are affected, the same sort of approach is now being thought to apply to autoimmune diseases. There are eight core diseases that appear to have strong interrelationships with each other genetically that are being extensively studied: rheumatoid arthritis, juvenile rheumatoid arthritis, systemic lupus, multiple sclerosis, autoimmune thyroid disease, Type I diabetes, psoriasis, and inflammatory bowel disease.

Not only does having a family member with autoimmune disease increase your risk of developing an autoimmune condition but your past history is relevant. Having an autoimmune disease yourself raises your risk of developing another condition. There are no specific calculations to precisely define that increased risk, but it's important to become familiar with the most common autoimmune diseases and their symptoms, and to be sure to include a personal and family history of autoimmune disease in your medical history and in discussions with your physician. Also, patients and their family members should be on the lookout for signs and symptoms of new autoimmune diseases that may develop.

One patient, Pat, who was first diagnosed with vitiligo at age 7, illustrates that several autoimmune diseases can appear over time in the same person and within the family:

Info was pretty scanty in 1957, so basically I was told vitiligo was a harmless condition, like male balding. It was difficult during my teen years and young adulthood, even though I had very few white patches on my hands and elbows and knees. After my children were born, this condition became more aggressive. It has increased considerably in the past few years around perimenopause. I also discovered I had thyroid disease after my first child was born, even though I am sure this condition was there much earlier than that, perhaps at puberty. I was 43 or so when I noticed that I could not get rid of blisters on my tongue. They would hurt so much . . . during this time I was plagued by loss of balance and numbness and tingling in my feet. When I walked, I couldn't seem to feel the ground and had trouble adjusting my footsteps as I walked on an uneven terrain. I complained to my endocrinologist that I thought something was wrong with my thyroid. He dismissed this as nothing. When I went to see a new doctor for my annual physical, she asked me to look at my tongue, she did several tests, and I went to see a hematologist, who confirmed the pernicious anemia. My son of 21 has diabetes, vitiligo, and thyroid disease. My daughters, 16 and 19, have both been diagnosed with thyroid disease.

■ Gender/Hormonal Status

According to the American Autoimmune Related Diseases Association, 75 percent of autoimmune diseases occur in women and most frequently during childbearing years. A study published in the September 2000 issue of the *American Journal of Public Health* reported that autoimmune diseases as a category are one of the ten leading causes of all deaths among U.S. women age 65 and younger, and the seventh leading cause of death by disease among females ages 45 to 65.

The disease that is most skewed toward women, Hashimoto's thyroiditis, shows up in women fifty times more often than in men. Lupus and Sjögren's syndrome both affect women nine times more often than men.

Interestingly, being pregnant or having had a pregnancy in the previous year also increases your risk of developing an autoimmune disorder. Pregnancy can worsen the symptoms of existing conditions. For example, lupus patients frequently experience flareups and worsening of symptoms during pregnancy, which has been especially correlated with the increased prolactin levels found close to delivery time.

In some cases, pregnancy actually has the opposite effect and ends up being protective in some women with autoimmune diseases. Women with rheumatoid arthritis or multiple sclerosis often find themselves with greatly improved symptoms or even a remission during pregnancy. In rheumatoid arthritis, for example, pregnancy improves the symptoms in about 75 percent of pregnant patients but relapses within six months postpartum in 90 percent of cases.

According to hormonal consultant, educator, and best-selling author Gillian Ford:

During pregnancy, the high levels of estrogen and progesterone and the tendency to be slightly hyperthyroid produce a steroid effect similar to taking cortisone. This cortisol effect generally boosts the immune system during pregnancy. A number of other hormones, including cortisol, are higher during pregnancy but mainly bound by protein, so they do not cause adverse side effects. Cortisol is actually high at delivery to help a woman cope with the stress and pain of childbirth.

Ford explains that many autoimmune diseases flare up or initially appear postpartum:

Delivery of the placenta and fetus lead to the precipitous drop in hormones, such as cortisol, estrogen, progesterone, and thyroid, at delivery. This drop causes what has been named an immune rebound. In the postpartum period, for example, thyroid disease can frequently occur, and there's even a temporary autoimmune form of thyroid disease known as postpartum thyroiditis.

Although the mechanism is not clearly understood, hormones in general definitely have a connection to autoimmune diseases. Since women typically have higher levels of estrogen and lower levels of androgens, such as testosterone, there seems to be a specific connection to estrogen, which can stimulate or suppress the immune system. Progesterone and androgens appear to suppress the immune system, whereas prolactin stimulates it. The onset of autoimmune diseases frequently occurs when women are in their 20s, a point during which estrogen levels are typically their highest.

Some experts believe that the risk for women may not be due to the presence or excess of estrogen but rather insufficient testosterone. In lupus, for example, use of the hormone dehydroepiandrosterone (DHEA), which is an androgen precursor to testosterone, has reportedly been helpful in the treatment of some patients.

Ford believes that the basic reason women have more complex immune systems, and therefore more susceptibility to autoimmune conditions, is due to the body's ability to adapt to pregnancy:

A baby is a foreign object, which under normal circumstances would be rejected by the mother's body. Women have more complicated immune systems to cope with pregnancy. Having a better immune system has its benefits and its detractions. Women tend to live longer, but they have a lot more immune system problems and the bulk of chronic metabolic disease.

In that vein, one theory behind why women are at higher risk centers on the recent finding that during pregnancy a mother and her baby exchange cells, and those cells can remain circulating in their bodies for years or even decades after the baby's birth. So the body may label those cells as nonself and mount an attack against them.

■ Nationality/Ethnicity/Origin Factors

It's believed that autoimmune diseases are more common in northern, more industrialized countries and colder climates, and less common in warmer, lesser-developed countries. This is called the hygiene hypothesis and holds that the growth of allergic and autoimmune disease in highly developed, industrialized nations may be partly due to the increasingly sterile environment and overuse of antibiotics and antibacterials. This sort of environment may prevent normal exposure to and development of healthy immunities to bacteria. Some experts suggest that when infants are exposed early to germs, their immune systems are redirected toward infection-fighting mode and away from the tendency to overreact to normally benign substances or to self. In particular, this lack of exposure to normal pathogens might weaken the gastrointestinal immune defenses, opening the pathways to various autoimmune diseases. Some evidence for this theory is also found in studies demonstrating that infants who have more colds and infections end up with a lower incidence of asthma as adults.

Other researchers are suggesting that infection with parasites such as roundworms, flatworms, and pinworms—more common in less industrialized areas—may prime the immune system and make it less likely to mistakenly target its own tissues.

According to Dr. Ronald Hoffman, best-selling author, radio host, and founder of New York City's Hoffman Center, a popular integrative medicine center:

> We do see a higher degree of autoimmune disease in populations not exposed natively to normal pathogens. The immune system doesn't get its boot camp through exposure in its early years to normal viruses and bacteria. That means that it's going to hyperreact to stimuli that it should be tolerant of normally.

Interestingly, a mechanism to explain some of this protective element may be found in recent findings by scientists in the United Kingdom that a protein produced by the *Escherichia coli* bacteria may actually ward off autoimmune diseases such as Type I diabetes and rheumatoid arthritis. *E. coli* occur naturally in the human intestines, but there are a variety of strains, many foodborne, that can cause diarrhea or other illnesses. The experts believe that treatments to deliver this nontoxic protein, if developed, could be given with an easy-to-use nasal spray early on in the course of a disease to help halt or slow the progression. Other researchers have speculated, however, that the recurrent medical visits and in some cases sophisticated tests involved in diagnosis of autoimmune diseases may make their diagnosis very unlikely in nations where basic health care is still not widely available.

Some countries, nationalities, and ethnic origins seem to have a higher prevalence of certain autoimmune diseases. People from northern Europe appear to have the highest incidence of Type I diabetes. In children, the highest incidence is found in the Scandinavian countries, particularly Sweden and Finland. Ulcerative colitis and celiac disease are more common in temperate climates. Irritable bowel disease overall is considered rare in Asia, Africa, and South America. Celiac disease and ulcerative colitis are more common in people of Ashkenazi Jewish descent (from eastern or central Europe). Multiple sclerosis primarily affects northern Europeans and those who have northern European ancestry. It's rare in East Asia and almost unknown among blacks in Africa. The rate of multiple sclerosis among African-Americans is half that of Caucasians. As many as 6 percent of Native Americans may develop rheumatoid arthritis, compared to only about 1 percent of the general population.

■ Work/Chemical Occupational Exposures

Although the mechanisms aren't clearly understood, there appear to be linkages between certain occupations, as well as occupational exposures to various minerals, solvents, and chemicals, and autoimmune disease. Workers in computer manufacturing who are exposed to certain chemicals have higher risks of autoimmune diseases, for example. Workers exposed to silica and quartz have a higher risk of scleroderma and the other connective tissue autoimmune diseases. According to researchers, scleroderma is also more common in workers exposed to vinyl chloride, epoxy resins, and solvents, among other chemicals. Even frequent use of or exposure to hair dye has been implicated as a risk for lupus and rheumatoid arthritis.

Perchlorate is a chemical that blocks iodine from entering the thyroid and prevents further synthesis of thyroid hormone. There is some evidence and concern that long-term exposure to concentrations of perchlorate—which is found in various water supplies around the nation, particularly in areas near rocket fuel or fireworks plants—can eventually interfere with proper thyroid function and cause increased rates of thyroid disease. There's also evidence that the thyroid can be damaged via exposure to other toxic chemicals, including dioxins, methyl tert-butyl ether (MTBE)—an oxygenate added to gasoline—and other chemicals that act as endocrine "disruptors."

On the occupational front, a study reported in the July 2001 issue of the *Journal of Rheumatology* found that teachers have a significantly higher risk of dying from an autoimmune disease. Researchers found that the teachers had almost double the mortality from some common autoimmune diseases than the general public, and secondary teachers had higher rates than elementary teachers. The researchers don't know exactly what mechanism is at work but suspect there may be a link with exposure to mononucleosis (acute Epstein-Barr virus infection), which is common among high school students. The researchers have theorized that teachers who have not yet been infected by the Epstein-Barr virus before they start their careers may face greater risk of developing infectious mononucleosis and could be at higher risk of an autoimmune response to that infection. A more detailed list of occupational and environmental exposures and their linkages to autoimmune diseases is featured in the checklist in Chapter 15.

■ Sun, Heat, and Cold Exposures

Temperature changes are quite common triggers of several autoimmune diseases. For example, exposure to sunlight can trigger a flare of lupus. A hot bath or shower, hot weather, or fever can trigger a flare of multiple sclerosis. Exposure to rapid changes in temperature, such as going from a heated house to the cold outdoors, and general exposure to cold can trigger Raynaud's phenomenon, the condition that causes pain, tingling, and numbness in fingers and toes.

■ Nuclear Exposure

Nuclear plants can release radioactive materials that are damaging to the thyroid. People who lived in or were visiting the area near the Chernobyl plant in the period after the nuclear accident that occurred on April 26, 1986, are at an increased risk for thyroid problems. The main countries at risk include Belarus, the Russian Federation, and the Ukraine. There is a risk, though reduced, to Poland, Austria, Denmark, Finland, Germany, Greece, and Italy. Those who lived near or in the area downwind from the former nuclear weapons plant at Hanford in south-central Washington state during the 1940s through 1960s, particularly 1955 to 1965, may have also been exposed to potentially thyroid-damaging radioactive materials. Hanford released radioactive materials that can cause autoimmune thyroid disease. During the 1950s and 1960s, approximately one hundred nuclear bomb tests were conducted at the Nevada Nuclear Test Site northwest of Las Vegas. The fallout from the tests was most concentrated in counties of western states located east and north of the test site, such as Utah, Idaho, Montana, Colorado, and Missouri. Exposure to this fallout increases the risk of thyroid cancer, particularly in the Farm Belt, where children drank fallout-contaminated milk. There are also cases of autoimmune thyroid problems in the United States that may be due to the iodine-131 released during these nuclear tests.

In the late 1990s, the newspaper *The Tennessean* presented the results of an effort to investigate a mysterious pattern of illnesses including autoimmune thyroid problems that seem to have been concentrated around the Oak Ridge nuclear facility in eastern Tennessee. This same pattern was, according to the newspaper, repeated at other nuclear facilities in Tennessee, Colorado, South Carolina, New Mexico, Idaho, New York, California, Ohio, Kentucky, Texas, and Washington state.

■ Metals Exposure

According to Dr. Rose, overexposure to mercury, gold, cadmium, and other heavy metals, coming from dental fillings, water supply, occupational exposures, and other sources, has been shown to induce autoantibodies and has been linked to the development of autoimmune disease.

■ Dietary Factors

A sensitivity or full intolerance to gluten, which is found in most wheat and many grain products, is a known trigger of autoimmune diseases. In fact, celiac disease is caused by the intake of gluten products in genetically susceptible individuals. People with autoimmune diseases are ten to thirty times more likely than the general public to also have celiac disease or gluten intolerance, and it's thought that having celiac disease increases the risk of developing other autoimmune disorders such as Type I diabetes, autoimmune thyroid, and other endocrine diseases. In some patients who have an increased risk of Type I diabetes, for example, a gluten-free diet can actually prevent or delay the onset of diabetes.

In addition to gluten, other food allergies and sensitivities are thought to create a propensity for development of autoimmune disease. It's thought that the constant irritation caused by exposure to an allergen inflames the intestinal lining. Ultimately, that lining becomes permeable, and a condition known as leaky gut develops. With leaky gut, the inflammation permits larger molecules and proteins, which normally would not be antigenic, to pass through the intestinal lining and directly into the bloodstream, where they are then perceived as invaders and trigger an autoimmune reaction.

There is a certain class of foods called goitrogens that can promote the development of goiters when eaten in large quantities, resulting in hypothyroidism. Goitrogens are a concern only for people who still have a thyroid, and are considered a problem when served raw. It's believed that thorough cooking may minimize or eliminate goitrogenic potential. Goitrogenic foods include brussels sprouts, rutabaga, turnips, kohlrabi, radishes, cauliflower, African cassava, millet, babassu (a palmtree coconut fruit popular in Brazil and Africa), cabbage, kale, and soy products.

Soy products, which have become increasingly popular due to a number of reported health benefits, are also being found to have a definite antithyroid and goitrogenic effect. This is of particular concern for infants on soy formulas, but it is also an issue for adults who regularly consume large quantities of soy products. Current research is beginning to show that long-term overconsumption of soy products can promote formation of goiters and development of autoimmune thyroid disease.

In general, obesity, particularly when combined with insufficient exercise, is a risk factor for diabetes.

Too much iodine—in the form of iodine supplements or iodine-containing herbs such as kelp, bladder wrack, or bugleweed—can increase the risk of autoimmune thyroid disease. A deficiency in iodine is a known cause of autoimmune hypothyroidism. But, Dr. Rose says, "Excess iodine can create an excess risk of autoimmune disease, but only in those with genetic predisposition."

Use of a particular type of food oil, denatured rapeseed oil, which had become toxic, caused an autoimmune "toxic oil syndrome" in more than 30,000 people in Spain in the 1980s. One idea gaining ground is the relationship between certain foodborne pathogens and their ability to trigger or even cause autoimmune diseases. A Greek study found evidence of a causative relationship between the bacteria *Yersinia enterocolitica* and Hashimoto's thyroiditis. Levels of antibodies to *Yersinia*—evidence of bacterial exposure—were fourteen times higher in people with Hashimoto's thyroiditis than in the control groups. These bacteria are found in the fecal matter of livestock, domesticated and wild animals. You can be exposed to *Yersinia* via contaminated meats (especially raw or undercooked products), poultry, unpasteurized milk and dairy products, seafood (particularly oysters) from sewage-contaminated waters, and produce fertilized with raw manure. Foods can also be contaminated by food handlers who have not effectively washed their hands before handling food or utensils used to prepare food. Improper storage can also contribute to contamination.

In a July 2000 study, doctors at the National Public Health Institute in Helsinki, Finland, reported that the more coffee consumed daily, the higher the risk of developing rheumatoid arthritis. The Finnish researchers found that, over time, those who drank eleven or more cups a day had almost a fifteen times greater risk of developing rheumatoid arthritis than noncoffee drinkers. The scientists suspect that something in the coffee may be triggering the production of rheumatoid factor (RF), the antibody that is a marker for rheumatoid arthritis and predicts the progression of the disease. Other dietary risk factors are detailed in the checklist in Chapter 15.

■ Drugs/Supplements

A long list of prescription drugs, supplements, and even the illegal drugs cocaine and heroin are all implicated as possible factors in particular autoimmune diseases. Some of the best known of these connections are between the disease lupus and the various drugs that can cause the form of the condition known as drug-induced lupus. The drugs that can induce lupus include D-penicillamine, interferon drugs and interleukin-2, hydralazine (Apresoline), isoniazid (Laniazid), procainamide (Pronestyl, Procanbid), methyldopa (Aldomet), and thorazine (Chlorpromazine), among others.

Occasionally, autoimmune diseases are identified that are triggered by exposure to a particular toxic or tainted substance. One fairly rare autoimmune disease estimated to affect several thousand people in the United States is eosinophilia myalgia syndrome (EMS). EMS causes debilitating muscle pain and a high eosinophilia count (a type of white blood cell that usually signifies infection). EMS results from past use of a particular brand of tainted L-tryptophan, a health food supplement that used to be available as a sleep aid in the 1980s. A specific list of some known drug/supplement triggers for common autoimmune conditions is featured in Chapter 15.

■ Bacterial and Viral Infections and Illnesses

Bacteria are implicated as the triggers, and perhaps even the cause, of some autoimmune diseases. As mentioned earlier, research has shown a linkage between exposure to the bacteria *Yersinia enterocolitica* and elevated levels of thyroid antibodies, a sign of autoimmune thyroid disease.

One known pathogen is mycoplasma. Mycoplasmas are simple types of parasitic bacteria, the smallest self-replicating bacteria, slightly larger than viruses but able to replicate on their own, which viruses cannot do.

With their lack of cell walls, mycoplasma can invade cells, bypassing the body's normal defense mechanisms, and once in the cell, drain off nutrients such as fats, vitamins, and other critical components of the cell, in particular, those components that allow for basic cellular energy. When they leave a cell, mycoplasma leave behind some of their own material, which can later trigger autoimmune reactions, in which the immune system starts to attack its own cells, because they are carrying the residue of the mycoplasma, which acts as an antigen.

Infection with the mycoplasma M. *pneumoniae,* for example, is known to frequently occur before development of certain autoimmune diseases. The organism M. *tuberculosis* has been shown in animal studies to potentially be involved in the development of rheumatoid arthritis. And a common mycoplasma, M. *fermentans,* may have a role in chronic fatigue syndrome, fibromyalgia, and rheumatoid arthritis.

In late 2000, findings published in the *Journal of Rheumatology* reported on Israeli research demonstrating that M. *fermentans* may have a specific role in triggering or worsening rheumatoid arthritis. The fluid from inflamed joints of RA patients contained this mycoplasma, as well as antibodies against it, whereas M. *fermentans* was not present in patients with other forms of arthritis.

Interestingly, mycoplasmas are thought to use molecular mimicry, a biological trick by which certain organisms can resemble their host to fool the immune system into thinking they are normal cells. This permits further infiltration into the body. The role of mycoplasmas in autoimmune disease is still being studied and should yield some interesting information.

Some experts, particularly more holistic-minded practitioners, believe that there are also so-called stealth pathogens—that is, pathogens that have changed their structure and activity in a way that makes them able to evade standard diagnosis, tests, and treatments. The concept of a stealth pathogen is based on the idea that, like mycoplasma, these bacteria have developed less structured cell walls, which enables them to move DNA between cells and infiltrate tissues and organs without detection. Some practitioners believe that infection with these stealth pathogens may be a key trigger in autoimmune disease.

Viruses are the smallest of all parasites. But viruses cannot reproduce on their own; they require other cells in order to reproduce. A virus is so small that it cannot be seen on a traditional microscope, only on an electron microscope. A virus requires cells (bacterial, plant, or animal) to reproduce. Viruses have an outside cover and a core composed of RNA or DNA. This core can frequently penetrate susceptible cells and trigger the infection. The body's exposure to a virus typically stimulates the production of antibodies against that virus.

There are several hundred different viruses that can infect people. The common cold, for example, is due to a virus—the rhinovirus—and many other common illnesses, such as measles, chicken pox, and influenza—the flu—and are also due to infection by a virus.

Viruses are most commonly spread by exposure to bodily fluids. Mononucleosis is often referred to as the kissing disease because it's frequently passed by saliva exposure. And it's considered common knowledge that you can catch a cold or flu by being exposed to an uncovered sneeze, or through hand-to-hand contact.

One unique feature of viruses is referred to as *latency,* the ability of a virus to go into a latent period—seemingly a remission—but then to recur. Viruses can, however, be spread during these latency periods. A good example of a virus that acts this way is the herpes virus, and herpes sufferers can still infect sexual partners when they themselves are not having an outbreak.

Diagnosing viruses can be tricky. Some viruses show up in characteristic ways that can be tested; for example, measles, rubella, chicken pox, and Epstein-Barr/mononucleosis all present with fairly identifiable features. Tests are available to identify certain antibodies against certain viruses, but they don't always show whether the virus is in a latent or active period, or whether a past exposure has conferred immunity.

A number of viruses have been associated with autoimmune diseases. The mechanisms of whether they are in fact the primary trigger, or whether the virus, in stimulating the immune system, sets into motion a chain of events leading to the autoimmune reaction, isn't known. But what is known is that Epstein-Barr virus, for example, seems to have some connection to rheumatoid arthritis, and Coxsackie B seems to have a connection to diabetes, among other links.

A particular type of virus, known as a retrovirus, may also be associated with autoimmune disease. According to researchers, a human endogenous retrovirus copies itself back into the DNA and inserts itself into the chromosomes of a newly infected cell. There, integrated into the genetic material of the cell, the virus becomes a permanent part of the genetic makeup of the cell. The retrovirus then moves on to infect a new cell, and replication continues. The human immunodeficiency virus (HIV) that causes AIDS (acquired immune deficiency syndrome) is a retrovirus.

Some experts theorize that the presence of detectable levels of RNA in the blood of individuals, which may be a by-product of retrovirus activity, may be a marker for certain forms of chronic disease. As more is understood about the relationship between RNA and particular diseases, this type of test may begin to become a more important part of the arsenal in autoimmune disease diagnosis.

Immunologists have long suspected that viral infections may be able to start off autoimmune responses, but it has been difficult to design an experiment that would clearly and convincingly differentiate the immune system's responses to a virus from those to self. According to the scientists, after an infection antibodies are normally produced against the antigen in large quantities, helping to clear the infection. In some cases, there may be a subset of these antibody-creating cells that can mount an even stronger defense against the targeted antigen. Those extra-strength cells may be so vigilant that they react with self, leading to a future autoimmune reaction.

Some viruses can actually cause cancer. One retrovirus is linked with the development of leukemia and lymphoma. Epstein-Barr virus has been tied to certain forms of lymphoma and Hodgkin's disease. And there are other viral/cancer connections established or being studied.

Persistent infection, such as having periodontal disease, can also be a general risk factor for autoimmune disease. At the same time, habits that can help prevent infection, such as regular handwashing or dental hygiene, can also decrease the risk of general infections and therefore decrease the risk of autoimmune disease.

A more comprehensive checklist of bacterial and viral linkages is featured in Chapter 15.

■ Smoking

If you are or were a smoker, you have an increased risk of developing autoimmune thyroid disease. Cigarettes contain thiocyanate, a chemical that adversely affects the thyroid gland and acts as an antithyroid agent. Researchers have found that smoking may increase the risk, severity, and side effects of hypothyroidism in patients with Hashimoto's thyroiditis, and smoking worsens the effects of thyroid eye disease, a complication of Graves' disease. Smoking also increases the risk of autoimmune oophoritis, lupus, and psoriasis.

■ Vaccinations/Immunizations

Some researchers believe that vaccinations may directly cause some autoimmune diseases via transmission of undetected mycoplasma or stealth pathogens. Indirectly, vaccinations may turn on the immune system and provide it with an antigen, or may cause the body to prevent the immune system from developing its own defense mechanisms.

Some scientists have theorized that when a developing immune system gets a heavy dose of antigens—even though they are inactivated in vaccines—the immune system can be harmed. There is speculation that exposure to inactivated viruses in vaccines may actually encourage autoimmune reactions against the proteins in those inactivated viruses, triggering autoimmune reactions or disease. In some studies, there have been links between use of hepatitis B, meningitis, and mumps vaccines and higher incidence of diabetes. The hepatitis B vaccination program in France brought with it a host of new reports of active multiple sclerosis. In 1998, the French government halted the program because of fears that the shots cause neurological disorders, including multiple sclerosis.

One of the most high-profile vaccines that has been suspected to have a role in autoimmune disease development is the controversial anthrax vaccine used by the military. Since the 1990s, there has been considerable debate about the vaccine's safety, and numerous reports associate anthrax shots with a variety of symptoms and side effects, including fatigue, nervous system problems, and autoimmune disease. In a 2000 Institute of Medicine report, the Committee on Health Effects Associated with Exposures During the Gulf War reviewed summaries of data from the Vaccine Adverse Event Reporting System (VAERS). In the ten-year period from 1990 to September 15, 2000, there were more than 1,500 reports of adverse events associated with use of the anthrax vaccine reported to VAERS. There were a number of reports of serious side effects, including aseptic meningitis, lupus, inflammatory demyelinating disease, and Guillain-Barré syndrome, among others, in some cases leading to death or permanent disability.

Dr. Rose admits that the vaccine/autoimmune disease connection is a theoretical possibility:

> A *number of people have raised vaccination as an issue, based partly on the issue of molecular mimicry. There may be antigens in the vaccine that resemble self-antigens, and as we induce immune response to a vaccine, we may induce autoimmune response. Some researchers have thought they have seen increases in Type I diabetes, for example, but when people did careful studies, no clear connection was shown.*

While the holistic health community tends to view vaccination with greater skepticism, according to Dr. Rose, "There's no firm evidence to support this claim or concern, and the cost-benefit ratio still strongly favors vaccinations."

■ Trauma/Physical Injury

Trauma to the body or to particular organs may be a trigger for autoimmune disease in some people. For example, workers with repeated hand-arm vibration injury, such as in jackhammer and chainsaw operators, are at greater risk of developing scleroderma-like conditions.

There is a link between neck trauma, such as whiplash or a broken neck, and the development of thyroid disorders, but such trauma-induced hypothyroidism has not been extensively studied. Anecdotally, some patients also report the rapid onset of some autoimmune diseases, such as multiple sclerosis or Graves' disease, following extreme physical trauma, such as in an automobile accident.

■ Stress

In one study of baboons, it was discovered that highly stressed animals—ones that were lower on the social hierarchy and subject to psychological harassment—had worse nutrition, more parasites, and shorter lives. Their resistance to infection was also lower.

Ultimately, it's clear that stressful conditions—whether imposed on us externally or created by our own mind–body connections—can overload the protective systems that are built into our nervous systems, through chronic elevation of stress hormones. Usually, production of stress hormones is supposed to shut down as a self-protective mechanism. But in the face of chronic stress, including chronic sleep deprivation, this mechanism can become stunted and doesn't shut off sufficiently.

One study found that people caring for family members suffering from dementia had slower healing of wounds than noncaregivers, taking 24 percent more time—an average of nine days longer—for similar-size wounds to heal. In another study, family members under the stress of caring for an Alzheimer's patient in five years showed a weakened immune system and significantly higher rates of infectious illnesses.

PART II

Key Autoimmune Conditions

4

Multiorgan Syndromes

Some of the most difficult autoimmune conditions to diagnose and treat are the multiorgan syndromes. These conditions can attack various and multiple organs, glands, and bodily systems, creating a cascade effect of symptoms. In this chapter, some of the more common autoimmune diseases in this category are discussed, including lupus, mixed connective tissue diseases, sarcoidosis, and Sjögren's syndrome.

■ Lupus

Lupus causes inflammation in the joints, the tendons, and other connective tissues and can cause inflammation in—and even destruction of—some organs. For most, lupus is considered a mild condition, affecting only a few organs. For others, however, it may not take such a simple course and may trigger serious—even life-threatening—conditions. Lupus generally affects the skin, joints, kidneys, lungs, heart, nervous system, blood, and/or other body organs or systems.

There are several types of lupus. Discoid lupus, also known as cutaneous lupus, affects the skin, causing a benign rash and disc-shaped lesions, usually across the face and upper part of the body.

Discoid lupus does not affect internal organs. It may be localized in a particular area such as the scalp, face, ears, arms, and so on, but can occasionally spread to other areas. Occasionally, if lesions become sufficiently inflamed, hair follicles and skin cells may be permanently destroyed, causing permanent scarring and hair loss. This type of lupus affects 10 percent of lupus patients and is more common in African-Americans.

Systemic lupus erythematosus (SLE) comes in two forms: non-organ-threatening and organ-threatening. Non-organ-threatening SLE affects approximately 35 percent of patients but does not typically threaten internal organs. When the organs—such as the kidney, heart, lung, liver, joints, or brain—are involved, it's considered organ-threatening SLE, which affects another 35 percent of patients.

Ten percent of lupus cases are considered drug induced, triggered by drugs including hydralazine (Apresoline), isoniazid (Laniazid), procainamide (Pronestyl, Procanbid), methyldopa (Aldomet), thorazine (Chlorpromazine), and D-penicillamine. When medication is discontinued, the lupus symptoms usually disappear.

The final 10 percent of lupus cases are considered crossover or overlapping cases seen with other autoimmune diseases.

Lupus is estimated to affect one million people in the United States, but some experts estimate that the actual number of sufferers is actually several million. According to Dr. Daniel Wallace, author of *The Lupus Book,* 10 million Americans have a positive lupus blood screen (called antinuclear antibody, or ANA), which may signal increased risk of developing lupus.

Approximately 90 percent of the sufferers are women, and almost all of them are in their childbearing years, as 80 percent of lupus sufferers develop the condition between the ages of 15 and 45. Onset after the age of 45 or after menopause is not common. Lupus seems to be more common among African-Americans, Latinos, and Asians, versus Caucasians. About 200,000 people are formally diagnosed with lupus each year in the United States.

In lupus, the immune system attacks the body's own joints, tendons, connective tissues, and organs. Lupus can be chronic and ongoing, but more commonly it is a relapsing/remitting condition that has periodic flare-ups, or "flares." Sunlight is known to trigger flares in many patients. Heat, infrared light, and, rarely, fluorescent light can also bring on flares.

Smoking is another trigger. One recent study conducted at the University of New Mexico Health Sciences Center in Albuquerque and reported in the *Journal of Rheumatology* found that current smokers were seven times more likely than nonsmokers to have lupus. Those who were former smokers were nearly four times more likely to develop lupus as those who never smoked.

Some other known triggers for lupus include hair-coloring solutions, silica and silicone, polyvinyl chloride, overconsumption of alfalfa sprouts, and the various drugs cited as causes of drug-induced lupus. Some drugs are also known to worsen lupus or trigger flares, including antibiotics and the nonsteroidal anti-inflammatory pain reliever ibuprofen (Advil or Motrin).

Symptoms

Lupus can be mild or it can be extremely serious, and how one experiences lupus will depend on the type of antibodies present and which tissues or organs are under attack. Because of the nature of symptoms, the slow appearance of some symptoms, and the remission/relapse patterns, lupus frequently is present a number of years before diagnosis.

In lupus cases where antibodies only affect the skin, symptoms may be mild, and staying out of the sun may be the only treatment needed. When tissues or organs are under attack, however, patients frequently experience profound fatigue, rashes, and joint pains, among other symptoms.

According to Dr. Wallace, the most common initial complaint in early lupus is joint pain or swelling, which occurs in about half of all patients, followed by skin rashes (20 percent) and malaise or fatigue, which affects 10 percent. Low-grade fever is present in as many as half of patients, and before any other symptoms begin, some patients have reported years of on and off fevers, accompanied by fatigue and malaise of unknown origin. Other experts indicate that Raynaud's syndrome, most frequently manifested by tingling, numbness, coldness, and color changes in hands and feet, is found in as many as one-third of lupus patients. Ultimately, some experts believe that 90 percent of lupus patients have joint inflammation, which can range from mild to severe multijoint arthritis.

Generally, lupus symptoms include:

- Fatigue
- Joint and muscle aches, pain, swelling, and stiffness, especially in legs and ankles
- Weight loss
- Low-grade fever, usually no more than 102°F
- Hair loss
- Butterfly-shaped rash on the nose and cheeks (rarely blisters and usually does not become raw)
- Discoid lesions (lesions that are disc shaped) on the scalp, face, neck, and ears
- Red-purple areas on palms and fingers
- Sun sensitivity (sunburn or rash after exposure to sunlight)
- Shortness of breath
- Chest pain
- Seizures
- Depression, psychosis
- Tingling, numbness, coldness, and color changes in hands and feet
- Tendency to bruise
- Dry eyes

- Dry mouth, mouth sores
- Swollen glands, swollen lymph nodes
- Headaches
- Difficulty thinking clearly

Diagnosis

The American College of Rheumatology has designated eleven specific criteria for a lupus diagnosis. To be officially diagnosed with lupus, you must have four or more of these criteria:

1. Facial rash: known as a malar rash, the flat or raised butterfly-shaped red rash that covers the cheeks below the eyes.
2. Discoid rash: red, raised disc-shaped patches that have scaling.
3. Sun sensitivity: rashes that develop specifically in response to exposure to the sun.
4. Sores/ulcers: usually painless sores in the mouth or nose.
5. Arthritis: swelling or tenderness in joints, especially affecting hands, knees, and wrists.
6. Inflammation: known as serositis, painful inflammation in sacs or membranes of the lung (pleuritis), heart (percarditis), and abdomen.
7. Kidney disease: Some lupus patients experience loss of protein in the urine, or urine samples show evidence of kidney inflammation.
8. Seizures and psychiatric problems: unexplained seizures, nerve paralysis, severe depression, and even psychosis.
9. Blood irregularities: Low blood counts of various blood components are known to occur, including low red blood cells (hemolytic anemia), low white blood cells (leukopenia or lymphopenia), and low platelets (thrombocytopenia).

10. Special testing: Special laboratory testing is done for lupus markers. For example, a particular syphilis test (VDRL) can show false positive in lupus patients and help confirm a diagnosis. Other markers can include the presence of antiphospholipid antibodies, lupus anticoagulant, or anti-DNA. Other immunological tests may indicate other findings.

11. Positive antinuclear antibody: A common test for the general presence of autoimmune disease is antinuclear antibody (ANA), but it can give false positives, and a positive ANA is not on its own indicative of lupus. Recently, however, it has been noted that when ANA is positive, a test for antibodies to double-stranded DNA can also be performed. A high level is more indicative of lupus, but absence of these antibodies does not exclude lupus.

Recently, researchers have also found that testing for antibodies known as serine arginine proteins can identify lupus in more than 50 percent of patients. Combined with other tests, researchers believe this new test will help speed up diagnosis.

Practitioners

Typically, rheumatologists are best trained to diagnose and treat lupus.

Treatment

Treatment for lupus depends on the extent of the symptoms and involvement. The first line of treatment usually includes non-steroidal anti-inflammatory drugs (NSAIDs) such as aspirin, ibuprofen, naproxen (Naprosyn), indomethacin (Indocin), nabumetone (Relafen), tolmetin (Tolectin), and many others. Acetaminophen, such as Tylenol, can help with mild pain, but it is not very effective for inflammation.

When inflammation becomes more serious, corticosteroids are frequently used. Side effects of steroids such as prednisone can include weight gain, puffiness and roundness in the face, acne, osteoporosis, elevated blood pressure, increased risk of cataracts, diabetes, infection, and increased appetite.

In some lupus patients, antimalarial drugs such as chloroquine (Aralen), hydroxychloroquine (Plaquenil), or quinacrine (Atabrine) are used, particularly for treatment of the skin and joint-related symptoms. These drugs can take months to work but have few side effects other than rashes and digestive disturbances. If you are prescribed antimalarials, there can be side effects to the eyes, however, and regular eye exams are essential, as is use of UV-protective sunglasses.

For some advanced cases of lupus, immunomodulating drugs may be used. Azathioprine (Imuran), cyclophosphamide (Cytoxan), methotrexate (Rheumatrex), and cyclosporine (Sandimmune, Neoral) can reduce inflammation but also suppress the immune system. These drugs can cause anemia, reduced white blood cell counts, and increased risk of infection. They are also linked to increased cancer risk.

For some patients with severe kidney or nervous system involvement due to lupus, a combination of corticosteroid and immunosuppressive drugs may be recommended. Occasionally, when clotting disorders are present, lupus patients are given anticoagulants, ranging from aspirin to drugs such as heparin or warfarin (Coumadin), which block clotting.

Numerous drugs and technologies are also being tested for lupus patients. While no one has found a surefire cure for the debilitating disease, it's clear that many lupus patients are now enjoying an increased quality of life, thanks to new drugs and treatments.

Dr. Rosalind Ramsey-Goldman, MD, DrPH, professor of medicine at Northwestern University, has said, "Just the fact that clinical trials are going on in lupus is a major breakthrough; the challenge has been to come up with a responder index that notes if a drug is effective or not." Dr. Ramsey-Goldman outlined some new studies that may prove beneficial, including the use of DHEA (done by Genelabs, currently under review by the FDA), the safety of hormones in lupus (oral contraceptives or replacement by NIH/NIAMS), a comparison of mycofenalate mofetil and cyclophosphamide for treatment of renal disease in lupus, and a treatment to reduce the rate of renal flare in lupus.

- *LJP 394:* One new product, LJP 394, an experimental drug to treat lupus, has had encouraging results in clinical trials. The drug, manufactured by La Jolla Pharmaceuticals, targets antibodies in double-stranded DNA that are linked to kidney failure, the primary cause of death in lupus. In an eighteen-month clinical trial of LJP 394, there were three times as many renal flares—an episode of inflammation that can damage the kidneys—in the group receiving a placebo as there were in the LJP-treated group. The drug, which has been granted Orphan Drug Status by the FDA, may offer further hope to patients who are hoping to prevent or delay renal flares and reduce the need for treatment with high-dose corticosteroids and/or chemotherapy drugs.
- *DHEA:* Research has found that DHEA (dehydroepiandrosterone) can improve the health of people with lupus. A regulated pharmaceutical-quality version of DHEA, known as Aslera, has been attempting to get FDA approval, and the Lupus Foundation has been actively supporting the approval of Aslera.

Ellen Ignatius, vice president of education and science information for the Lupus Foundation, presented results in which lupus patients were treated over long periods of time with DHEA, an androgen much weaker than testosterone and thus less likely to have unpleasant masculinizing side effects. Although not cured by any means, the patients on DHEA reported feeling more energetic and less symptomatic, and less likely to need an immune-suppressant drug such as prednisone than the group taking dummy pills.

Things to Know

Lupus is frequently difficult to diagnose, and many patients see numerous practitioners before an accurate diagnosis is made. Dr. Marie Savard, patient advocate and author, says patients can play a role in that process:

> There is perhaps no other illness that requires detailed collection of all prior tests, symptoms, etc., as the tests and symptoms can fluctuate and confuse people. Sometimes blood tests are positive, other times not so. The vague symptoms of fatigue are written off by patient and doctor as stress only. Trust your gut that something is wrong on this one!

As many as 10 percent of lupus patients may also have other autoimmune disorders such as scleroderma, rheumatoid arthritis, or mixed connective tissue disease (MCTD), so patients should be alert for the appearance of symptoms of other autoimmune disorders.

Lupus and hormones are linked. Pregnancy can be difficult for lupus patients, and miscarriage is more common in lupus patients. Flares after childbirth are also common and can be particularly debilitating. Flares occur far less often, however, after a woman reaches menopause.

People with lupus should learn to recognize early symptoms of a flare so that they can help their doctor know when a change in therapy is needed. Regular laboratory tests can also be valuable because sometimes lab results will start to change before symptoms begin. And, generally, the earlier a flare is detected, the more easily it can be controlled. Also, early treatment may decrease the chance of permanent tissue or organ damage and reduce the time spent on high doses of drugs. For people with sun-sensitive lupus rashes, appropriate use of ultraviolet-blocking sunscreens and protective clothing is critical.

■ Mixed Connective Tissue Disease

Mixed connective tissue disease (MCTD) is a chronic inflammatory autoimmune disease characterized by joint pain, muscle weakness, cardiac, lung, and skin manifestations, kidney disease, and dysfunction of the esophagus. MCTD describes a collection of symptoms that may have similarities to lupus, scleroderma, and other connective tissue diseases but is not strictly diagnosable as one of those conditions because signs and symptoms overlap.

Diagnosis of MCTD can be difficult, as it may feature simultaneous symptoms of lupus, scleroderma, and rheumatoid arthritis. Sometimes, MCTD is a precursor to a later diagnosis of one of these conditions. In other cases, it's considered a condition on its own and never progresses to full lupus, scleroderma, or rheumatoid arthritis.

MCTD can occur at any age, with the average age of onset in the teens to 30s. Eight out of ten patients are women. The disease occurs in all races and is found worldwide. The prevalence is not known, but it's thought to be somewhat less than lupus, which affects 15 to 50 people in 100,000.

Symptoms
Symptoms of MCTD usually include

- Raynaud's phenomenon, causing increased sensitivity of the fingers and toes to the cold, changes in skin color, pain, and occasionally ulcers of the fingertips or toes
- Arthritic pain and aches in joints, and weakness and pain in muscles, especially in the shoulders and hips

- Swollen hands, sausage-like fingers, swollen or red patches over the knuckles
- Lung disease, including pleuritis, shortness of breath on exertion, or, more rarely, pulmonary hypertension
- Lupus-like rashes, including a butterfly-shaped, purple-colored rash on the cheeks and nose bridge
- Spider veins on the face and hands
- Small patches of hair loss or thinning hair
- Shortness of breath
- Fever
- Swollen lymph nodes
- Abdominal pain, heartburn
- Hoarseness, difficulty swallowing
- Dry eyes and dry mouth

In a small percentage of patients, kidneys can be affected, but damage is usually mild.

Diagnosis

MCTD is diagnosed when lupus, scleroderma, and rheumatoid arthritis symptoms overlap. Bloodwork in MCTD patients may reveal

- High levels (often greater than 1:1,000) of antinuclear antibodies (ANAs)
- Positive rheumatoid factor
- High levels of anti–U1-RNP antibodies
- Presence of anti-RNP antibodies
- Presence of anti–U1-70 kD
- Antiphospholipid antibodies (including anticardiolipin antibodies and lupus anticoagulant)
- Moderate anemia

In the long term, as symptoms evolve, eventually lupus, sclero-derma, or rheumatoid arthritis may be diagnosed.

Practitioners

A rheumatologist experienced in the diagnosis and treatment of MCTD should be involved in treatment of this condition. Other specialists, such as a pulmonologist, may be called in to help coordinate treatment, especially in the case of lung-related complications.

Treatment

Treatment for MCTD is similar to lupus. Nonsteroidal anti-inflammatory agents (NSAIDs) are given to help reduce pain and inflammation, and may be the only drugs needed in mild MCTD. Low-dose oral corticosteroids or low-dose methotrexate is reserved for more serious and debilitating joint inflammation.

- Naproxen (Naprosyn, Naprelan, Aleve, Anaprox) can be used for inflammation and swelling.
- Celecoxib (Celebrex) and rofecoxib (Vioxx) are frequently used to treat muscle and joint pain related to MCTD.
- Calcium channel blockers such as nifedipine (Adalat, Procardia XL) may be recommended for Raynaud's phenomenon.
- Omeprazole (Prilosec) is used for esophageal reflux.
- Antimalarial drugs such as hydroxychloroquine (Plaquenil) can be prescribed to help prevent disease flares.
- Corticosteroids such as prednisone (Deltasone) are used for active or severe disease.
- Cytotoxic agents such as cyclophosphamide (Cytoxan) are prescribed for major organ involvement.

Things to Know

With MCTD, symptom-free periods can last for years. In around 13 percent of people, MCTD can progress and become more serious or life-threatening. Secondary Sjögren's syndrome occurs in 25 percent of patients with MCTD and may cause eye symptoms and dry mouth.

■ Sarcoidosis

Sarcoidosis is a chronic autoimmune disease that affects multiple systems of the body. In sarcoidosis, abnormal collections of dead tissue, known as granulomas, form in many organs, including the lymph nodes, lungs, liver, eyes, skin, and other areas.

Sarcoidosis doesn't follow the same course for each person. Some patients will have very minimal symptoms, whereas others can have severe implications. In some people, sarcoidosis may go away, even without treatment. In others, sarcoidosis will go into remission and then relapse over time, but the majority of people with sarcoidosis will have it for their lifetime.

Sarcoidosis is an uncommon condition and occurs predominantly between the ages of 20 and 40. There are an estimated 25,000 cases in the United States, mostly women, and it's most commonly found in the southeastern part of the country. In the United States, sarcoidosis is ten times more common among African-Americans than Caucasians, and it occurs most often in people of northern European ancestry. In Sweden, for example, the disease affects 6.5 people in 10,000. The condition is almost unknown among Native Americans, Australian aborigines, and southern Asians.

As with many other autoimmune diseases, there's no clear cause or trigger for sarcoidosis, but a slow viral- or toxic-triggering process is suspected. Genetic predisposition also appears to play a role.

Symptoms

In about 60 percent of patients, sarcoidosis typically develops over a period of several weeks, with symptoms such as

- Fever/night sweats
- Fatigue, malaise
- Weight loss, loss of appetite
- Shortness of breath, sometimes with exertion
- Hoarseness, dry cough, tonsillitis
- Chest discomfort
- Tachycardia (fast heartbeat)
- Parotid gland inflammation and enlargement
- Abnormal lung x-ray showing possible pleural effusion (small amounts of fluid on the lungs)
- Rashes, lesions on the face or extremities, raised pink or purplish areas or rashes
- Painful nodules and lesions under the skin, on the shins and lower extremities
- Dry eyes, blurry vision, tearing eyes, red eyes, double vision, or light sensitivity
- Muscle pain or weakness
- Aching joints and arthritic symptoms
- Arthritis
- Enlarged lymph nodes
- Headaches
- Dizziness

The eyes are affected in 15 percent of patients.

In 40 percent of patients, onset of sarcoidosis is rapid and acute. Some of those patients fall into two syndrome categories: (1) Lofgren's syndrome, which includes swollen lymph nodes and joint symptoms; and (2) Heerfordt-Waldenstrom syndrome, which includes fever, enlarged parotid glands, eye inflammation, and facial nerve involvement.

Diagnosis

Sarcoidosis can affect many organs and tissues, but most often it affects the lungs. Diagnosis of sarcoidosis is, therefore, usually made by a chest x-ray, which can show inflammation or fluid in and around the lungs. Other blood test results that can potentially aid in a sarcoidosis diagnosis include

- Elevated erythrocyte sedimentation rate (ESR)
- Hypercalcemia (excessive calcium)
- Elevated alkaline phosphatase
- Elevated antinuclear antibodies (ANAs)
- Elevated rheumatoid factor (RF)
- High immunoglobulin levels, known as hypergammaglobulinemia
- Elevated creatine phosphokinase (CPK) and CPK-MB levels
- Low white blood cell counts

Other helpful tests may include

- Whole body scan looking for abnormal patterns in lungs or lymph nodes
- Pulmonary function tests to reveal reduced lung capacity
- Elevated liver enzymes, especially alkaline phosphatase

Practitioners

A rheumatologist is the practitioner best qualified to diagnose and treat sarcoidosis, although some pulmonologists may specialize in autoimmune diseases that affect the lungs.

Treatment

Sarcoidosis is generally treated with steroids. Topical steroids may be used for eye and skin problems. Joint and muscle symptoms are generally treated with NSAIDs or oral corticosteroids such as prednisone to reduce inflammation.

The small percentage of people who fail to respond to corticosteroids are frequently switched to the immunosuppressive drug methotrexate (Folex, Rheumatrex) or the antimalarial drug hydroxychloroquine.

Physical therapy for improved breathing and interval exercise training to improve aerobic capacity are both important therapies for sarcoidosis.

Things to Know

Diabetes is more common in sarcoidosis patients and can result from the pituitary gland being affected by the sarcoidosis, so it's important for patients to be on the alert for diabetes symptoms.

Sarcoidosis may sometimes be misdiagnosed as tuberculosis.

Some granulomas resulting from sarcoidosis can produce vitamin C, which enhances calcium absorption and leads to high calcium levels. Symptoms of excess calcium include loss of appetite, nausea, vomiting, thirst, and excessive urine production. They should be evaluated and treated quickly, because over time, excess calcium (hypercalcemia) can lead to kidney stones or kidney failure. It is important for sarcoidosis patients to avoid getting lung infections, so an annual flu shot is typically recommended.

The prognosis for sarcoidosis is good. Enlarged lymph nodes and lung inflammation may disappear over a few months or years. In low-level sarcoidosis, some patients may have a full remission within two to five years after onset. More than 75 percent of those with only enlarged lymph nodes and more than half of those with lung involvement recover after five years. More than two-thirds of people with lung sarcoidosis have no symptoms after nine years. About half of those diagnosed have periodic relapses, and only 10 percent develop serious disability or life-threatening complications.

■ Sjögren's Syndrome

Sjögren's syndrome is a chronic condition in which the immune system produces white blood cells, which then produce antibodies that attack the exocrine glands that secrete fluids, such as the salivary and tear glands. The glands become injured, resulting in dry mouth (xerostomia) and dry eyes (xerophthalmia), as well as the presence of lymphocytes in these exocrine glands. These symptoms are collectively known as the sicca complex or sicca syndrome.

While the majority of cases affect the tear ducts, salivary glands, and vagina, other mucous membranes that can become dried out in Sjögren's syndrome include the gastrointestinal tract and windpipe.

Sjögren's syndrome can affect both men and women at any age; however, the majority of patients are women (nine women to every man), and the onset is most common in the 40s and 50s. In the United States, it's estimated that Sjögren's syndrome is the second most common rheumatologic disorder, following lupus.

Sjögren's syndrome can occur by itself, or it frequently shows up as secondary Sjögren's syndrome, alongside other autoimmune diseases such as lupus, rheumatoid arthritis, scleroderma, thyroid disease, and other conditions. It's suspected but not proven that the autoimmune reaction seen in Sjögren's syndrome is set in motion by a viral infection. Suspected viral agents include herpes, retroviruses, hepatitis C, cytomegalovirus (CMV), Epstein-Barr, and human herpes virus type 6 (HHV-6).

Symptoms

Sjögren's syndrome symptoms include

- Dry, sore, or burning sensation in mouth
- Difficulty chewing and swallowing
- Recurrent cavities
- Enlarged salivary or parotid glands

- Dry cough
- Reduced tears, dry eyes, sensitivity to light, air, and smoke
- Burning sensation, itchiness, sandy feeling or pain in eyes
- Ghosting (visual disturbance where you get a visual sense of a ghost image as your eyes move)
- Joint and muscle pain, morning stiffness
- Nausea, stomach pain
- Raynaud's phenomenon, most frequently manifested by tingling, numbness, coldness, and color changes in hands and feet
- More frequent infections, including bladder infections, cold sores, and vaginal yeast infections
- Increased thirst/drinking a lot of fluids

Dryness of eyes can cause damage to the cornea, and dryness of the trachea and lungs make them more susceptible to infection.

Diagnosis

One of the key tests for the condition is the Schirmer test, in which a small strip of paper is inserted into the lower lid of the eye to measure the level of tears. Normal results are tears of fifteen millimeters or more after fifteen minutes. A positive test for Sjögren's is considered less than 5 millimeters after five minutes. Some other tests that can help confirm a diagnose include

- Erythrocyte sedimentation rate (ESR): 80 percent of Sjögren's patients have elevated ESRs.
- Rheumatoid factor: More than two-thirds of patients will test positive for it.
- Anti-SS-A and anti-SS-B antibodies: A majority of primary Sjögren's patients test positive for these antibodies.
- Antisalivary duct antibodies: Secondary Sjögren's patients frequently test positive for these antibodies.

- Anemia: A third of Sjögren's patients will show some evidence of anemia.

Practitioners

In many cases, an ophthalmologist may be the first to suspect Sjögren's syndrome and can conduct Schirmer's test. General practitioners, rheumatologists, and internists can frequently recognize and treat Sjögren's as well.

If you have Sjögren's syndrome, plan to have regular checkups by both your ophthalmologist and dentist.

Treatment

Treatment of Sjögren's syndrome mainly involves lubricating the dry areas. This includes

- Medications such as pilocarpine HCI (Salagen) and cevilimine HCI (Evoxac), which flood the body with moisture
- Eye lubricants, such as daytime formulas of artificial tears for use throughout the day, with a thicker, longer-acting lubricant gel or cream at bedtime
- For oral dryness, sugarless gum, candies, or lozenges specifically designed to help increase saliva
- Carrying water with you
- Avoiding windy or dry climates, avoiding air-conditioning with low humidity
- Avoiding dust and smoke
- Good oral hygiene

According to Dr. Frederick Vivino, a rheumatologist at Thomas Jefferson University, a Sjögren's expert, and a medical consultant to the Sjögren's Syndrome Foundation:

The current medicines we have can stimulate the endocrine system to start producing saliva again, and they've literally been lifesavers for many patients. However, they don't address the autoimmune aspect of the disease—they merely treat the symptoms, rather than address the underlying issues—and they don't help every patient. Some people are too far advanced in their disease to receive any benefit.

There are several other new treatments on the horizon. A Japanese study of an alpha-interferon lozenge that was sucked by the patient three times daily showed promising results in reducing the inflammation and stimulating salivary flow. An American company, Amarillo Biosciences, Inc., completed the third phase of clinical trials using alpha-interferon lozenges in 2001 and they are undergoing further study. The trial was a double-blinded, placebo-controlled study in which 256 patients were treated three times daily with a lozenge containing either 150 International Units of natural interferon alpha (IFN-a) or with a placebo for 24 weeks. An improvement rate—more than twice that of the placebo group—in saliva production was noted in the group given IFN-a.

Other developments have centered on finding hormonal clues to the disease. Harvard Medical School's Dr. David Sullivan discovered that Sjögren's patients have lower than normal levels of testosterone. Low levels of the hormone are linked to inflamed and dysfunctional eye glands. Sullivan's lab has developed testosterone eye drops to treat these symptoms. Allergan, Inc., has been testing the drops in clinical trials for the treatment of dry eyes due to Sjögren's disease, aging, and menopause.

The popular rheumatoid arthritis drug etanercept (Enbrel) is being examined by researchers at the National Institute of Health to see if it can be used to treat Sjögren's. And thalidomide, once off the market due to the risk of birth defects, is also being cautiously studied for its use in Sjögren's syndrome.

Dr. Bruce Baum of the National Institute of Health is investigating the development of artificial salivary glands. In the high-tech world of gene therapy, tissue may be engineered to grow artificial saliva-producing glands. Under this scenario, new genes could be placed into the damaged glands of Sjögren's patients, thus restoring saliva flow and preventing further destruction.

Other treatments involve medications that lessen the symptoms of Sjögren's, including dry eyes. The National Eye Institute (NEI) of the National Institutes of Health (NIH) is conducting a study on the use of an anti-inflammatory medication, cyclosporine, in the treatment of dry eyes. Occasionally, particularly difficult cases of Sjögren's are sometimes treated with oral corticosteroids.

Things to Know

Wear glasses or sunglasses to help shield eyes when you're going to be in a windy environment. The best sunglasses are wraparound ones that protect from wind.

Non-Hodgkin's lymphoma, which strikes about 50,000 people each year in the United States, is forty-four times more common in people who have Sjögren's syndrome, so it's important to be on the alert for these symptoms, which include enlarged lymph nodes; difficulty swallowing; rashes; vomiting; fluid retention; shortness of breath and difficulty breathing; facial swelling; abdominal pain or distention; swelling in legs; weight loss, diarrhea; thickened, dark, itchy areas of skin; fever; night sweats; and severe fatigue.

Sjögren's is relatively common in people with other autoimmune diseases, particularly chronic fatigue syndrome and rheumatoid arthritis. In fact, as many as 30 to 50 percent of Sjögren's syndrome patients also have rheumatoid arthritis. Sjögren's syndrome patients should probably have their thyroid tested to find undiagnosed thyroid abnormalities, as there is a higher incidence of subclinical thyroid disease in these patients as well.

Endocrine Conditions

The endocrine system is a prevalent target for autoimmune disease. Some of the most common autoimmune diseases—insulin-dependent diabetes, Graves' disease, and Hashimoto's thyroiditis—for example—are all autoimmune endocrine conditions. Other lesser-known conditions also target the endocrine glands, such as autoimmune Addison's disease and autoimmune oophoritis.

Endocrine autoimmune conditions affect the various endocrine glands, which are glands that secrete hormone and metabolic substances, and include the thyroid, ovaries, testes, pituitary, pancreas, and adrenals. There are also endocrine gastric cells lining the stomach. The endocrine system is the body's hormonal regulator, releasing and then slowing and stopping production of different hormones, in response to various external and internal triggers. While hormones circulate around the body, they act on particular cells. Some cells have receptors that recognize particular hormones. When these cells come into contact with their matching hormones, they bind to each other, and further processes can occur.

With autoimmune endocrine conditions, you can also produce antibodies to a variety of hormones, including the form of estrogen known as estradiol, progesterone, and others. Women with antibodies to hormones may have erratic ovulation or insufficient production of uterine lining, which can prevent successful implantation and pregnancy, and create erratic or abnormal menstrual periods.

■ Thyroid Disease

With an estimated 20 million sufferers—and a vast 13 million of them undiagnosed—thyroid disease is the most common autoimmune condition in the United States today. Thyroid disease prevalence increases with age, and generally women are seven times more likely than men to develop it. Thyroid problems are also common in many other countries, particularly areas covered at one time by glaciers, where iodine is not present in the soil and in foods. In many of these countries, an enlarged thyroid, known as goiter, is seen in as many as one in five people, and is usually due to iodine deficiency. Around the world, an estimated 8 percent of the population have goiter, most commonly women. A woman faces as high as a one in five chance of developing a thyroid problem during her lifetime. The risk of thyroid disease increases with age, and by age 74, the prevalence of subclinical hypothyroidism in men, 16 percent, is nearly as high as the 21 percent rate seen in women.

Your thyroid is a small bowtie- or butterfly-shaped gland located in your neck, wrapped around the windpipe and below the Adam's apple area. The thyroid, which is considered the master gland of metabolism, produces several hormones, of which two are most critical: triiodothyronine (T3) and thyroxine (T4). The thyroid has the only cells in the body capable of absorbing iodine. It takes in the iodine obtained through food, iodized salt, or supplements and combines it with the amino acid tyrosine. The thyroid then converts the iodine/tyrosine combination into the hormones T3 and T4. The "3" and the "4" refer to the number of iodine molecules in each thyroid hormone molecule.

When it's in good condition, of all the hormones produced by your thyroid, 80 percent will be T4 and 20 percent will be T3. T3 is considered the biologically more active hormone—the one that actually functions at the cellular level—and is also considered several times stronger than T4. Once released by the thyroid, T3 and T4 travel through the bloodstream. The purpose is to help cells convert oxygen and calories into energy and serve as the basic fuel of your metabolism. As mentioned, the thyroid produces some T3. But the rest of the T3 needed by the body is actually formed from the mostly inactive T4 by a process sometimes referred to as *T4 to T3 conversion*. This conversion of T4 to T3 can take place in some organs other than the thyroid, including the hypothalamus, a part of your brain.

The thyroid is part of a huge feedback process. The hypothalamus in the brain releases thyrotropin-releasing hormone (TRH). The release of TRH tells the pituitary gland to release thyroid-stimulating hormone (TSH). This TSH, circulating in your bloodstream, is what tells the thyroid to make thyroid hormones and release them into your bloodstream.

There are actually two different autoimmune diseases that target the thyroid: Graves' disease, which causes an overactive thyroid (hyperthyroidism), and Hashimoto's thyroiditis, which causes an underactive thyroid (hypothyroidism). In Graves' disease, autoantibodies bind to the thyroid gland and cause the thyroid to overproduce thyroid hormone. Graves' disease is more common in women and most frequently appears between the ages of 20 and 30. It's estimated that 3 million people have Graves' disease worldwide, with around 1.5 million in the United States. Rarely, Graves' disease is asymptomatic, but usually, Graves' disease triggers hyperthyroidism, causing the gland to produce too much thyroid hormone. When hyperthyroid, your body goes into overdrive, causing increased heart rate, increased blood pressure, and the burning of calories at an increased rate.

Hashimoto's thyroiditis can also be referred to as autoimmune thyroiditis or chronic lymphocytic thyroiditis. In Hashimoto's, antibodies are reacting against proteins in the thyroid, causing gradual destruction of the gland itself and its ability to produce the thyroid hormones the body needs. According to the American Autoimmune Related Diseases Association, as many as 25 percent of patients with Hashimoto's may develop additional conditions such as pernicious anemia, diabetes, adrenal insufficiency, or other autoimmune diseases.

Most people with autoimmune thyroid disease end up hypothyroid—that is, the thyroid is either underactive, totally unable to function, or has been surgically removed. Hashimoto's thyroiditis usually slowly destroys the thyroid. Treatments for hyperthyroidism, such as radioactive iodine (RAI) treatment and surgical removal of the thyroid, also usually result in hypothyroidism. Besides the treatments already mentioned, there are other factors that can contribute to the development of various autoimmune thyroid problems:

- Exposure to radiation, such as occurred after the Chernobyl nuclear plant accident
- Overconsumption of isoflavone-intensive soy products, such as soy protein, soy capsules, and soy powders
- Overconsumption or shortage of iodine in the diet (also applies to iodine-containing supplements such as kelp and bladder wrack)
- Radiation treatment to the head, neck, or chest; radiation treatment for tonsils, adenoids, lymph nodes, thymus gland problems, or acne
- Nasal radium therapy, which took place during the 1940s through 1960s as a treatment for tonsillitis, colds, and other ailments, or for military submariners and/or pilots who had trouble with drastic changes in pressure
- Overconsumption of uncooked "goitrogenic" foods, such as brussels sprouts, broccoli, rutabaga, turnips, kohlrabi, radishes,

cauliflower, African cassava, millet, babassu (a palm-tree coconut fruit popular in Brazil and Africa), cabbage, and kale

- Excess exposure to chemicals in water, such as fluoride or perchlorate
- Excess exposure to metals, such as mercury
- Excess exposure to environmental estrogens such as pesticides

There is a higher risk of onset of Graves' disease right after pregnancy, and one study found that two-thirds of women had been pregnant before the onset of Graves' disease. Pregnancy also seems to be a factor triggering Hashimoto's disease. Infection is thought to be a trigger in susceptible people. The foodborne bacteria *Yersinia enterocolitica* infection, for example, has been associated with production of thyroid antibodies, as have allergies or sensitivity to gluten.

People who have been treated for hyperthyroidism, have a history of neck irradiation, have suffered postpartum thyroiditis, or have other autoimmune disorders, especially Type I diabetes, are at higher risk for subclinical hypothyroidism.

Symptoms

Common Hashimoto's symptoms that typically accompany an underactive thyroid include

- Fatigue, exhaustion
- Depression, moodiness, sadness, difficulty concentrating, difficulty remembering
- Sensitivity to cold, cold hands and feet
- Inappropriate weight gain, or difficulty losing weight
- Dry, tangled, or coarse hair, and hair loss, especially from the outer part of the eyebrow
- Brittle fingernails
- Muscle and joint pains and aches

- Tendinitis in arms and legs, carpal tunnel syndrome
- Plantar's fasciitis—pain in the sole of the foot
- Swelling or puffiness in the eyes, face, arms, or legs
- Heart palpitations
- Low sex drive
- Infertility, recurrent miscarriages
- Heavy, longer, more frequent or more painful menstrual periods
- High cholesterol levels, especially unresponsive to diet and medication
- Worsening allergies, itching, prickly hot skin, rashes, hives (urticaria)
- Chronic infections, including yeast infections, oral fungus, thrush, and sinus infections
- Shortness of breath, difficulty drawing a full breath
- Constipation
- Full or sensitive feeling in the neck
- Raspy, hoarse voice

Common Graves' disease symptoms manifesting as hyperthyroidism include

- Rapid weight loss, or increased appetite without weight gain
- Insomnia, difficulty falling asleep or staying asleep
- Anxiety, erratic behavior, nervousness, irritability, nervousness, or panic attacks
- Difficulty concentrating, short attention span
- Palpitations, irregular heartbeat, high pulse and heartbeat
- Atrial fibrillation
- Feeling hot, sweating more than usual
- Hand tremors
- Diarrhea
- Fatigue
- Dry skin, even thickened patches on shins and legs

- Fine, brittle hair
- Infertility
- Lighter menstrual periods, less frequent or they stop altogether
- Muscle weakness, especially in the upper arms and thighs
- Eye problems, including double vision, scratchy eyes, bulging, sensitivity to light

Diagnosis

One self-test you can do is a thyroid neck check. Hold a mirror so that you can see the area of your neck just below the Adam's apple and right above the collarbone. This is the general location of your thyroid gland. Tip your head back while keeping this view of your neck and thyroid area in your mirror. Take a drink of water and swallow. As you swallow, look at your neck. Watch carefully for any bulges, enlargement, protrusions, or unusual appearances in this area when you swallow. Repeat this process several times. If you see anything that appears unusual, see your doctor right away. You may have an enlarged thyroid or a thyroid nodule, and your thyroid should be evaluated. Be sure you don't get your Adam's apple confused with your thyroid gland. The Adam's apple is at the front of your neck; the thyroid is further down and closer to your collarbone. Remember that this test is by no means conclusive and cannot rule out thyroid abnormalities. It's just helpful to identify a particularly enlarged thyroid or masses in the thyroid that warrant evaluation.

Another possible sign of thyroid abnormality is a low basal body temperature. Some practitioners even believe that a low basal body temperature (taken upon awakening, in bed, before getting up and before any substantial movement) can be indicative of hypothyroidism. Typically, basal body temperatures lower than 97.8 to 98.2°F are thought to potentially indicate hypothyroidism. This self-testing method was popularized by the late Dr. Broda Barnes. Again, this test is not considered conclusive by many practitioners and does not either definitively diagnose or rule out thyroid abnormalities.

Blood tests are another key way of identifying thyroid problems. The most commonly performed test is the thyroid-stimulating hormone (TSH) test. Although ranges vary from lab to lab, the general normal range for TSH is from 0.5 to 5.5. Levels above 5.5 are evidence of hypothyroidism, and levels below 0.5 are indicative of hyperthyroidism. *Note:* Increasing numbers of doctors are finding that a TSH of around 1 to 2 is optimal for most people to feel well and avoid having hypothyroid or hyperthyroid symptoms. There is now research that provides some scientific basis for this, saying that values above 3 may in fact represent subclinical hypothyroidism and that borderline low TSH levels may be indicative of subclinical or subtle hyperthyroidism.

- If your doctor runs a test called total T4 or total thyroxine, the normal range is approximately 4.5 to 12.5. If you had a low reading and a high TSH, your doctor might consider a diagnosis of hypothyroidism. If you had a low reading and a low TSH, your doctor might investigate a pituitary problem.
- If your doctor runs a test called free T4 or free thyroxine, the normal range is approximately 0.7 to 2.0. If your result was less than 0.7, your doctor might consider a diagnosis of hypothyroidism.
- If your doctor runs a test called total T3, the normal range is approximately 80 to 220. If your result was less than 80, your doctor might consider a diagnosis of hypothyroidism.
- If your doctor runs a test called free T3, the normal range is approximately 2.3 to 4.2. If your result was less than 2.3, your doctor might consider a diagnosis of hypothyroidism.
- Thyroid antibody tests can also detect the antibodies that signal the presence of Hashimoto's or Graves' disease, even when TSH levels are normal.

A diagnosis of thyroid disease can be difficult, particularly when you have borderline thyroid conditions, or when antibodies are present and causing symptoms, but bloodwork has yet to reflect the TSH abnormalities. There are practitioners who believe that you do not need to have an elevated TSH level in order to actually be diagnosed and treated for hypothyroidism. Increasingly, innovative doctors are also viewing high-normal or normal TSH levels as possible evidence of low-level hypothyroidism. One thyroid expert, Dr. John Dommisse, has said that "the so-called normal range is way too high."

In more difficult-to-diagnose cases, a test called thyrotropin releasing hormone (TRH) can be performed. This ultrasensitive test can detect very subtle thyroid function abnormalities, but because of the time and expense of the test, it's been abandoned by most practitioners in favor of the faster, less costly TSH test.

If you don't have insurance or prefer to start with self-testing, you can do a home TSH test. A company called Biosafe markets an accurate, affordable (less than $50) home TSH test. Biosafe's test kit requires an almost painless finger prick using a special finger lancet. All you need are a couple of drops of blood, which you put into the collection device and send to Biosafe's lab for analysis. Results are mailed back to you quickly. For information or to order a test, you can call Biosafe at 1-800-768-8446, extension 123, or find out more at this book's website, http://www.autoimmunebook/biosafe.

Another option is more conventional blood testing that requires a blood draw from a laboratory, but a doctor and prescription for the bloodwork are not required for testing. HealthCheckUSA offers online and telephone ordering of three different test options: a standard TSH test; the Comprehensive Thyroid Profile, which includes T3 uptake, T4 total, T7, and TSH; and Comprehensive Thyroid Profile II, which includes T3 (triiodothyronine) free, T4 (thyroxine) free, and TSH. The tests are extremely affordable, and HealthCheckUSA doctors sign off on bloodwork requests. You receive the results online or by mail. You can order tests by calling 1-800-929-2044 or by visiting the website at http://www.autoimmunebook.com/healthcheckusa/.

Ultimately, a complete clinical evaluation of your thyroid is required, including an examination of the thyroid by a professional, who will feel for enlargement, nodules, and masses. Your reflexes will be checked—sluggish reflexes can be a sign of hypothyroidism, and hyperresponsive reflexes are more common in hyperthyroidism. Other clinical details will be observed, and family history will be discussed. The clinical observation, in combination with symptoms and the results of blood tests, should all be considered together for a diagnosis.

Practitioners

Endocrinologists are doctors who specialize in diseases of the endocrine system. They typically have FACE after their names, standing for Fellow, American College of Endocrinology. The two main issues that endocrinologists typically deal with are diabetes and thyroid problems. Some endocrinologists, however, have subspecialties such as reproductive endocrinology (fertility), nuclear medicine, growth disorders, or osteoporosis. It is important to find one who actually focuses on thyroid disease, as the vast majority concentrate almost exclusively on diabetes and treat thyroid problems as a sideline, if they even treat them at all.

Internists and general practice doctors sometimes provide diagnoses and ongoing treatment for thyroid disease. When you are having difficulty getting diagnosed, or you don't do well with a conventional approach, or when you want to understand more about the many side effects and symptoms of hypothyroidism, the fairly conventional focus of most internists and general practice doctors may fall short of what you need. That's when you should consider an osteopathic, holistic, or metabolically oriented physician with expertise in thyroid disease, metabolism, and hormonal medicine.

Treatment

If you have a milder case of Graves' disease/hyperthyroidism, your doctor may initially prescribe antithyroid drugs such as methimazole (Tapazole) or propylthiouracil (PTU), as these drugs offer some chance of a remission. Despite the fact that as many as 40 percent of patients treated with antithyroid drugs can achieve a permanent remission, radioactive iodine (RAI) treatment is still preferred in the United States, whereas antithyroid drugs are the primary treatment in other countries. In this treatment, radioactive iodine, known as I-131, is given in the form of a drink or capsule. The thyroid absorbs this radioactive iodine in the same way that it attracts and concentrates other forms of iodine, allowing the radiation ultimately to disable all or part of the thyroid and treat the hyperthyroidism. By partially or fully disabling the thyroid, RAI eliminates hormone overproduction. RAI is typically followed by an elevation in thyroid antibodies, which can further aggravate the autoimmune-related symptoms. According to experts, the majority of patients do become hypothyroid after RAI, and while sometimes it is due to radiation-induced follicular damage, there is some suggestion that this promotion of antibodies worsens the underlying thyroiditis and causes hypothyroidism. Some innovative practitioners recommend a technique known as block replace therapy (BRT), which involves simultaneous use of antithyroid drugs to disable the overproduction and thyroid hormone replacement to suppress function. Surgery, known as thyroidectomy, is typically done when antithyroid drugs cannot be tolerated or if the person is not a good candidate for RAI (such as in the case of life-threatening hyperthyroidism during pregnancy).

For hypothyroidism, doctors typically prescribe the synthetic T4 hormone known as levothyroxine. Popular brands include Levoxyl, Unithroid, Levothroid, and Synthroid. Research reported in the *New England Journal of Medicine* in February 1999, however, found that a majority of patients may feel better on a combination of hormones. On the basis of that study, more doctors are also adding synthetic T3 (liothyronine)—the popular brand in the United States is Cytomel. Alternative physicians tend to prefer Thyrolar (a synthetic T4/T3 combination), or the natural desiccated thyroid drugs, Armour, Naturethroid, and Biotech, which also include T4 and T3.

Some patients find they feel best on the natural form of thyroid hormone replacement. One patient, Penny, had dramatic improvements on Armour after some of her doctors would only prescribe Synthroid. Penny explained:

> I am ready to live again! I have even lost half of the weight that I had gained since being on Armour . . . it makes me so mad to hear that others have had the same ignorant, narrow-minded, pompous, uncaring doctors like the first two I had the displeasure to come into contact with.

In Hashimoto's disease, around 10 percent of patients can have a spontaneous remission, typically from four to eight years after starting thyroid hormone replacement. This remission is also associated with the disappearance of antibodies. It's not clear whether these remissions are permanent.

Things to Know

Hypothyroidism is more common in people with rheumatoid arthritis, so be on the alert for signs and symptoms that you may have an undiagnosed case of this disease. In Hashimoto's thyroiditis, frequently during the initial phase of the condition, and periodically, you may actually have hyperthyroid phases, as the thyroid overcompensates for its reduced capacity to produce thyroid hormone. This can create the confusing situation where you have hyperthyroid symptoms but hypothyroid blood test results.

If you have infertility, get your thyroid checked. Says patient advocate Dr. Marie Savard:

A woman came to me with years of infertility for a simple checkup. She said she had tons of bloodwork from the infertility and didn't need to be tested. I insisted on a TSH because I felt her thyroid was a little enlarged. Her TSH was very high, in the 80s or more, and ultimately she got treated . . . and had five healthy kids of her own without fertility drugs. Her problem, after years of expensive and invasive infertility treatment, was a simple thyroid problem. Everyone pointed the finger at someone else, assuming the other person had checked the thyroid.

Lotus Biochemical is currently researching a new thyroid drug that includes both T4 and T3 but delivers thyroid hormone in a time-released pill form. This delivery form is meant to simulate the way the body actually releases thyroid hormone, avoiding the ups and downs in energy, pulse/heart rate, and side effects some patients experience from their thyroid drugs. This drug could be an improvement on the current thyroid hormone replacement treatments currently available.

Diabetes

It's important to start the discussion of diabetes by differentiating between its two types. The autoimmune type is Type I diabetes—also known as insulin-dependent diabetes, juvenile diabetes, and diabetes mellitus—which is frequently diagnosed in childhood or young adulthood. The more common type of diabetes, Type II, or non-insulin-dependent diabetes, is the form that typically develops in adulthood and is almost overwhelmingly associated with obesity. There is some evidence that autoimmunity may contribute to a tendency to develop Type II diabetes, and it is more common in patients with other autoimmune conditions.

Each year, as many as 800,000 people are diagnosed with diabetes, and currently, according to the Centers for Disease Control, approximately 16 million already have the condition. According to the Joslin Diabetes Center, each year 13,000 new cases of Type I diabetes are diagnosed in children and teenagers, making it one of the most common chronic diseases in American children. More than 90 percent of diabetics are Type II, and more than one-third of these people do not know they have diabetes. In August 2000, the CDC reported that diabetes jumped 33 percent nationally, to 6.5 percent, between 1990 and 1998. The rise crossed races and age groups but was sharpest—about 70 percent—among people ages 30 to 39.

Diabetes alone is the sixth leading cause of death in the United States and a major cause of cardiovascular disease, blindness, visual impairment, and amputations. Total costs of this disease have been estimated to be in excess of $92 billion annually.

Type I diabetes is more common in colder climates—northern Europe has the highest incidence—and the incidence appears to increase with distance from the equator. Caucasians have the highest reported incidence of Type I diabetes; Chinese, the lowest. American Caucasians are 1.5 times more likely to develop Type I diabetes than African-Americans or Hispanics in the United States. For relatives, there's a 6 to 8 percent risk of having Type I diabetes if you have a first-degree relative—parent, sibling, or child—with the condition. Identical twins have a 60 percent lifetime risk of also developing Type I diabetes, and 30 percent of identical twins will develop diabetes within ten years of their twin's diagnosis. In fraternal twins, there is an 8 percent risk, equivalent to the risk between other siblings.

In Type I diabetes, which is slightly more common in women than in men, the immune system makes the mistake of thinking insulin-producing cells are foreign invaders, and T cells activate an attack against them, killing off the healthy insulin-producing islet cells of the pancreas. Since insulin is required by the body to keep the blood sugar (glucose) level under control, high levels of glucose result. Typically, symptoms only develop after most of the insulin-producing cells are destroyed.

In Type I diabetes, it's thought that the autoimmune reaction may be triggered by a viral infection. Finnish researchers reported in September 2001 that babies infected with common viruses known as enteroviruses are at an increased risk of developing Type I diabetes. Enteroviruses include polio, echoviruses, and the more common Coxsackie A and B, which are frequently the cause of many childhood illnesses. Researchers found that among children who had Type I diabetes, 24 percent had enterovirus infections in infancy or higher levels of antibodies to the virus. Only 16 percent of the healthy infants had enterovirus infections in infancy. The researchers also found that there is a higher incidence of the development of Type I diabetes–associated antibodies within six months of an enterovirus infection.

Breastfed infants have a lower risk for Type I diabetes, and a direct relationship exists between per capita cow milk consumption and incidence of diabetes. The reason for this connection seems to be related to the fact that some cow milk protein antigens may be similar to islet cell antigens.

Another factor that appears to lower the risk of developing Type I diabetes is ensuring that infants receive the recommended daily dose of vitamin D. A study found that babies who received at least 2,000 international units (IU) of vitamin D daily, which is the recommended daily allowance, were 80 percent less likely to develop Type I diabetes over the following thirty years, compared with infants who did not meet daily requirements of vitamin D.

A single gene has been identified that causes a high rate of a hereditary form of Type I diabetes, along with other autoimmune symptoms. The disorder caused by this genetic defect, which is called X-linked autoimmunity allergic dysregulation syndrome (XLAAD), causes diabetes, as well as diarrhea and eczema. Because XLAAD causes severe wasting, it often kills babies during the first months of life. Researchers are now attempting to use this information to help identify ways that diabetes might be better treated or even prevented.

In Type II diabetes, which is sometimes also called adult-onset diabetes, or the more old-fashioned term, sugar diabetes, the body either fails to make enough insulin or the cells ignore the insulin completely. This is typically due to increasing insulin resistance, which results from obesity and overconsumption of simple carbohydrates. About 80 to 90 percent of Type II diabetics are obese. African-Americans and Hispanics have a two- to threefold increased risk of developing Type II diabetes. While researchers don't quite know what the mechanism is, younger women who have long or irregular menstrual cycles are also at higher risk of developing Type II diabetes as they reach middle age. Specifically, women whose cycles lasted 40 days or more had double the risk of being diagnosed with diabetes, compared with women whose cycles lasted 26 to 31 days. The risk was even higher for women with long cycles who were obese.

There is some evidence that a tendency toward autoimmunity may increase the risk of developing Type II diabetes, and having a family member with Type II diabetes increases the risk of developing the condition. Having an autoimmune disease, particularly one of the endocrine conditions such as thyroid disease, or adrenal problems, can also increase the chances of developing Type II diabetes.

In some patients with Type II diabetes, insulin eventually becomes necessary. It's theorized that the constant stimulation of beta cells may destroy the cells, and the proteins associated with these cells builds up, triggering an autoimmune reaction that attacks the remaining healthy cells. When this occurs, it's referred to as Type I and one-half diabetes, or transitional diabetes.

Symptoms

Symptoms of Type I diabetes typically include

- General malaise, weakness, drowsiness
- Headache
- Urinary frequency, high volume of urine
- Increased thirst, even insatiable thirst
- Slower healing of cuts or abrasions
- Frequent infections (such as urinary tract infections)
- Weight loss, even with good appetite
- "Pins and needles" or deadened sensation on the feet or legs
- Abdominal pain
- Vomiting
- Babies or children may become ill-tempered
- Children may appear to be bedwetting

Symptoms of ketoacidosis—a life-threatening situation that can develop with advanced and untreated Type I diabetes—include all the symptoms just listed plus:

- Deep, rapid breathing
- Breath that smells like nail polish remover
- Abdominal pain, particularly in children
- Mental confusion
- Seizures

Type II symptoms are slow to develop, and the typical patient has this condition for five to seven years before being diagnosed. According to the American Diabetes Association, the most common symptoms of Type II diabetes include

- Blurred vision
- Extreme fatigue

- Extreme hunger
- Unusual thirst
- Unusual weight loss
- Frequent urination
- More frequent infections of bladder, gums, skin, or vagina
- Irritability
- Itchy skin
- Slow healing of cuts and bruises
- Tingling or numbness in legs, feet, or hands
- Mental confusion

Diagnosis

Diabetes is diagnosed by testing of blood sugar. A random blood glucose test with a result over 200 can be considered indicative of likely diabetes. In some cases, a fasting glucose test is done. After ten to twelve hours of fasting, blood is taken, and a level of more than 125 can be indicative of diabetes.

A glycosylated hemoglobin A1C (HA1C) test may be done. It can show average blood glucose levels over three to four months. The HA1C test does not diagnose people who have borderline diabetes or prediabetes, but it can detect full diabetes, and it is also used by diabetics to monitor blood sugar.

You may have some difficulties getting diagnosed. With sometimes vague symptoms such as fatigue, it may be difficult to get a physician to put together the symptom picture to identify diabetes. This is more likely with Type II diabetes. Paula Ford-Martin, a diabetes activist and webmaster, explains, "I have heard from many members of my community who have had trouble getting a proper Type II diabetes diagnosis simply because so many physicians tell them 'You just need to lose weight and you'll be fine.' "

An affordable self-testing option is HealthCheckUSA's Master Chemistry test, which determines if you have elevated glucose levels. This test also looks at cholesterol levels, kidney function, liver function, and other key measurements. HealthCheckUSA doctors sign off on the bloodwork requests, and you receive the results online or by mail. You can order tests by calling 1-800-929-2044 or by visiting this book's website at http://www.autoimmunebook.com/healthcheckusa.

If you suspect diabetes, self-testing is not really the best course of action, particularly in the case of Type I diabetes. Rapid diagnosis and medical treatment is important to ward off any potentially dangerous or even life-threatening side effects of diabetes. Self-testing is mainly useful for diabetics who wish to more frequently monitor blood sugar control after treatment. However, in the absence of options, a low-cost self-test for blood glucose can be a first step toward diagnosis, particularly in the case of slow-onset Type II diabetes.

Practitioners

Although general practitioners can frequently diagnose diabetes, it's important to consult with an endocrinologist for more in-depth assessment and recommendations. This is particularly important in Type I. Says Paula Ford-Martin:

Because Type 1 is typically diagnosed in childhood when kids are already going through such significant developmental changes, it's important to find a good pediatric endocrinologist. The American Diabetes Association keeps a database of physicians who are "Recognized Providers" on their website: http://www.diabetes.org/recognition/physicians/i_ prvstate2. asp. This status indicates they are meeting certain quality care standards in their practice. Anyone who takes part in a support group or attends a diabetes education class also has an excellent opportunity to network with other patients (and parents of patients). This can be one of the best ways to find a doctor, and also to learn the details that a physician locator

*service just won't tell you (such as communication style, bed-
side manner, willingness to try new treatments, etc.).*

Because diabetes and its related complications can have such different effects on the body, Paula Ford-Martin also advises that
patients pursue a team care approach, with an endocrinologist or
experienced GP overseeing and coordinating treatment strategies in
conjunction with you. Says Ford-Martin:

*You'll need endocrinologists, certified diabetes educators
(CDE), registered dietitians (RD), ophthalmologists, podia-
trists, nephrologists, exercise physiologists, and on and on,
as members of your team. I stress the patient participation
element. It's essential for patients to remember that effective
diabetes management requires that they take an active role in
their own care. Patients often tell me that they know something is wrong, or that their current treatment just isn't working right, but say: "Maybe I should just be quiet and follow
directions. After all, they're the doctor." It isn't always appar-
ent to them that it should be a two-way street; their doctor
should take the time to really* hear *what they are saying to
provide effective treatment. After all, no one is going to manage health care, or the health care of their children, but them.*

Treatment

In the cases of Type I and transitional diabetes, you'll need to
take insulin by injection. Your doctor will work out the specifics of
how, when, and in what quantity to best take your insulin for optimal blood sugar control. The different types of insulin include

- Quick-acting insulin: starts working in five to fifteen minutes,
  greatest effect on blood sugar in forty-five to ninety minutes,
  finishes working in three to four hours

- Short-acting regular insulin: starts working in thirty minutes, greatest effect in two to five hours, finishes working in five to eight hours
- Intermediate-acting insulin: starts working in one to three hours, greatest effect in eight to twelve hours, finishes working in sixteen to twenty-four hours
- Long-acting insulin: starts working in four to six hours, greatest effect in eight to twenty hours, finishes working in twenty-four to twenty-eight hours

Patients taking injectible insulin usually require blood glucose monitoring during the day. This can be done using glucose monitoring with finger pricks, meters that eliminate finger sticks by testing the arm or thigh, and even a new device that provides continuous monitoring from a wristwatch-like instrument that reads blood sugar levels through the skin.

An innovative form of delivery for injectable insulin is the insulin pump. An insulin pump is a small mechanical device, about the size of a deck of cards, which delivers insulin directly into the body, traveling by a long, thin plastic tube attached to a small flexible needle, collectively called an infusion set. The pump is worn outside the body, in a pouch or on a belt holder. The infusion set is moved every two to three days. A computer enables the pump to deliver insulin at programmed times, and blood sugar still must be monitored multiple times a day. The main reason for using a pump is flexibility. Working with only short-acting insulin, diabetics can eat whenever they want, unlike when on longer-acting insulin. Pumps can also be helpful in managing diabetes in children, who may not eat consistently. They are also very precise in terms of dosage delivery, better blood sugar control, convenience, and reduced number of injections. Pumps are best for those who are most dedicated about managing their blood sugar and who have family support and education.

According to Paula Ford-Martin, insulin pumps offer patients more flexibility in what and when they eat. They're also an excellent option for people with "brittle" diabetes (diabetics who experience large swings in blood glucose levels and have difficulty maintaining tight control). Says Ford-Martin:

Pumps are a particular godsend for kids, who are often put on pumps to give them greater flexibility, more efficiently manage their diabetes, and provide them with some measure of normalcy. Several companies are even working on units that can also constantly monitor glucose levels and dispense insulin accordingly.

For Type II diabetics, several categories of oral medications are usually given. The first category of drugs stimulate the beta cells to release more insulin. These include

• Sulfonylureas, which stimulate the pancreas to make more insulin, thereby lowering blood sugar. Chlorpropamide (Diabinese) is a first-generation sulfonylurea still in use today. Second-generation sulfonylureas include glipizide (Glucotrol), glyburide (Micronase, Glynase, and Diabeta), and glimepiride (Amaryl). These drugs are typically taken one to two times a day, before meals.
• Megilitinide, which causes a rapid, short-lived release of insulin. At press time, the only megilitinide available is repaglinide (Prandin), but others are being developed. These drugs are usually taken before each meal to affect blood sugar levels after eating.

The second category of drugs sensitize the body to the insulin that is already present.

• Biguanide drugs, such as the popular metformin (Glucophage), lower blood sugar by helping insulin work better, mostly in the liver. These drugs reduce the sugar the liver releases during fasting, so less insulin is needed to transport sugar from the blood to individual cells. They are usually taken twice a day and are frequently prescribed for those with Type II diabetes who are overweight and have elevated cholesterol.

• Thiazolidinediones reduce blood sugar by making tissues more sensitive to insulin, resulting in less sugar in the bloodstream and preventing the liver from overproducing glucose. Pioglitazone (Actos) and rosiglitazone (Avandia) are the drugs in this category. Because of rare but serious liver side effects, liver function is monitored closely in patients taking these drugs.

The third class of oral drugs slow or block breakdown of starches and certain sugars, and are also known as alpha-glycosidase inhibitors. Acarbose (Precose) and meglitol (Glyset) block the action of enzymes in the digestive track that break down carbohydrates into sugar, and slow the rise in blood sugar levels after a meal. They should be taken with the first bite of a meal. Side effects can include gas and diarrhea.

In some cases, doctors will prescribe oral drugs in combination. This can be expensive and present more side effects, however, so ideally one drug is the optimal treatment.

Diet and exercise are important in both Type I and Type II diabetes. Diet should focus on low-glycemic (low-sugar) foods, with an emphasis on vegetables, some fruits, low-fat proteins, and good fats, and minimizing or avoiding simple carbohydrates such as bread, pasta, rice, many grains, cereals, desserts, and sugary drinks. Exercise also helps with control of blood sugar in many diabetics.

New drugs are in the works. Nateglinide (Starlix) is designed to mimic the body's natural response to food by helping the pancreas cells to secrete insulin rapidly and reduce the large increase in blood glucose that diabetics experience at mealtime. It then shuts down that production, preventing any overproduction and drops in blood sugar levels.

Since diabetes is one of the most expensive health problems in the United States, costing an average of $92 billion each year for treatment and research, it's a hot area for research and development, and many new developments are on the horizon:

- **Diabetes vaccine:** In December 2001, the *British Medical Journal* reported that scientists have developed the world's first drug that can successfully stop the immune system's destruction of pancreatic cells in humans, which can act as a vaccine against diabetes. The drug, called DiaPep277, may be able to prevent Type I diabetes in those who have a genetic risk of the disease but have not yet developed the condition. It's anticipated that this promising drug will be submitted to the FDA for approval sometime in 2004.
- **Stored insulin:** One very exciting development was reported by scientists at the University of California at San Diego. The researchers were able to modify the insulin, making it dormant until activated by a special antibody. Researchers believe that this development may represent a new type of treatment for diabetes, and practical applications will be seen in the next decade.
- **Salicylates:** The Joslin Diabetes Center recently reported that high doses of salicylates—salicyclates are the active ingredients in aspirin—can reverse high blood sugar, high insulin, and high blood fat levels in animals. Their research suggests that aspirin-like drugs may offer potential for new drugs for Type II diabetes. High-dose aspirin is not currently used as a long-term treatment for diabetes because it causes serious side effects.
- **Oral insulin for prevention of Type I diabetes:** The National Institute of Diabetes and Digestive and Kidney Diseases (NIDDK) found that injections of insulin do not prevent Type I diabetes in high-risk people. Researchers are still attempting to determine, however, via the Diabetes Prevention Trial–Type I, whether insulin

taken orally can prevent or delay Type I diabetes in people with a lower risk—25 to 50 percent—of developing diabetes in five years. The study is also looking at those who have evidence of autoimmunity but no loss of ability to produce insulin. The theory is that oral insulin stimulates a protective immune response that may counteract the destructive process that causes Type I diabetes.

• **Synthetic antioxidant:** Researchers are currently studying a synthetic antioxidant from Incara Pharmaceuticals that may be able to slow or prevent Type II diabetes.

• **GLP-1:** A synthetic version of a natural intestinal hormone, glucagon-like peptide 1 (GLP-1) is currently being studied as a possible treatment to normalize insulin response and treat Type II diabetes.

• **CFA:** In one study, researchers were able to cure Type I diabetes in mice, through a 40-day course of injections with a drug called CFA. CFA triggers the production of tumor necrosis factor alpha (TNF-a), which then causes the dysfunctional autoimmune cells to self-destruct, in a process known as apoptosis. Once rid of the errant autoimmune cells, the mice regrew healthy islet cells, which allowed the pancreas to function normally and cured the diabetes.

• **Insulin pill as treatment:** It's likely that within the next decade diabetics will be able to take their insulin orally rather than by injection. Purdue University researchers recently demonstrated a unique method of pill production that protects the drugs from being broken down by the enzymes in the stomach before being absorbed. Special particles built into the drug anchor to the upper small intestine long enough for the medication to be absorbed, rather than passing through into the lower intestine. The harmless particles are then flushed out by the natural digestive process.

• **Islet cell transplants:** After transplanting insulin-producing islet cells, if the transplant works, the new cells produce insulin, essentially curing the diabetes. Patients receiving the transplants also have to take antirejection drugs, to make sure they don't reject the transplanted cells. To date, more than a dozen Type I diabetes patients have gone through the clinical trials of this procedure, and almost all of them are now cured, with normal blood sugar levels and no need for insulin. Because antirejection drugs carry risks and side effects of their own, these treatments are still reserved for only the most seriously ill diabetics, but researchers hope to make this treatment safer and more available in the future.

• **Diabetes sensor:** Since Type I diabetics typically have to prick their fingers numerous times a day to check blood sugar, a new device, the Diasensor 2000, is a promising development for patients. Using near-infrared light transmitted through the skin, the device can measure the blood sugar changes on a cellular level, with no pricks and no pain. Studies found it measured blood sugar levels within 15 percent of traditional monitors. The Diasensor has already been approved for use in Europe, and the accuracy is now being studied at ten centers in the United States.

Things to Know

Diabetics are twice as likely to suffer from depression as those without the disease, and the rate is even higher in women. While it's not hard to understand why diabetes would affect mental state, it's also thought now that depression could contribute to development of diabetes. Inactivity and overeating may be one component. Treatment for the depression has been shown to help diabetics control blood sugar, so it's important that changes in mood not be overlooked or undertreated.

Programs that help diabetics to manage stress can help lower blood sugar levels significantly. Even small reductions in blood sugar can reduce the long-term risks of medical complications such as kidney disease and blindness.

Alcohol and some diabetes pills may not mix. Discuss whether you can drink at all on the drug regimen recommended by your physician. Occasionally, chlorpropamide, and more rarely other sulfonylureas, can interact with alcohol to cause vomiting and flushing. Ask your doctor if you are concerned about this effect.

You should have your doctor annually perform a complete foot check for sores or ulcers, and your eye doctor should screen you for retinopathy, a complication of diabetes that can lead to blindness.

Diabetics should wear a medical alert bracelet or necklace and carry a medical data card.

In addition to daily self-monitoring of blood sugar as directed by your doctor, you should get an HA1C blood test at least once a year. If you don't have insurance, or prefer self-testing, or want to test more frequently, you can do a home HA1C test using Biosafe's kit. Results are mailed back to you. For information or to order a test, you can call Biosafe at 1-800-768-8446, extension 123, or find out more at this book's website, http:/www.autoimmunebook/biosafe.

For diabetics who are monitoring their own care, HealthCheck-USA also offers the Diabetes Management Test, which includes both an HA1C test and a glucose test. For both tests, HealthCheckUSA doctors sign off on the bloodwork requests and you receive the results online or by mail. You can order tests by calling 1-800-929-2044 or by visiting this book's website at http://www.autoimmune book.com/healthcheckusa.

Because diabetes raises the risk of high cholesterol, every year you should have a complete blood lipid panel (total cholesterol, HDL, LDL, and triglycerides) to assess heart disease risk. Again, in addition to testing through your own practitioner, affordable self-tests are available at Biosafe, and lab tests are available via HealthCheckUSA.

British researchers found that celiac disease—sensitivity or intolerance of wheat gluten products—is common in Type I diabetes, so screening for celiac disease should be part of routine examinations. In a diabetic with celiac disease, the benefits of a gluten-free diet include control of symptoms, better stabilization of diabetes, and prevention of celiac complications. Some diabetics may not be gluten intolerant but rather gluten insensitive. Researchers have found that people with diabetes often have various gastrointestinal symptoms, including nausea, heartburn, bloating, vomiting, diarrhea, and constipation. The more acute symptoms were reported in those diabetics who had poor glycemic control and who were not controlling blood sugar optimally. For more information on celiac disease, see Chapter 8.

■ Addison's Disease

Autoimmune Addison's disease is a fairly rare condition, estimated to occur in 5 people out of every 100,000 in the United States. In Addison's disease, the adrenal cortex, the outer layer of the adrenal gland—small glands that are located above each kidney—does not function properly. Adrenal glands produce glucocorticoid hormones, which help the body use and store carbohydrates, protein, fat, and sugar. In Addison's, also known as primary adrenocortical insufficiency, not enough of these glucocorticoid hormones are produced. This results in the release of sodium, a buildup of potassium, low blood pressure, severe dehydration, and dangerously low blood sugar, which can all eventually lead to shock.

There are some physical irregularities, such as tumors, tuberculosis, sarcoidosis, histoplasmosis, hemochromatosis, acquired immunodeficiency syndrome (AIDS), or overuse of steroids, which can lead to Addison's disease. The most common cause of Addison's, however, is a chronic autoimmune process.

The onset of Addison's is typically between ages 30 and 50, but it can occur in younger people, particularly with other autoimmune diseases. Addison's strikes women and men fairly equally. It can develop slowly and chronically, but in as many as 25 percent of cases, a more dangerous, rapid, acute onset of Addison's can occur, usually triggered by infection, trauma, surgery, emotional stress, or other stressors. In patients who are already taking cortisone drugs, the failure to increase the dosage as required during periods of high stress can also trigger an acute adrenal crisis.

Addison's disease can be found alongside other conditions as part of several known syndromes. For example, Addison's disease with an underactive parathyroid gland and candidiasis (chronic yeast overgrowth) is considered part of a syndrome called poly-glandular autoimmune syndrome type I. When Addison's is found with Type I diabetes and either Hashimoto's thyroiditis or Graves' disease, the syndrome is known as polyglandular autoimmune syndrome type II. And Addison's disease and Hashimoto's thyroiditis together are known as Schmidt's syndrome.

Symptoms

Chronic Addison's can develop with a variety of symptoms, including

- Hyperpigmentation (areas of skin coloration, such as tan or freckles) in the skin and mucous membranes, particularly the sun-exposed areas of the skin, knuckles, elbows, knees, hands, nail beds, mouth, and vaginal area
- Vitiligo, patches of no pigmentation, white spots on the skin
- Fatigue, general feeling of weakness
- Poor appetite, weight loss
- Nausea, vomiting, diarrhea
- Intolerance to cold
- Orthostatic hypotension—a drop in blood pressure when standing up or getting out of bed that may result in dizziness or fainting
- Dizziness, fainting, disturbances in balance and walking
- Muscle weakness, muscle and joint pains
- A heightened sense of smell, taste, and hearing

- Cravings for salt
- Impotence and decreased sex drive in men
- Lack of menstrual periods
- Decreased body hair in women
- Difficulty thinking or concentrating, mood changes
- Behavioral problems

In an acute adrenal crisis, symptoms will frequently develop quickly. The most common symptoms of rapid-onset Addison's disease include

- Nausea, vomiting
- Shock
- Confusion
- Abdominal or flank pain
- Extremely high temperatures
- Coma
- Dehydration
- Low blood pressure

Diagnosis

In chronic-onset Addison's, early blood tests may show low cortisol levels, low sodium, or high potassium. To diagnose Addison's, a common test is the rapid ACTH (adrenocorticotrophic hormone) stimulation test, which is done using various medicines, including cosyntropin (Cortrosyn) or synthetic ACTH (Synacthen). Blood is drawn in two separate tubes to measure baseline levels of cortisol and aldosterone. Then an injection of synthetic ACTH is given. Thirty or sixty minutes after the ACTH injection, blood samples are drawn again for cortisol and aldosterone. The baseline and thirty- or sixty-minute samples can usually diagnose a full-scale case of Addison's, or rule it out entirely. Milder, subclinical forms of autoimmune adrenal insufficiency that may present with some of the classic Addison's symptoms are not easily diagnosed or ruled out with the rapid ACTH stimulation test, however.

With Addison's, an abdominal CT scan (CAT scan) may show some enlargement, atrophy, or changes to the adrenal glands. Measures of kidney function, such as blood urea nitrogen (BUN) and creatinine, may show that the kidneys aren't functioning as well as they should.

Some thyroid-related irregularities may show up in bloodwork. Some people with Addison's disease will have elevated TSH levels, with or without low T4/thyroxine levels, and with or without symptoms of an underactive thyroid. Many Addison's patients also have thyroid antibodies, specifically antithyroglobulin (anti-Tg), and antimicrosomal and antithyroid peroxidase (anti-TPO) antibodies. Borderline high levels of prolactin, the hormone that causes milk production in new mothers, may also be seen in Addison's disease.

Practitioners

Because Addison's is not a very common condition, an endocrinologist should absolutely be involved in helping to properly diagnose, treat, and manage this condition.

Treatment

The main treatment for Addison's disease is use of corticosteroid drugs as replacement therapy. In very acute situations, high doses of hydrocortisone drugs (i.e., Cortef or Hydrocortone) are used. For ongoing treatment, a longer-acting corticosteroid such as prednisone is used. In some cases, fludrocortisone (Florinef) may also be recommended to help restore the sodium/potassium balance. Your doctor may also advise you to increase your intake of salt in hot weather.

When you are on steroid replacement therapy, you need to be closely followed by your practitioner. In particular, you want to watch for any signs that you are not taking enough of the corticosteroid, such as morning headaches, weakness, and dizziness. You also need to be alert for any signs that you are taking too much, which can include the classic symptoms of Cushing's disease, including a puffy, rounded face, fat pads creating a "buffalo hump" on your shoulders, easy bruising, abdominal stretch marks, and elevated blood pressure.

Talk to your doctor about when and how much to increase your dose of steroids if you are going through a stressful situation, such as having a cold or flu, or you have a stressor coming up, such as a tooth extraction or surgery. Your doctor may also teach you how to do an intramuscular injection and give you a prescription for injectable hydrocortisone that you can take in the event of emergency, when oral intake may not be possible, or in situations of marked vomiting or diarrhea.

In pregnancy, you need to continue taking your steroids, and you may need an adjustment in your dosage. Extensive morning sickness may increase your dosage requirements. You should also talk to your doctor about increased dosage requirements during labor and delivery or cesarean section.

Things to Know

If you have Addison's, you should wear an emergency medical alert bracelet.

When you have Addison's disease, you should have a periodic bone DEXA study to monitor for osteoporosis, which is a risk for patients taking corticosteroid drugs.

If you are diagnosed as having Addison's disease and asymptomatic hypothyroidism, the hypothyroidism may clear up once you are receiving corticosteroid treatment, and you may not need to even be started on any thyroid treatment. If you have substantial thyroid symptoms, thyroid hormone replacement may help and may be needed only temporarily. Thyroid testing should be redone once the corticosteroid treatment has been regulated.

■ Autoimmune Oophoritis

Autoimmune oophoritis is an autoimmune attack on the ovaries. Starting with inflammation of the ovaries, autoimmune oophoritis can result in premature ovarian decline and premature ovarian failure—conditions in which the ovaries do not function optimally, or fail completely, leading to early menopause. While the average age of menopause is approximately 51 years, and generally ranges from 45 to 55 years, premature ovarian failure describes failure of ovarian function before age 40. Premature ovarian decline refers to premature deficiencies in key hormones and an accompanying reduction in fertility in younger women.

It's estimated that 1 in 1,000 women between ages 15 and 29 and 1 in 100 women between ages 30 and 39 have full premature ovarian failure. Other studies estimate that 3 percent of women between ages 15 and 39 suffer from premature ovarian failure. Many more may experience the intermittent symptoms of premature ovarian decline. These conditions appear most frequently in a woman's late 20s.

Women all begin life with around the same number of follicles and begin their first menstrual period with a fixed number of follicles. During each cycle, menstruation begins with low estrogen levels. The hypothalamus then tells the pituitary gland to secrete follicle-stimulating hormone, known as FSH. FSH then stimulates development of a number of follicles. Follicles produce estradiol—the key estrogen. As menstruation ends, the pituitary gland also begins to release luteinizing hormone (LH). Follicles develop on the ovary, but one becomes dominant, matures, and on approximately day 12 of the cycle, estradiol levels reach their highest, a surge of LH is released, and within twenty-four to thirty-six hours ovulation occurs—the follicle finishes maturing and the egg is released into the abdominal cavity.

The fallopian tubes then pick up the egg and lead the egg down toward the uterus. Meanwhile, the abandoned follicle turns into the corpus luteum, which remains on the ovarian wall and produces progesterone, thickening the lining of the uterus. After ovulation, the increasing progesterone and lower estrogen tell the pituitary to signal a slowing in production of FSH and LH. These hormones then drop and stay low until the end of the cycle. If the egg is not fertilized, the corpus luteum disintegrates, and progesterone and estrogen drop sharply, triggering the disintegration of the endometrial wall and the start of the menstrual period.

When the ovaries come under autoimmune attack, it's thought that women produce antibodies to their own FSH or to their own ovarian substances. If a follicle isn't stimulated, or if there isn't enough estrogen, the body will continue to produce FSH, making the level rise.

Autoimmune reactions are a common cause of premature ovarian failure, and it's thought that up to two-thirds of the women with premature ovarian decline or failure may have it due to an autoimmune disorder. In the case of premature ovarian failure, you may have antibodies to your own ovarian tissue, to your endometrium, or to one or more of the hormones regulating ovulation. These antibodies attack your reproductive system, and may interfere with and ultimately destroy your ovarian function.

One factor we know can trigger premature ovarian failure is smoking. Researchers have linked premature ovarian failure to exposure to certain types of chemicals called polycyclic aromatic hydrocarbons in tobacco smoke that accelerate the death of egg cells in the ovaries.

Symptoms

The symptoms of premature ovarian decline include

- Irregular, heavier, or more painful periods
- Reduced sex drive

- Vaginal dryness
- Sleep disruptions, insomnia
- Painful sex
- Infertility
- Depression, mood disturbances, poor concentration

The symptoms of premature ovarian failure are essentially the same, except periods may stop completely, and there may be hot flashes and night sweats as well.

Diagnosis

Diagnosis takes into account the menstrual history. The main diagnostic tool is the FSH test, and levels above 40 are usually indicative of premature ovarian failure. High-normal levels (above 15 to 20) during the first days of the cycle after menstruation can be indicative of premature ovarian decline.

It's not always easy to diagnose premature ovarian failure, according to patient advocate and author Dr. Marie Savard, so a family history is particularly important. Says Dr. Savard:

A 35-year-old patient stopped getting her period abruptly. Her family doctor and gynecologist reassured her that it was just stress. No one asked her a detailed family history—she didn't have a genogram filled out, which would have revealed that her mother and maternal grandmother had mild thyroiditis and osteoporosis and were on thyroid replacement, and her grandmother also had pernicious anemia—a B12 deficiency—that is not only autoimmune but common in the elderly. Her gynecologist believed that since her family doctor have checked her FSH level . . . the family doctor just assumed the gynecologist was doing his part. No one actually reviewed the bloodwork to see that only the bare minimum was done. She received no treatment, simply suffering through the symptoms of menopause with sleep disturbance, dry vagina, etc., believing it was only stress. At age 44 she experienced a number of rib fractures after a minor automobile accident and was diagnosed by an astute doctor with osteoporosis. It turns out her premature ovarian failure meant no estrogen for almost ten years, rapid bone loss since she received no treatment, and now osteoporosis. Had she brought to her doctors a family genogram, done her own research on why she wasn't getting periods, brought her bloodwork to each doctor to see how little was actually done, and kept a journal detailing her sleep disturbance, hot symptoms, dry vagina, etc., the diagnosis could have been suspected and tests/treatment started sooner.

Practitioners

When it comes to diagnosing and treating autoimmune ovarian problems, there's not necessarily one particular specialty that is best at diagnosing or treating this condition. The best possible practitioner may be a reproductive endocrinologist, general endocrinologist, or gynecologist, or even a general practitioner, ob-gyn, or internist who specializes in women's hormonal medicine. Generally, however, reproductive endocrinologists and gynecologists may have the best ability to diagnose, and then properly treat, these types of women's hormonal imbalances.

Treatment

The main conventional treatments include hormone replacement therapy. Typically, this involves both estrogens and progestins. The conventional method is sometimes birth-control pills, or the estrogen drug Premarin. Alternative practitioners usually recommend use of oral or transdermal (patch) estradiol, along with natural progesterone in pill form. There is some evidence that the negative effects attributed to estrogen (increased risk of stroke and certain cancers) are minimized when synthetic estradiol is used, versus the pregnant mare's urine used to produce the most widely prescribed brand of estrogen replacement, Premarin.

According to hormonal expert Gillian Ford, author of the best-selling book *Listening to Your Hormones,* when women experience premature ovarian failure with an autoimmune cause, this is not necessarily a permanent problem: "Giving women estrogen replacement (with progesterone in the second half of the cycle) can bring FSH levels down, and it is a treatment that has restored the menstrual cycle and permitted pregnancies to take place."

Things to Know

When infertility is the issue and pregnancy is desired, it's useful to look at some of the successes that have been enjoyed by reproductive medicine experts such as Dr. Alan E. Beer of the Chicago Medical School's Reproductive Medicine Program. Dr. Beer has found success with several treatments for autoimmunity-related infertility. His research has found that this sort of treatment is required prior to successful pregnancy in some women. The treatments include lymphocyte immune therapy (LIT), which was initially a treatment for recurrent miscarriages but is now used to help kidney transplant patients, as well as being a treatment for diabetes, rheumatoid arthritis, autoimmune encephalomyelitis, and autoimmune thyroiditis. The LIT produces antibodies against T cells and B cells that help to calm down autoimmune responses. Dr. Beer has stated in research findings that this is the first line of therapy for women with immune infertility and reproductive failure. The other treatment, intravenous immunoglobulin G (IVIG)—also known as gammaglobulin—is given to women to prevent them from developing a negative immune response to pregnancy.

6

Pain/Fatigue Syndromes

Chronic fatigue immune dysfunction syndrome (CFIDS) and fibromyalgia syndrome are still labeled as "fad" diagnoses by some less-enlightened practitioners, but these two related conditions, suspected to be autoimmune in nature, can cause varying degrees of muscle and joint pain, fatigue, exhaustion, and depression, and are very real for a combined total of at least 8 million sufferers. Both CFIDS and fibromyalgia can share some similar symptoms: fatigue, pain, concentration difficulties, and sleep disturbances. They are also both difficult to diagnose and treat. Some practitioners suspect they are related, or are perhaps even manifestations of the same metabolic dysfunction.

■ Chronic Fatigue Immune Dysfunction Syndrome

Chronic fatigue immune dysfunction syndrome (CFIDS)—sometimes referred to as chronic fatigue syndrome (CFS), or by the British-European name, myalgic encephalomyelitis (ME)—is a chronic inflammatory illness of undetermined origin. There is some medical evidence that CFIDS is autoimmune in nature. The American Autoimmune Related Diseases Association has identified it as autoimmune, due to the inflammatory nature of the condition, coupled by the fact that more than half of those with CFIDS who are tested are positive for circulating antinuclear antibodies (ANAs), a marker for autoimmune disease. There is no definitive test for CFIDS, and the diagnosis is more of an exclusionary process of ruling out all the other possible causes of chronic fatigue, while documenting markers and common CFIDS symptoms.

While CFIDS affects an estimated one to two million people, it's thought to strike more than twice as many women as men. All ages, races, and income levels can be affected. It's not considered to be a "contagious" condition in the traditional sense, although there have been cases where CFIDS appears to have struck groups of people geographically. The theory is that a viral trigger, combined with a genetic susceptibility, may be the cause of CFIDS.

Initially, there was a theory that CFIDS was caused by Epstein-Barr (the virus that causes mononucleosis), because the symptoms were so similar to mononucleosis. Subsequent research, however, has been unable to establish a direct cause-effect relationship between the Epstein-Barr virus and CFIDS. There are also researchers who suggest that *Chlamydia pneumoniae* may be responsible for CFIDS. Other infectious agents that have been studied as potential triggers for CFIDS include human herpes virus 6 (HHV-6), Coxsackie virus B, spumaviruses, and even human T-cell leukemia virus (HTLV) strains. Overall, while viral triggers are thought to play a role, the exact mechanisms are not understood.

What we do see, however, is that CFIDS frequently starts with some sort of infection and illness—in some cases, Epstein-Barr infection, mononucleosis, cytomegalovirus, pneumonia, diarrhea, or an upper respiratory tract infection. While fatigue is not uncommon in most of these conditions, after the infection seems to resolve, in CFIDS the fatigue remains.

According to CFIDS/FMS patient advocate Lisa Lorden, director of communications for the National Fibromyalgia Awareness

Campaign, there is no consensus regarding the epidemiology of chronic fatigue syndrome and fibromyalgia. Says Lorden, who has studied the issue extensively and communicated with thousands of patients:

> My opinion is that any of these can serve as "triggers" (in addition to other forms of physical injury/trauma, such as an auto accident). What is unique and still not understood about CFIDS/FMS is why the body does not recover from these triggers as it normally would. In other words, many people contract bacterial and viral infections, for example, and do not develop CFIDS/FMS. I believe that with CFIDS/FMS something happens to the systems of the body—whether immune, central nervous system, etc.—that perpetuates the systemic dysfunction even after the trigger is removed. In essence, the body is fighting something that is no longer there.

A number of studies have suggested that CFIDS may represent a dysfunction in the hypothalamic-pituitary-adrenal (HPA) axis. Since physical or emotional stress is common in many CFIDS patients before the onset of the condition, it's been thought that the HPA axis is activated, causing cortisol levels to drop, not so significantly that levels become abnormal, but to low-normal levels, or levels that are low relative to an individual's previous readings. Since proper levels of cortisol suppress inflammation and the immune system, these reduced levels may allow for inflammation and imbalances in the immune system.

Some experts believe that a number of different factors, which could include stress and viral infection, combine in a susceptible person to trigger the release of cytokines, but again, the relationship seems complex and is not direct. According to a consensus panel convened by the Centers for Disease Control and Prevention, and the Chronic Fatigue and Immune Dysfunction Syndrome Association of America, stress is not a direct cause of CFIDS. It can worsen existing CFIDS, however, and may be one factor increasing susceptibility.

Some investigators have observed common autoimmune antibodies, as well as immune complexes, in many CFIDS patients, both of which point to some autoimmune nature of the condition. However, most autoimmune diseases are associated with tissue destruction or organ damage (i.e., the thyroid in Graves' disease, or the joints in rheumatoid arthritis), but in CFIDS there is no specific damage identified. So the autoimmune mechanism behind CFIDS is suspected though not clear.

Dr. John Lowe, in his book *The Metabolic Treatment of Fibromyalgia*, proposed that the immune abnormalities found in CFIDS and fibromyalgia patients are actually secondary to hypothyroidism or thyroid hormone resistance:

> *Some patients with primary hypothyroidism due to autoimmune thyroiditis have elevated thyroid antibodies but so-called "normal" TSH levels. Some of these patients have symptoms commonly diagnosed today as fibromyalgia/ CFIDS. Many doctors don't recognize that these supposed symptoms are classic symptoms of hypothyroidism. The doctors may dismiss any possibility of hypothyroidism when they find that the patients have "normal" TSH levels. If the doctors don't order thyroid antibody tests, they fail to identify the autoimmune thyroiditis as the cause of the FMS/CFIDS symptoms.*

According to Dr. Lowe, one study found that 16 percent of patients with chronic, widespread musculoskeletal pain had elevated thyroid antibodies, and thyroid function tests show that about 12 percent of fibromyalgia patients have primary hypothyroidism. Dr. Lowe says, "Most of the other 88% of patients have lab results indicating either thyroid hormone resistance or central hypothyroidism."

Symptoms

Primarily, the main symptom is unusually debilitating fatigue that lasts at least six months and forces you to reduce your activity level substantially. CFIDS expert Dr. Jacob Teitelbaum describes the onset of the condition as frequently starting with a bout of flu-like illness, which then converts to extreme fatigue. Other symptoms found in CFIDS include

- Prolonged fatigue after physical activity, known as a post-exertional malaise, usually lasting more than 24 hours
- Fatigue with or after normal activity, or fatigue after sleep ("unrefreshing" sleep)
- Mild, low-grade fever or chills
- Dry, inflamed, sore throat
- Swollen or tender lymph nodes in neck or armpits
- General muscle weakness and pain
- Generalized headaches, particularly headaches of a new type, pattern, or severity
- Pain that moves from one joint to another without swelling or redness
- Forgetfulness, difficulty remembering or saying words, excessive irritability, confusion, or inability to concentrate, to the extent that it interferes with your job, education, social or personal activities
- More frequent illness, with susceptibility to infections, viruses, or worsening of allergies
- Neurally mediated hypotension—when you stand up, your blood pressure drops, which can make you feel faint, dizzy, nauseous, your heart rate drops, and you can even pass out

- Reactivity to environmental exposures (i.e., increased sensitivity to chemicals, perfumes, odors, bug sprays, etc.)
- Night sweats
- Hypersensitivity to temperatures, sounds, sensations, confusion
- Gastrointestinal problems, such as diarrhea, constipation, bloating
- Feeling cold

One chronic fatigue patient, Lara, described the condition as feeling like "having the flu for twenty years." Or having such fatigue that after a shower you feel "as though you accomplished a new world's record. Then, calling it a day."

Diagnosis

After ruling out all the possible causes of chronic fatigue—including lupus, multiple sclerosis, Lyme disease, adrenal disorders, HIV or AIDS, thyroid disease, rheumatoid arthritis, depression, cancer, and other conditions—specific criteria are applied to make a CFIDS diagnosis. These criteria include new onset of fatigue lasting six months and reducing activity to less than 50 percent of usual, plus at least eight of the following symptoms:

- Mild fever or chills
- Dry, inflamed, sore throat
- Swollen or tender lymph nodes in neck or armpits
- General muscle weakness
- General muscle pain
- Prolonged fatigue after physical activity, known as a post-exertional malaise, usually lasting more than 24 hours
- Generalized headaches, particularly headaches of a new type, pattern, or severity
- Pain that moves from one joint to another without swelling or redness

- Forgetfulness, excessive irritability, confusion, or inability to concentrate, to the extent that it interferes with your job, education, social or personal activities
- Sleep disturbances, unrefreshing sleep (waking up exhausted after sleep)

Some practitioners also feel that certain tests may help to confirm a CFIDS diagnosis, and in CFIDS patients, the following are more common:

- Very low erythrocyte sedimentation rate (ESR)
- Elevated IgM/IgG Coxsackie virus B titer
- Elevated IgM/IgG HHV-6 titer
- Elevated IgM/IgG *Chlamydia pneumoniae* titer, detected by enzyme-linked immunosorbent assay (ELISA) tests
- Decreased natural killer (NK) cells, either the percent or their activity

Practitioners

In CFIDS, you can really go in two directions. There are rheumatologists who specialize in treating CFIDS. They run the various bloodwork and antibody tests, and are familiar with some of the cutting-edge approaches to diagnosing and treating CFIDS. Some of the CFIDS patient support organizations can provide good referrals to these doctors.

There is also a subgroup of general practitioners, holistic doctors, and osteopaths who specialize in some of the conditions that are more difficult to diagnose and treat, such as CFIDS, fibromyalgia, candidiasis, environmental allergies, chemical sensitivity, subclinical hypothyroidism, and Lyme disease. Some of these practitioners are innovative in working with both alternative and conventional approaches for diagnosis and treatment of CFIDS. These doctors can be a bit harder to find, but Appendix A offers some referral sources for the best holistic and alternative physicians.

Patient advocate Lisa Lorden believes that finding a good practitioner who understands how to diagnose and treat CFIDS and FMS is one of the most important responsibilities of a CFIDS/FMS patient:

> *It's essential to have a partner in your quest to find answers and improve your quality of life. Accurate diagnosis is essential; if CFIDS/FMS is misdiagnosed, you may actually have another illness that is treatable. So it's important to make sure that all other conditions that could be causing your symptoms be ruled out. In addition, some medical professionals don't like to diagnose CFIDS/FMS even when they can't find another cause because there is little they can do to "fix" it— or worse, they say they don't "believe" in CFIDS/FMS. I recommend getting several opinions. Once a diagnosis is reached, you'll need someone who listens to and understands your symptoms and does his/her best to help you minimize them or cope with them. Trust your instincts. If a practitioner makes you feel uncomfortable, or shares information you know from other sources is questionable, look elsewhere. Since many practitioners don't understand CFIDS/FMS or are unwilling to treat it, the best way to find an appropriate provider is through referrals from other patients. Support groups and online resources can help.*

Treatment

Conventionally, some physicians would say that there is no actual treatment for CFIDS. Since they don't really know what metabolic, immune, or infectious mechanism is at work to cause it, there's no specific treatment.

Some physicians, however, have successfully used amphetamine-type drugs, including methylphenidate HCI (Ritalin)—the drug typically used to treat children with attention deficit hyperactivity disorder—with some success. Some practitioners have tried the appetite suppressant phentermine HCI (Fastin) or phantermine resin (Lonamin). Again, the stimulatory effect seems to help in some cases of CFIDS.

PolyI:polyC12U (Ampligen), which may be approved in the United States by the time this book is released, is a drug shown to boost immunity and restore cognitive functioning. It has gone through clinical testing in the United States and is available by prescription in Canada. However, it's an expensive intravenous drug.

In patients with elevated IgM *Chlamydia pneumoniae* titers, a two- to three-week course of doxycycline antibiotics can have a positive effect in terms of helping to restore energy and reduce the memory and mental impairment associated with CFIDS. The response is typically fast and fairly dramatic if it's the right treatment. Surprisingly, the benefits frequently continue even after treatment ends.

Another treatment that has been helpful in some patients who do not have elevated IgM chlamydia titers is high-dose beta-carotene, at 50,000 units per day for three weeks. If a positive response is seen, another three-week course of beta-carotene can be given six months after the initial three-week course.

Some practitioners believe in intravenous gamma globulin (IVIG) for CFIDS patients. This therapy is very expensive, with a monthly dose costing up to $1,000. Since this treatment is rarely covered by insurance, it's not often pursued, but some practitioners and patients claim that it offers substantial improvement of symptoms.

When a "stealth" bacteria such as mycoplasma is suspected as a possible underlying infectious trigger for CFIDS, antibiotic therapy—usually with erythromycin, doxycycline, minocycline, or the quinolone antibiotics such as Cipro—can be helpful in some patients.

Massage, especially craniosacral therapy or myofascial therapy, has been recommended for the joint and muscle pain associated with CFIDS. Hydrotherapy, fifteen to thirty minutes, two or three times weekly at 85°F, is also a commonly recommended approach for joint and muscle pain. If there is no access to a warm pool, a soak in a tub at home in slightly warmer water can substitute.

Patient advocate Lisa Lorden finds that there are thousands of different therapies for CFIDS and FMS, but because the cause of the illness is not yet understood, treatment focuses on relieving symptoms:

> A wide variety of medications, alternative remedies, and other treatment strategies are used because they have been found to be somewhat effective in some patients. The goal here is improving symptoms, not a cure. The most important thing to keep in mind is that everyone is different. What is helpful to one patient may make no difference to another, while making someone else actually feel worse. It's essential to communicate with your health care provider about what new treatments you might decide to try, and methodically introduce these one at a time. There are a lot of remedies out there advertised as "cutting-edge," claiming to cure CFIDS/FMS or alleviate various symptoms. My best advice is buyer beware. Some of these may actually be dangerous, and not just to your wallet. Remember, there is as of yet no cure for CFIDS/FMS. Those who claim to have a "secret cure" are most certainly worth steering clear of.

Things to Know

Researchers have found that CFIDS tends to be more common in perfectionist, high-achieving, type A people who work hard and typically are trying to fulfill multiple roles. A history of allergies is also a risk factor.

Drinking sufficient fluid is considered absolutely essential for

CFIDS patients. Some practitioners have speculated that insufficient blood volume may contribute to some of the CFIDS symptoms, and insufficient intake of fluids can contribute to this problem. The absolute minimum daily starting point for fluid intake should be 64 ounces of water (eight glasses). Caffeine-free herbal tea, club soda, and flavored, unsweetened seltzers can be substituted, but water is best.

■ Fibromyalgia/Fibromyositis

Fibromyalgia has only recently been recognized as an actual condition, when formalized criteria for diagnosis were established in 1990. Fibromyalgia, also known as fibromyalgia syndrome (FMS), fibromyositis, fibrositis, and myofibrositis, is characterized by widespread joint and muscle pain and tenderness, fatigue, and exhaustion after sleep and after exertion. While the alternate names ending in "itis" usually suggest inflammation, no specific inflammation is associated with FMS. But pain is definitely associated with the condition, and a diagnosis is typically confirmed by examining the pain felt in a specific set of trigger points on the body.

Fibromyalgia has not been identified as an autoimmune disorder itself. However, it is well known that it often accompanies other endocrine and rheumatic autoimmune disorders, and AARDA has designated it as autoimmune. It is a common and perplexing clinical condition characterized by the constant presence of widespread pain so severe that it is often incapacitating; it is also characterized by the total absence of any definable pathophysiologic or laboratory abnormality, even under the most intense scrutiny.

Fibromyalgia affects 4 to 6 million people in the United States, occurring mainly in women of childbearing age. Symptoms usually arise between ages 20 and 55, but the condition may be diagnosed in childhood. It's estimated that as many as 3 to 6 percent of the general population, including children, meet the criteria for diagnosis of fibromyalgia. This would make fibromyalgia over twice as common as rheumatoid arthritis. Fibromyalgia strikes women seven times more often than men, according to a 1998 National Institutes of Health report.

Symptoms

- Feeling of pain, burning, aching, and soreness in the body
- Headaches, tenderness of the scalp, pain in the back of the skull
- Pain in the neck, shoulder, shoulder blades, and elbows
- Pain in hips, top of buttocks, outside the lower hip, below buttocks, and the pelvis
- Pain in the knees and kneecap area
- Fatigue, unrefreshing sleep, waking up tired, morning stiffness
- Insomnia, frequent waking, difficulty falling asleep, or falling asleep immediately
- Raynaud's phenomenon (hands feel cold, numb, or turn blue when exposed to temperature changes)
- Irritable bowel syndrome, diarrhea, constipation, bloating, cramping
- Balance problems
- Neurally mediated hypotension—when you stand up, your blood pressure drops, which can make you feel faint, dizzy, nauseous, your heart rate drops, and you can even pass out
- Restless leg syndrome
- Sense of tissues feeling swollen
- Numbness, tingling and feeling of cold in the hands and feet
- Chest pain, palpitations
- Shortness of breath
- Painful periods

- Anxiety, depression, and "fibrofog" (i.e., confusion and forgetfulness, inability to concentrate, difficulty recalling simple words and numbers, transposing words and numbers)
- Frequent urination
- Muscle twitching
- Dry mouth

The pain of fibromyalgia can be truly debilitating for some patients. One fibromyalgia patient, Cathy, suffered for years before finally being diagnosed:

My second child was born when I was 38 years old. After one year, I began to have chronic pain episodes for no particular reason. They would come in January with the flu season and not leave until after the pollen season in June. I could hardly walk. My insomnia became worse. I had to sleep with ice packs on my back. The doctors sent me to a chiropractor, but the relief was temporary. Sometimes I had to crawl across the floor. No one seemed to understand how much pain I was in. One doctor told me to take ibuprofen. I eventually needed twenty-four per day.

Diagnosis

Unfortunately, no medical test or x-ray can provide a definitive diagnosis of fibromyalgia. Since 1990, guidelines to aid in diagnosis of fibromyalgia have existed, but they are not definitive. To be diagnosed with fibromyalgia, you must have pain in all four quadrants of your body, as well as in the skeleton, for at least three months. The second main determinant is the presence of at least eleven of eighteen specific tender points, which exist as nine pairs of points, including

- Base of the skull, where it meets the neck
- Between neck and shoulder

- Back shoulder-blade area
- Hip level/top of buttocks
- Outside lower hip, below buttocks
- Front of neck
- Front shoulder blade
- Elbows
- Outer kneecaps

There are some bloodwork findings that may help in a diagnosis. One common abnormality associated with fibromyalgia patients is unusually low serotonin levels. These low levels may be due to low levels of both the serotonin precursor tryptophan and low levels of 5-hydroxyindole acetic acid.

Other studies show that FMS patients have elevated levels of substance P, a neuropeptide found in spinal fluid. Substance P is a neurotransmitter that increases sensitivity to and awareness of pain.

Researchers also have found the existence of low levels of adenosine triphosphate (ATP) in red blood cells of patients with fibromyalgia. Other abnormalities that may be observed in fibromyalgia patients include

- Low free cortisol in twenty-four-hour urine
- Elevated evening cortisol
- Hypoglycemia
- Low levels of growth hormone

Treatment

Much like CFIDS, there is no agreed-upon standard treatment for fibromyalgia. Rather, there is a collection of various approaches that address different symptoms, each approach having varying levels of success.

In a recent analysis, nearly fifty studies involving people with fibromyalgia found that nondrug approaches generally were superior to pharmacological treatments in reducing symptoms and improving daily function. According to recent research reported in *Arthritis Care Research,* a Canadian study documented that patients with fibromyalgia find that exercise is more effective in alleviating symptoms—including pain, depression, and disrupted sleep—versus medication or alternative treatments. A third of the patients reported that they had approximately a 30 percent improvement in pain symptoms. Over time, many patients reduced the amount of pain medications, antidepressants, and tranquilizers they used.

Dr. Andrew Weil recommends that patients build up some moderate aerobic activity such as cycling, water aerobics, or walking from even five minutes a day, three times a week, to thirty minutes most days of the week. He also recommends adding some form of Eastern exercise, such as yoga, tai chi, or qigong.

Drug treatments are, however, often the only treatments offered by conventional practitioners, and they may be part of the overall program offered by an alternative practitioner. For example, if you're suffering from sleep problems and depression, some practitioners may prescribe antidepressants, such as trazodone, selective serotonin reuptake inhibitors (SSRIs), and tricyclics. Some brand names you might recognize include Prozac, Welbutrin, and Paxil. Some studies have found that they help approximately 25 percent of people with fibromyalgia who take them. Keep in mind that these drugs can also have a variety of side effects, including weight gain, loss of sex drive, and others.

Sleep problems are sometimes treated with low-dose tranquilizers such as clonazepam (Klonopin) or even mild muscle relaxants. For pain, nonsteroidal anti-inflammatory drugs (NSAIDs) are frequently recommended, including over-the-counter products such as ibuprofen (Motrin, Advil) or ketoprofen (Aleve), or prescription versions such as vicoprofen. Analgesics may be recommended, including acetaminophen (Tylenol) and aspirin, as well as prescription painkillers such as hydrocodone. Cyclo-oxygenase-2 (Cox-2)–specific inhibitors such as Vioxx or Celebrex may also be recommended.

Botulinum toxin type A, known as botox, is a cutting-edge treatment for some of the pain associated with fibromyalgia. Some patients have reported several months of relief in their tender points after botox injections. The effects of botox injections take about a week to be felt, and the highest point of relief is typically within four weeks of receiving the injection. Botox can be expensive, costing as much as $400 per shot, and is often not covered by insurance.

Another promising fibromyalgia treatment is cranial electrotherapy stimulation (CES). Low-level currents of electrical stimulation are passed across the head, delivered via electrodes that are clipped to the ear lobes. In a double-blind, peer-reviewed study, those treated with CES had a 28 percent improvement in tender point scores and a 27 percent improvement in self-reported levels of pain. Those patients reporting that their quality of sleep was poor dropped from 60 percent at the beginning of the study to only 5 percent.

One small study conducted by Dr. Joel S. Edman of the Center for Integrative Medicine at Thomas Jefferson University Hospital in Philadelphia, Pennsylvania, found that people with fibromyalgia may have a reduction in symptoms when they eliminate allergenic foods from their diet. Patients removed common allergens from their diet, and after two weeks without eating any of the allergens, almost half of the patients reported a significant reduction in pain, and more than three-fourths had a reduction in symptoms such as headache, fatigue, bloating, heartburn, and breathing difficulties.

Yet another effective approach may be acupuncture. Researchers at the Federal University of Sao Paulo, Brazil, showed that acupuncture can help relieve symptoms such as pain and depression in fibromyalgia patients.

Although few practitioners believe there is a cure for fibromyalgia, Dr. John Lowe believes that most fibromyalgia patients can fully recover with a treatment regimen called metabolic rehabilitation:

For all patients, the regimen involves a wholesome diet, nutritional supplements, exercise to tolerance, the proper form and dosage of thyroid hormone, balancing of sex and adrenal hormones, and avoidance of metabolism-impeding drugs. Some patients, however, have other metabolism-impairing factors that we must identify and correct. Most patients require careful, systematic guidance to achieve normal metabolism and symptom relief. Some have never known what is necessary to achieve and maintain optimal health, and others lost sight of this during their illness. Through proper guidance, they learn either for the first time or once again. This regimen is a time- and energy-consuming process for both patients and doctors, but this is the nature of rehabilitation.

Things to Know

Patients with fibromyalgia usually see many physicians before receiving a correct diagnosis, and some experts estimate that patients seek medical attention for five years before a correct diagnosis is made. Some practitioners continue to believe that fibromyalgia is some sort of psychiatric or psychosomatic problem.

According to research in the *Journal of Rheumatology*, there is a higher incidence of antibodies against enteroviruses in patients who have an acute onset of fibromyalgia. This may indicate that acute-onset fibromyalgia has a viral basis.

Up to 70 percent of those with fibromyalgia also meet the criteria for chronic fatigue syndrome. One study found that fibromyalgia sufferers have more intense and longer-lasting pain than people without the syndrome when touched with a hot instrument for a brief moment. The study suggested that people with fibromyalgia have a lower pain threshold than people without the disorder, and that the nerve cells responsible for firing in response to pain—part of the body's warning system—stay activated for too long in fibromyalgia patients.

Fibromyalgia patients may have difficulty tolerating regular doses of most medications and supplements; they can be very sensitive to medications, and side effects are common. To avoid these problems, use the lowest dose available or perhaps half to a quarter of the lowest recommended dose.

Several medications should be avoided or used very carefully. Most investigators recommend using narcotics sparingly. In fibromyalgia without concomitant rheumatic illnesses, steroids are not helpful and should be avoided.

Avoid complications and confusion by asking for written instructions and drug information. If you're in the midst of "fibrofog," you may need to have things written down.

7

Hair and Skin Conditions

Sometimes, autoimmune conditions attack the hair and skin. The effects can range from the emotionally devastating but otherwise benign hair-loss syndrome alopecia, to the potentially debilitating condition known as scleroderma.

■ Scleroderma/CREST Syndrome

Scleroderma is a chronic disease in which the immune system attacks the skin (localized scleroderma), or blood vessels and connective tissue (systemic scleroderma). The word *scleroderma* means "hard skin" in Greek. Tightened, thickened, leather-like skin is a common sign, and in people with scleroderma, thickening of skin and blood vessels can result in loss of movement and shortness of breath, or, more rarely, in kidney, heart, or lung damage or failure.

Systemic scleroderma can be a progressive form, known as systemic sclerosis, or CREST syndrome, which stands for calcinosis (accumulation of calcium under the skin), Raynaud's phenomenon, esophageal dysfunction, sclerodactyly (stiffness/tightening of fingers), and telangiectasia (dilation of blood vessels, creating lesions). CREST has a better prognosis than other forms of scleroderma.

Pulmonary hypertension is considered the most dangerous complication of scleroderma. While scleroderma is one of the most serious autoimmune diseases, the best assessment of long-term survival is based on the type of scleroderma. Localized scleroderma affecting the hands has a good survival rate after ten years, whereas scleroderma that affects the trunk of the body presents a more uncertain prognosis.

Scleroderma can affect both men and women, but women are eight times more likely to get it, with the peak of onset occurring during childbearing years in the 20s through early 40s. In the United States, the prevalence of scleroderma is approximately 2.4 per 10,000 people, with an estimated 70,000 to 125,000 people with the condition. The number of scleroderma patients also seems to be on the rise, likely due to better diagnosis, earlier detection, and increased survival of patients. There is a slightly higher risk for African-Americans compared to Caucasians.

According to autoimmune disease expert Dr. Noel Rose in his textbook *The Autoimmune Diseases*, there are a variety of environmental exposures implicated as triggers in the development of scleroderma, including

- Silica exposure, typically in those who work as miners and stone masons
- Vinyl chloride exposure, for nuclear reactor workers
- Epoxy resins exposure, for chemical industry workers
- Exposure to solvents such as perchlorethylenes, naphtha, benzene, trichloroethylene, benzene, carbon tetrachloride, toluene, diesel fuel
- Certain drugs, such as fenfluramine (the fen in the phen/fen weight-loss drugs) and cocaine
- Rapeseed oil that has gone bad
- Silicone, such as in implants

- Vibration, such as in those who operate jackhammers and chainsaws

It's also thought but not proven that a virus can trigger or accelerate scleroderma, with cytomegalovirus and human herpes virus 5 identified as the most likely prospects.

Symptoms

Key signs of scleroderma are the unique hardening of the skin, known as tissue fibrosis, and Raynaud's phenomenon, a spasming and dilation of the blood vessels of the fingers and toes that makes these body parts numb and tingling, sensitive to cold, occasionally painful, and subject to changes in skin color. Scleroderma symptoms include

- Thickening and swelling of the ends of the fingers, sores on fingertips and knuckles
- Skin pigment changes (hyper- or hypopigmentation), taut, shiny darker skin, may appear to be tanned
- Raynaud's phenomenon in fingers and toes in response to cold or stress (*Note:* 70 percent of patients will initially present with this complaint, but almost everyone with scleroderma eventually develops it)
- Spider veins or dilated blood vessels on fingers, chest, face, lips, and tongue
- Calcium deposits causing bumps on fingers, bony areas, joints
- Diffuse itching
- Aches and pains in joints, including shoulder pain, elbow pain, knee pain, wrist and finger pain
- Fingers, wrists, and elbows become frozen in flexed position
- Hoarseness, cough, difficulty swallowing
- Shortness of breath
- Heartburn

- Constipation alternating with diarrhea
- Carpal tunnel syndrome symptoms
- Fatigue, muscle weakness
- Headache, facial pain
- Chest pain, palpitations and irregular heartbeats
- Erectile dysfunction
- Dry eyes, dry mouth, loosening of teeth
- Hypothyroidism
- Increased blood pressure
- Ultimately, scarring that can damage the lower end of the esophagus, causing heartburn and making it difficult to swallow, leading to weight loss

In its most serious form, scleroderma can cause scar tissue to accumulate in the lungs, esophageal blockage or cancer, kidney disease, and ultimately, life-threatening heart abnormalities, including heart failure and abnormal rhythms.

Diagnosis

The three key diagnostic criteria for scleroderma include

1. Tissue fibrosis (hardening of the skin)
2. Blood vessel involvement, almost always involving Raynaud's phenomenon, which is a spasm of the blood vessels of the fingers and toes
3. Presence of scleroderma autoantibodies

Some other characteristic lab test results include

- Elevated creatine phosphokinase (CPK)
- Elevated aldolase
- Elevated erythrocyte sedimentation rate (ESR)
- Absence of anti-Ro and anti-La antibodies

- Antinuclear antibodies present in about 95 percent of scleroderma patients
- Anticentromere antibodies present in about 60 to 90 percent of patients with limited scleroderma
- Fibrillarin antibodies (antibody to U3 ribonucleoprotein) may occur
- Other antibodies that may be present: anti-U3RNP, anti-ThRNP, and anti-PM-Scl

Pulmonary function testing is particularly important for scleroderma patients, since it can help to monitor lung damage, or possible pulmonary hypertension. High-resolution CT scans can be used to help evaluate lung status.

Practitioners

While scleroderma frequently manifests in skin symptoms, an experienced rheumatologist who has a full understanding of the disease, the complications of the therapies, and the frequently serious side effects may be the best practitioner for diagnosis and management of this complex condition. When lungs are involved, a pulmonologist may also be an important part of the health team. You may need to be seen by other specialists (i.e., cardiologist for heart involvement, or nephrologist for kidney involvement) depending on your symptoms.

Treatment

There is no official treatment for scleroderma. But the first line of treatment typically includes nonsteroidal anti-inflammatory drugs (NSAIDS) and corticosteroids such as prednisone for muscle and joint pain and inflammation.

Azathioprine (Imuran) is sometimes prescribed to reduce autoimmune activity, methotrexate (Folex, Rheumatrex) to suppress the immune system, and cyclophosphamide (Cytoxan,

Neosar) to interfere with the reproduction of lymphocytes and reduce the progression of scleroderma. D-penicillamine (Cuprimine, Depen) is sometimes prescribed for its ability to prevent the formation of collagen.

Dr. James Dauber, a pulmonologist at the University of Pittsburgh Medical Center, believes that the effects of scleroderma can be reversed by cyclophosphamide. This very toxic cancer drug has a variety of side effects, but has had some significant results. If given before lung damage has become too advanced, some patients have been able to resume a fairly normal lifestyle. In an interview with Ivanhoe news service, Dr. Dauber discussed the treatment:

> *I think what we're hoping—that it's going to at least arrest the disease at a stage where people still have enough function that they can do most everything they need to do. I think there have been isolated incidences where there's been a 25 percent or 30 percent or 40 percent improvement in lung function—nearly restoring lung function to normal—but that's probably the exception, and we really want to try to treat people at a relatively early stage in their disease, stabilize the inflammatory process, and prevent progression.*

Studies of cyclophosphamide are now going on in a variety of centers around the country.

Discomforts such as itching can be treated with moisturizers, antihistamines, and antidepressants. Raynaud's phenomenon symptoms can be treated with calcium blockers, aspirin, blood thinners such as warfarin (Coumadin), and other drugs. In the event of blood clots, additional drugs such as heparin may be necessary.

Heartburn can be treated with antacid and histamine-blocking drugs (e.g., Pepcid and Tagamet), and you should eat smaller, more frequent meals to inhibit acid production. Also, consider sleeping with the head of your bed elevated. High blood pressure and kidney involvement are frequently treated with ACE (angiotensin-converting enzyme) inhibitor blood pressure drugs.

Surgery may be called for in the rare cases of severe Raynaud's phenomenon that threaten loss of fingers, in severe acid reflux problems, or when there is an esophageal blockage. Some practitioners treat scleroderma with antibiotics. Tetracycline can help malabsorption and bacterial overgrowth in intestines, and some practitioners believe that antibiotic therapy addresses some underlying infectious mechanism to the disease.

One patient, Julie, was so short of breath that she could barely walk when she first consulted her doctor in early 1999. Her doctor referred her to a heart and lung doctor, who declared her fine. Then, Raynaud's phenomenon symptoms appeared, and a new blood test showed scleroderma. She found a cutting-edge doctor who put her on the antibiotic minocycline (Minocin). Says Julie:

I did this faithfully for two years. We used to dance twice a week and I walked 4 miles a day before this happened. Well, I am now dancing (jitterbugging) and trying to walk a little further every day. I can do all my own housework activities and have no trouble with my joints. I am now wearing my rings and all my shoes. This June I went to see the doctor and he said I was in remission!

Things to Know

Frequently, Raynaud's phenomenon may be the first symptom of scleroderma, but it may be months or years before other symptoms develop. About 10 percent of scleroderma patients will face renal crisis, in which kidneys are at risk of failing. The main symptoms include high blood pressure, headache, fatigue, swelling, and a rising serum creatinine level. Most often, when renal crisis occurs, it takes place within four years of diagnosis, but it can occur as much as twenty years after diagnosis. African-Americans are slightly more at risk than Caucasians to develop renal crisis, and men have a greater risk than women. This crisis requires aggressive treatment, or there is a risk of renal failure, which can lead to dialysis, or rarely even be fatal. As many as half of the patients who require dialysis may be able to go off the dialysis within eighteen months, however.

Pregnant women with scleroderma have a higher risk of miscarriage and complications. In one study of these women, 18 percent miscarried, 26 percent had premature deliveries, and 55 percent delivered full term. During pregnancy, scleroderma symptoms may worsen.

Many practitioners advise scleroderma patients to avoid high-dose vitamin C (i.e., more than 1,000 mg per day) because of the risk of collagen formation.

■ Alopecia

Alopecia results in hair loss, and the autoimmune reaction appears to be the body's attack on its own hair follicles. Hair can be lost from any part of the body. Although the main impact is cosmetic, and alopecia doesn't usually involve any specific medical or disease symptoms, the loss of hair can make it a particularly stressful and upsetting condition for sufferers, especially women.

Hair loss may be in round bald patches on the scalp (alopecia areata) or can involve the loss of all facial and scalp hair (alopecia totalis). Alopecia universalis is the loss of all body hair.

With or without treatment, most people will spontaneously regrow hair within several months to a year. Once you've had an episode of alopecia, you're likely to experience a relapse, however. One study found that 90 percent of patients had a recurrence of alopecia within five years. In a small percentage, hair loss is permanent.

Alopecia is frequently seen alongside other autoimmune conditions. In some studies, 10 percent of alopecia patients had lupus, compared to less than 0.5 percent of the general population. Vitiligo tends to be more common in patients with alopecia. And there's a definite connection to thyroid disease. Some researchers have found evidence of thyroid antibodies in alopecia patients. In various studies, from 3 percent to approximately 16 percent of alopecia patients test positive for the presence of microsomal antibodies, and these patients also tend to have a substantially higher risk of subclinical thyroid problems, as evidenced by abnormal TRH tests.

Alternatively, diabetes is actually less common in patients with alopecia than in the general public. However, as with other autoimmune diseases, the relatives of people with alopecia are at higher risk of some autoimmune diseases, particularly Type I diabetes.

According to the American Autoimmune Related Diseases Association, alopecia is "found equally in both men and women. The disease can occur at any age, including the childhood years. It has been estimated that approximately 2 million people have some form of alopecia." Although alopecia can occur at any age, the prime period is between ages 15 and 30.

If a family member has alopecia, you have a 10 to 20 percent chance of developing it, versus less than 2 percent in the general public. If a family member has more widespread alopecia, then your risk is almost 20 percent. Genetic mapping has identified particular human leukocyte antigens (HLAs) that may indicate susceptibilities to various types of alopecia.

Some experts believe that alopecia may be triggered after exposure to a virus—cytomegalovirus is one that is frequently cited—or exposure to bacteria. No clear relationships have been established, however. In as many as 15 percent of patients, alopecia seems to be triggered by a major life event, such as an illness that involved fever, death of a family member, certain drugs, pregnancy, or physical trauma.

Symptoms

The primary symptom is hair loss, usually round or oval hairless patches. Typically, in 80 percent of cases, alopecia will present as only one patch, usually around the size of a quarter. Approximately 12 percent will have two patches, and 8 percent will have a number of patches of hair loss. The most frequent location is the scalp, which affects from two-thirds to almost all alopecia patients. In men, around 33 percent lose hair in the beard. Rarely, hair is lost from eyebrows and extremities. In only 7 percent of cases, alopecia is extensive, involving loss of more than half of the body's hair. Only a very small percentage of those cases will have total hair loss. Other less common symptoms include

- Pitting in nails
- Burning sensation
- Itching

Diagnosis

Diagnosis of alopecia is usually made by a doctor's clinical observation. Occasionally, if the doctor suspects that the hair loss may be due to some other condition, a scalp biopsy may be conducted. It's important to have hair loss evaluated, however, to rule out any sort of infectious or disease-based origin.

Getting a diagnosis can be frustrating. One alopecia patient, Rachel, described her experiences:

I am 29 years old and had my first experience with alopecia areata at the age of 19. I woke up one morning with a bald spot about the size of a quarter in the crown of my head and

*freaked out! I immediately went to my doctor. He said, "Your
scalp looks very healthy. I don't see anything wrong. You
must have been born with it." I looked at him as if he were
from outer space. Come on now! I obviously was not born
with a bald spot; otherwise it would not have taken me nine-
teen years to discover it! Needless to say, I have never gone
back to that particular doctor. After several doctors and many
years, I have now found a doctor that at least recognized it is
an autoimmune disease. My current doctor has suggested that
I try steroid injections into my scalp when these bouts occur.
These bouts usually occur every two to three years and range
from the size of a dime to the size of a half dollar, and usually
I get one spot and then another shows up shortly thereafter.
So far, my hair has always grown back.*

Practitioners

The practitioners with the greatest experience in dealing with
hair loss are dermatologists.

Treatment

Some practitioners do not believe in even treating alopecia,
because the condition is not considered medically dangerous, and
because remission and hair regrowth can be expected in the majority of cases. In alopecia patients with extensive disease, as many as
8 to 45 percent have some positive regrowth using the 5 percent
solution of minoxidil (Rogaine), but the treatment needs to be continuous in order to promote and maintain regrowth.

Drug treatments include injected corticosteroids into the
affected area. While this treatment hasn't been extensively studied,
one study found that 92 percent of patients with small amounts of
hair loss had some regrowth, and 61 percent of patients with total
alopecia had some regrowth. Topical steroids are also used in some

patients. Fluocinolone acetonide cream 0.2 percent (Synalar) and betamethasone dipropionate cream 0.05 percent (Diprosone) had some regrowth results in studies.

Occasionally, in cases where alopecia comes on suddenly and extensively, oral corticosteroids may be used, in order to attempt to slow or stop the alopecia. Some practitioners, however, have found no results with this treatment, and even when success has been reported, patients relapse after stopping the therapy. The doses needed to obtain results are high enough that adverse side effects can also be experienced.

Oral cyclosporine is used in some patients, and all patients experienced some regrowth taking this drug, with half having cosmetically acceptable regrowth. Stopping the drug almost always triggers a relapse, however, and there's no evidence that oral cyclosporine can slow or prevent hair loss.

In cases of severe alopecia, topical immunotherapy may be beneficial. In this therapy, allergic irritation of the skin is triggered by topically applying strong allergens. These include squaric acid dibutylester (SADBE) and diphencyprone (DPCP). These products are, however, not approved by the Food and Drug Administration, and their long-term safety is not known, although the treatment has been used for almost twenty years with no major adverse effects reported. Anthralin is another immunotherapy agent that is used. Some studies have shown no response to this treatment, whereas others have shown varying response rates for patchy alopecia, with lesser response for severe alopecia. How immunotherapy works is not clearly understood.

Another common treatment is psoralen plus UVA light therapy (PUVA). The initial response rate varies from 20 to 73 percent, but patients usually relapse after treatment is stopped. PUVA is generally not considered an effective long-term treatment for alopecia.

Things to Know

There's a significant link between alopecia and an increased risk of stress and mental health problems. People with alopecia are at higher risk for developing anxiety, personality disorders, depression, and paranoia. As many as three-fourths of all alopecia patients may suffer from some sort of mental health condition.

Patients who have extensive hair loss tend to have less spontaneous remission than patients who have small patches of hair loss. In one study of fifty patients, 24 percent experienced spontaneous complete or nearly complete regrowth at some stage over a three-year period.

■ Psoriasis

Psoriasis is a common, chronic autoimmune skin disease. New skin cells grow abnormally and too rapidly, creating inflamed, painful, and scaly patches of skin, called plaques, where the old skin has not shed quickly enough. Occasionally psoriasis affects the eyes, nails, and joints, and in a small percentage of patients a mild form of arthritis will develop.

According to the National Psoriasis Foundation, psoriasis affects more than 7 million Americans. As many as a quarter-million people are newly diagnosed each year. Psoriasis is more common in women, in colder climates and lighter-skinned people, particularly Caucasians. Although as many as one in ten cases start in children under 10, the median age of psoriasis onset is 28 years. Psoriasis also tends to run in families.

Psoriasis can flare up for no reason, but certain conditions appear to trigger attacks: some drugs (e.g., lithium, beta-blockers, or medicated ointments and creams), sunburn, climate, hormonal factors, and smoking. Bacterial infections and pressure or trauma to the skin can also aggravate psoriasis.

Symptoms

The symptoms of psoriasis are primarily the skin involvement, which can take a number of forms.

- In plaque psoriasis, plaques most commonly show up on the knees, elbows, scalp, and trunk. Typically, plaques are raised, inflamed lesions, covered with a silvery white scale. The scale may be scraped away to reveal inflamed skin beneath. The scalp is one of the most common areas for psoriasis, affecting as many as 50 percent of patients, with small silvery scales that may be mistaken for dandruff. The way to tell if it's psoriasis is that there are flaking areas alongside normal ones.
- Guttate psoriasis shows up as small red dots on the trunk, arms, and legs. The dots may have scales.
- Inverse psoriasis occurs in the armpit, groin, under the breast, and in the folds of the skin. These lesions typically are smooth and inflamed, with no scaling.
- Pustular psoriasis presents as blistery pustules on the hands and the soles of the feet.
- Erythrodermic psoriasis includes swelling, itching, pain, and scaling on most parts of the body.
- Nail psoriasis can cause pitting, yellowing, and thickening of the nails.

About one in ten psoriasis patients has some stiffness, pain, and joint damage, usually to the hands, feet, and other joints. This is known as psoriatic arthritis.

Diagnosis

Diagnosis of psoriasis is usually made by observation from a doctor, but to rule out other conditions, occasionally a practitioner may want to do a small skin biopsy.

Practitioners

Dermatologists typically have the most experience in diagnosing and treating psoriasis.

Treatment

Most treatments for psoriasis focus on topical skin care to relieve the inflammation, itching, and scaling. For simple, limited psoriasis, topical creams are typically used, including moisturizing emollients, vitamin D cream, corticosteroid ointments, and creams containing salicyclic acid. Sun exposure and sunbathing can help clear up plaques, and some physicians will recommend time in the sun.

For more severe cases, oral medications are used. Researchers found that alefacept (Amevive) had positive results in clinical trials. The drug targets the T cells that cause psoriasis and hones in on the disease without causing immune suppression. Of the patients studied, a majority saw greater than a 50 percent reduction of symptom severity with use of alefacept versus a placebo. One-third of patients studied had a greater than 75 percent reduction in symptoms.

Another potentially successful new drug is efalizumab is (Xanelim), from the developer Genentech. Xanelim, which is given by injection, is an antibody designed to block certain immune cells from entering and binding to skin tissue. Research has shown that Xanelim cut the incidence of psoriasis by at least 75 percent in 58 percent of patients receiving the drug weekly for six months. The main side effects include headaches and body aches after the first couple of injections, as well as some nausea and chills. Patients not only experienced dramatic improvement of symptoms but remained symptom-free for periods averaging 10 months and lasting as long as 18 months.

In some cases, retinoids such as isotretinoin (Accutane) and acitretin (Soriatane) are recommended. Infliximab (Remicade), which is typically used for irritable bowel syndrome, Crohn's disease, and rheumatoid arthritis, is also being investigated for use in psoriasis. Infliximab blocks the production and activity of tumor necrosis factor alpha (TNF-a), thus reducing the body's inflammatory response. In a research study, 80 to 90 percent of patients given varying doses of infliximab responded to treatment. The drug may gain more widespread use in psoriasis as more studies are conducted.

Another treatment used in more serious psoriasis is UV light therapy. It combines the drug psoralen, which makes skin sensitive to ultraviolet light, with exposure to UV light. The treatment is known as PUVA. It's used sparingly, however, as it may increase the risk of skin cancer.

In rare cases of severe arthritic involvement, immunosuppressive drugs such as methotrexate and cyclosporine are sometimes used. But a recent study has found that etanercept (Enbrel), used for treating rheumatoid arthritis, can also be effective in treating psoriatic arthritis. In one study, 59 percent of patients taking the drug saw significant improvement in arthritis and psoriasis symptoms.

Things to Know

Current drug treatments provide short response periods and can be extremely toxic, leading to an increased risk of liver and renal failure, as well as an increased risk for melanoma. As a result, there is a high rate of dissatisfaction and noncompliance among patients. A recent survey by the National Psoriasis Foundation (NPF) found that almost 80 percent of patients expressed frustration with current treatments due to lack of efficacy. To address these concerns, a variety of new immunotherapies are in development. These new drugs will work to help psoriasis without targeting the entire immune system.

■ Vitiligo

Vitiligo is an autoimmune skin disease in which the absence of melanocytes (pigment-producing cells) causes a decreased pigmentation (coloration) in the skin. The body creates antibodies directed against the melanocytes themselves. Vitiligo has a tendency to run in families and may follow unusual trauma, especially to the head. The disease may also be referred to as leukoderma.

Pigment cells give color or tint to the skin. The loss of pigment causes depigmentation, or loss of color, which results in blotches and two-toned patches of skin. Vitiligo is temporary in one-third of those diagnosed with it.

Vitiligo can be localized in one particular area, or generalized, affecting the body more broadly. Generalized vitiligo is more common. Vitiligo strikes the face, neck, and scalp. Other common sites are the elbows, knees, ankles, shoulders, and other bony areas; the forearms, wrists, hands, and fingers; and body orifices such as the lips, genitals, gums, and nipples.

Vitiligo can show up as a patch or streak of white or gray hair on the scalp, or, in some cases, it can turn all of the scalp hair white or gray. Vitiligo can affect eyebrow, pubic, and underarm hair.

Vitiligo alone is considered primarily a cosmetic problem, as it is not life-threatening, and on its own, it does not usually come with medical symptoms. It is, however, frequently emotionally difficult, because of the visibility of the depigmentation.

The disorder can also be a warning sign for future development of other autoimmune conditions, such as thyroid disease or diabetes. Vitiligo is ten to fifteen times more common in patients with other autoimmune diseases, such as Addison's disease, diabetes mellitus, pernicious anemia, alopecia areata, discoid lupus, and abnormal thyroid function.

Vitiligo is considered fairly common, with as many as 1 to 2 percent, or approximately 3.5 million people, suffering from this condition. In approximately 30 percent of patients, there is "cluster-ing" among family members. It affects women and men fairly equally, and may be somewhat more common in blacks and some Jews of Moroccan or Yemeni descent. Vitiligo can strike at any age but rarely starts in infancy or old age; the most common age of onset is between 10 and 30 years.

Symptoms

The main symptoms are white spots on the skin, which are more noticeable in those with darker complexions or when the skin is tanned. Typically, vitiligo begins with only a few small spots, but then more spots appear, borders can become defined and outlined, and they can grow in size, taking on more unusual shapes.

Diagnosis

Vitiligo is typically diagnosed by observation of a practitioner. If your physician is attempting to clarify a diagnosis and rule out other pigmentary disorders, a skin biopsy may be ordered.

Practitioners

Most dermatologists should be able to recognize the telltale depigmentation of vitiligo fairly easily.

Treatment

There is no single, agreed-upon treatment for vitiligo. Treatment is usually specific to each case and depends on the response. Pho-tochemotherapy, combining UVA light treatment with certain oral drugs, can cause the return of color (repigmentation) in as many as 70 percent of early or localized cases. Several treatments a week are needed over many months before results are seen, and the best results are usually enjoyed on the face. Vitiligo on the hands and feet is frequently the most resistant to treatment.

In some cases, oral steroid drugs such as prednisone may be used for vitiligo. Practitioners are reluctant to use these over time because their side effects are not considered warranted for what doctors feel is not a medically life-threatening condition.

Topical steroid drugs are frequently recommended for localized vitiligo. Some of these include triamcinolone (Aristocort), which is available as an ointment or stronger cream, or topical hydrocortisone creams, which are stronger than over-the-counter hydrocortisone creams. Topical psoralen plus UVA (PUVA) is of benefit in some patients with localized patches. Psoralen cream is applied thirty minutes prior to UVA radiation and is usually done once or twice a week. This treatment can have risks, however, and sun and UVA exposure should be avoided during treatment. There is also a risk of burns.

The last-resort treatment for vitiligo is depigmentation, in which a cream is used to eliminate all pigment from the skin to eliminate the spotted effects. A cream that contains hydroquinone is applied for up to a year and results in permanent depigmentation. Typically, this process is only performed after a complete assessment, including discussions with a mental health professional.

For very small areas of vitiligo, some patients may be good candidates for surgical transplants, including punch grafts, in which a small biopsy sample from a donor site is transplanted into a depigmented area. Other patients get minigrafts, which are larger transplants. A technique known as micropigmentation, which is actually a form of tattooing, can be used to repigment skin in dark-skinned individuals. You can't get a very exact match, however, and the tattooed area tends to fade.

Things to Know

Vitiligo is more common in people who have other autoimmune diseases, especially thyroid conditions and diabetes. Anyone who starts out with vitiligo should become educated regarding the symptoms of thyroid disease, diabetes, pernicious anemia, Addison's disease, alopecia areata, and other autoimmune conditions.

Sunscreens should be given to all patients with vitiligo to minimize risk of sunburn or repeated solar damage to depigmented skin, with the understanding, however, that most sunblocks have a limited ability to screen UVA light. Tanning of surrounding normal skin exaggerates the appearance of vitiligo, and this is prevented by sun protection.

■ Pemphigus

Pemphigus is a rare, incurable, and frequently debilitating autoimmune disease in which the immune system attacks the skin and mucous membranes, causing nonhealing, burn-like blisters. In some extremely serious cases, sores can cover substantial areas of the body. Pemphigus vulgaris, or common pemphigus, is the most frequently diagnosed type and usually starts with painful sores and blisters in the mouth. Pemphigus foliaceus usually begins with itchy but less painful crusted sores or blisters on the face and scalp, and later, the chest and back. Paraneoplastic pemphigus is the rarest but most serious form of the disease, and usually occurs only in someone who has been diagnosed with cancer. This condition involves painful sores in the mouth, lips, and esophagus, as well as skin lesions.

Pemphigus is most common in adulthood, especially in seniors. Its prevalence is not known, but it's a good example of an autoimmune condition that is frequently misdiagnosed.

Symptoms
The main symptoms include

- Clear, soft, fluid-filled blisters of various sizes
- Blisters that rupture and do not heal
- Scaly patches

- Ruptured mouth blisters that form ulcers
- Mouth pain

Diagnosis

Diagnosis is typically done clinically, but because of the rarity of the condition, many practitioners may not be able to recognize pemphigus. When it is suspected, a skin specimen can be examined for specific antibodies that confirm the disorder.

Practitioners

Dermatologists and oral surgeons would offer the best chance of a diagnosis of pemphigus, although some specialists may not recognize it because the condition is so rare.

Treatment

The first course of treatment is to prevent new blisters. Typically, an oral corticosteroid drug such as prednisone is used at high dose, then tapered down. To keep pemphigus in check, the corticosteroid may need to be taken for months or even years.

In severe cases, immunosuppressive drugs such as methotrexate, cyclophosphamide, and azathioprine (Imuran) may be prescribed along with steroids. Since immunosuppressive drugs also have their own side effects, plasmapheresis may be recommended to filter antibodies from the blood.

Pemphigus foliaceus sometimes responds to topical steroid creams, and in some cases, the antimalarial drug hydroxychloroquine (Plaquenil) is prescribed. In addition, the exposed skin surface of open blisters needs particular care to avoid infection.

Things to Know

If you have any persistent skin or mouth lesions, consult your dermatologist. Early diagnosis of pemphigus may permit treatment with low levels of medication.

Pemphigus may be particularly difficult to diagnose, since it's not common. One patient, Rick, who was diagnosed more than three years ago, underwent an odyssey that began after a dentist discovered a lesion in his mouth, and a sore appeared on his cheek. A dermatologist didn't recognize early pemphigus and diagnosed a yeast infection. At that point, his crotch and buttocks became covered by blistering sores and his fingernails and toenails had fluid building up to the point where they started to fall out. After months of suffering, a series of dermatologists diagnosed his condition as a staph infection. Finally, he saw another dermatologist who was able to diagnose the open sores over a third of his body as pemphigus vulgaris. After six weeks of high-dose steroids, he started Imuran to help reduce the steroid dosage. Says Rick:

Four months later and I was able to crawl into my bed for a few hours sleep a night. After many trials and tribulations and a year and a half of treatment, I stopped taking steroids; another nine months and I was off of the Imuran. I was lucky and responded to these drugs well. I've had a few small flare-ups and preventatively take prednisone before and after dental appointments.

8

Gastrointestinal Conditions

Autoimmune diseases affecting the gastrointestinal system are quite common and can be debilitating. Given that the digestive tract can be a front-line defender in the immune system, it's no surprise that it is often the target of autoimmune diseases.

■ Inflammatory Bowel Disease

The inflammatory bowel diseases (IBDs) are autoimmune diseases that involve a reaction against the body's own intestinal tract. The intestines are a front-line defense in the body's immune system. Their mucosal barrier is designed to recognize and protect against pathogens, while dealing with various bacteria that are meant to populate the intestines. The intestines are supposed to be acting as a barrier against bacteria and toxins, while allowing for absorption of nutrients. When this complex process fails, or when intestinal permeability increases, allowing greater exposure to antigens, then IBDs can develop.

There are two major IBDs: ulcerative colitis and Crohn's disease. While ulcerative colitis involves the inside lining of the colon—the large intestine—or the rectum, Crohn's disease can affect any part of the gastrointestinal tract, from the mouth to the anus. Crohn's disease may be referred to as chronic ileitis, regional enteritis, or granulomatous colitis. Although there are some differences in the IBDs, many of the symptoms and treatments tend to be similar.

Both ulcerative colitis and Crohn's disease are considered remitting and relapsing conditions, with periods of active intensity—known as flares—and periods of remission, with minimal inflammation and a reduction in symptoms. Over a four-year period, approximately one-quarter of Crohn's disease patients remain in remission, one-quarter have frequent flares, and one-half have remitting and relapsing Crohn's. Both conditions are aggravated—but not likely caused—by stress.

Both conditions can cause diarrhea, nausea, vomiting, abdominal cramps, and pain, but bloody diarrhea and incontinence are most often associated with ulcerative colitis, and fatigue, diarrhea, abdominal pain, and weight loss are more often linked to Crohn's disease. Some IBD patients also have inflammatory reactions involving the skin, joints, eyes, and liver.

Approximately 1 to 2 million people in the United States are estimated to have ulcerative colitis or Crohn's disease. Ulcerative colitis was more common than Crohn's disease prior to 1960. Recently, however, the incidence of Crohn's disease is approaching that of ulcerative colitis.

IBDs are most common in developed countries. Colder climates have a greater rate of IBD, and urban areas have a greater rate. The incidence has been reported to be highest in the American Jewish population—which has a prevalence from four to five times that of the general population—followed by non-Jewish Caucasians. Ulcerative colitis seems to be more common in women and is thought to affect 30 percent more females than males.

Most frequently, IBDs are diagnosed from late adolescence to the 30s. There appears to be a family connection, and a parent with IBD has approximately a 4 percent chance of having a child develop IBD; 10 to 25 percent of IBD patients are thought to have first-degree relatives with IBD.

The cause of IBD is being actively studied. But there are many theories:

- Growing up in an "overclean" environment leads to an underexposure to intestinal pathogens in childhood and an overreaction to them later in life.
- Modern diets heavy on refined sugars and low in fiber make people more prone to IBD.
- IBD is an immune response to an antigen such as protein from cow's milk. Consumption of milk and milk products is a known factor in worsening ulcerative colitis. Lactose intolerance is also common in Crohn's disease and ulcerative colitis, and this relationship may hold some key toward understanding the cause.

Some experts believe that IBD is a chronic inflammatory response to an unrecognized infection by a pathogenic organism. Bacterial triggers mentioned by researchers have included streptococcus, listeria, and in particular *Escherichia coli.*

In an article in *The Scientist,* John Hermon-Taylor, chairman of the Department of Surgery at St. George's Hospital Medical School, London, implicated *Mycobacterium avium* subspecies paratuberculosis (MAP) in 50 to 70 percent of all Crohn's cases: "I am certain that paratuberculosis is present in the guts of people with Crohn's disease. [But] the correct methods haven't been used to detect and study it. It's a tough bug." Hermon-Taylor says that he has treated 150 Crohn's cases with a combination of drugs, including rifabutin and clarithromycin, which are more active against MAP. About 70 percent of these cases, he says, went into remission after the intestine was healed.

Symptoms: Ulcerative Colitis

- Bloody diarrhea
- Pain
- Fatigue
- Anemia
- Bowel urgency
- Abdominal cramps
- Weight loss in severe cases
- Joint inflammation
- Irritation of eyes
- Mild fever
- Rapid heart rate
- Dehydration
- Abdominal tenderness

Symptoms: Crohn's Disease

- Abdominal pain, most frequently in the lower abdomen or right lower quadrant
- Diarrhea
- Fatigue
- Intestinal strictures, obstructions, and fistula
- Low-grade fever
- Weight loss
- Anemia
- Growth retardation in children
- Gallstones and their symptoms, including indigestion, right quadrant abdominal and back pain

Skin lesions and inflamed patches of skin can be complications of IBD. Usually as the IBD is treated, these symptoms lessen. In rare cases, joint aches and inflammation can occur.

Diagnosis

Some lab tests helpful in diagnosing IBD include

- Stool studies to rule out other infections
- Blood tests for iron levels, to show anemia, a common sign of IBD
- Erythrocyte sedimentation rate (ESR), known as a "sed rate"; elevated ESR is a marker for inflammation
- Serum vitamin B12, as deficiency can occur in some Crohn's disease patients
- Abdominal x-rays to show evidence of obstruction and inflammation of the colon
- A barium enema, as results can exclude or diagnose ulcerative colitis
- Small bowel series x-rays to sometimes diagnose Crohn's disease in the small intestine
- Abdominal/pelvic computerized tomography (CT) scans to sometimes find abcesses and fistula
- Colonoscopy, which can diagnose many cases of IBD
- Flexible sigmoidoscopy, which can diagnose some ulcerative colitis cases but rarely Crohn's disease
- Upper endoscopy, which can evaluate some cases of Crohn's disease

Patient advocate and author Dr. Marie Savard says that diagnosis of IBD can be tricky:

I have found that patients diagnosed with irritable bowel either get too much testing (each doctor repeats the same x-ray tests and patients get too much radiation, rather than the doctor simply checking old records and films themselves) or patients get too little testing, and doctors assume everyone else before them did all the necessary tests (in this instance

*other diseases such as giardia and cancer have all occurred,
yet the patient thought it was just irritable bowel syndrome).
I have also found with this condition that lactose intolerance
is so common, but people don't think of it . . . diet history is
so important; keeping a diet journal can be very helpful linking the diet and symptoms.*

Practitioners

According to patient advocate Amber Tresca, anyone with a
digestive condition really needs a medical care team:

*Gastroenterologists are going to be the main source for treat-
ments and tests. They are the best trained to offer a diagnosis
using tests such as colonoscopies or other endoscopy procedures. Anyone with a chronic condition may also want to see
a therapist, particularly when first diagnosed. A chronic illness is a great burden that these professionals can help
unload. A nutritionist or dietitian will also be helpful in
developing a proper diet. The glue that holds them all
together is a general practitioner, who should aid in getting all
the members of the team talking together.*

Treatment

• The first step in medication usually is aminosalicylates. The
oral aminosalicylates available in the United States include sulfasalazine (Azulfidine), mesalamine (Rowasa, Asacol, Pentasa), and
olsalazine (Dipentum). These are typically available in enema and
suppository form. Aminosalicylates can treat flares of the IBD
and maintain remission.

• Another concurrent step sometimes taken for Crohn's disease
is use of the antibiotics metronidazole (Flagyl) or ciprofloxacin
(Cipro). Antibiotics are not frequently used with ulcerative colitis.

• If IBD fails to respond to the preceding treatments, the next step is corticosteroid drugs. Depending on severity, corticosteroids may be given intravenously, orally, by enema, suppository, or topical foam. They are not typically used long-term to control or treat IBD, however. In late 2001, the FDA approved budesonide (Entocort EC) capsules for the treatment of mild to moderately active Crohn's disease. Entocort EC is an orally administered steroid that is released in the intestine, where it works locally and topically to decrease inflammation. Entocort causes less side effects than steroids such as prednisone because most of the drug is not absorbed into the body.

• If a patient can't go on a low dose or taper off corticosteroids, the next step is immunosuppressants, such as azathioprine (Imuran) or 6-mercaptopurine (6-MP). These are used for long-term treatment in steroid-dependent cases, or for those who do not respond to aminosalicylates or corticosteroids.

• For Crohn's disease, another drug option is available: infliximab (Remicade). In one study, patients with Crohn's disease–related arthritis who were unresponsive to conventional treatment improved very rapidly and safely with the use of infliximab, the antibody-based drug that is directed against tumor necrosis factor alpha. The patients were able to stop or significantly decrease other antirheumatic medications after the infliximab infusions.

• The last step for IBD treatment involves drugs with efficacy levels that have been less well demonstrated, but they have been shown to be useful in some patients. For ulcerative colitis, cyclosporine (Neoral, Sandimmune) and nicotine patches fall into this category. For Crohn's disease, methotrexate may fall into this category.

Total removal of the colon (total colectomy) may be called for in severe cases of ulcerative colitis where there is evidence of cancer or precancerous conditions, a chronic and severe ulcerative colitis that is not responding to medicines, or other systemic complications. Colectomy eliminates the disease and the increased risk for colon cancer.

Surgery for Crohn's is mainly done for complications such as blockages or fistula, rather than for the disease itself, as surgery does not typically resolve the underlying condition. As many as a third of Crohn's disease patients who have surgery will require surgery again within five years, and two-thirds require surgery again within fifteen years.

Things to Know

Patients with ulcerative colitis are much more likely than those without the disorder to have a history of depression or anxiety. It is possible that by suppressing the immune system, depression might put certain people more at risk of bowel disease. The results showed prior depression and anxiety were both significantly more common in patients with ulcerative colitis than in the general population. British researchers report that left-handed people are twice as likely to suffer from IBD as right-handed people, which suggests some sort of genetic and/or environmental linkage.

Ulcerative colitis carries with it a risk of colon cancer, and after someone has had the condition for eight years, experts recommend surveillance colonoscopy every one to two years. Ulcerative colitis can also be accompanied by inflammations of the eye, known as iritis or uveitis. If untreated, these complications can lead to vision loss, so high-dose systemic steroids are frequently used.

The average patient with ulcerative colitis has a 50 percent probability of having a flare during a two-year period. A liquid/predigested formula has been found to reduce inflammatory activity in Crohn's disease. There is a fair amount of controversy over whether aspirin or nonsteroidal anti-inflammatory drugs (NSAIDs) can cause flares of IBD. Some practitioners tell all IBD patients to avoid these drugs; others suggest that only if an episode occurs after taking one of these drugs should patients avoid them.

Infliximab (Remicade), the immune-suppressing drug used to treat rheumatoid arthritis and Crohn's disease, was found to be behind seventy reported cases of tuberculosis—four of them fatal—among U.S. patients who received the medication between 1998 and May 2001. Patients should be tested and treated for inactive, or latent, TB prior to infliximab therapy. Up to 15 million Americans are estimated to have latent TB infections. When the immune system is suppressed—as it is in patients on infliximab—latent TB can become active.

■ Celiac Disease/Celiac Sprue Dermatitis

Celiac disease, also known as celiac sprue, celiac sprue dermatitis, or gluten intolerance, is a chronic disease of the digestive system that prevents absorption of nutrients from food. People who have celiac disease have an allergic sensitivity to gluten, a protein that is found in grains such as wheat, rye, barley, and possibly oats. Eating these foods causes damage to the mucosal lining of the intestine, which leads to an inability to properly digest and absorb nutrients.

Celiac sprue has a strong hereditary component. When one identical twin has the condition, there is a 70 percent chance that the other twin will develop it. An estimated 1 in 4,700 Americans has been diagnosed with celiac disease, which would put the total at less than 100,000 in the United States. But recent studies suggest that the number is actually closer to 1 in 250, according to the National Institute of Diabetes and Digestive and Kidney Diseases (NIDDK). That would mean that more than a million people in the United States currently have celiac disease.

Although it is the most commonly diagnosed genetic disease in Europe and is very prevalent among people of European descent, celiac disease is rarely diagnosed in people of African and Asian descent. It can affect both men and women but is slightly more common in women.

Celiac disease can first appear in infants when they begin to eat gluten products. However, it may not be diagnosed at that time, and symptoms flare and diminish through adolescence and into adulthood, when symptoms reappear again. Most cases are diagnosed in the 30s and 40s.

Symptoms

Symptoms of celiac disease include

- Diarrheal, watery, odorous, semiformed, tan, gray, oily, or frothy stools
- Abdominal bloating, cramps, excessive or explosive gas
- Weight loss in some patients
- Failure to gain weight and growth retardation in infants and children
- Weakness, fatigue, including muscle weakness
- Bone pain
- Tingling and numbness in hands and feet
- Skin lesions, known as dermatitis herpetiformis, which primarily appear on elbows, knees, and buttocks
- Absence of menstrual periods, delayed start of menstrual periods in adolescents
- Infertility in women and men
- Impotence
- Orthostatic hypotension, where blood pressure drops when you stand up after being in bed or sitting, which can cause dizziness or fainting

Diagnosis

In addition to the symptoms, tests to help make a diagnosis of celiac disease include

- Blood tests for anemia (which is more common in celiac disease)
- Blood tests to measure circulating antibodies to gliadin
- Evaluation for signs of bone disease (such as scoliosis or compression fractures)
- Dental examination (celiac disease can cause changes in the enamel of the teeth)
- Endoscopic examination
- Small-bowel biopsy
- Symptom evaluation during and after a test of a gluten-free diet

Many adults spend years being misdiagnosed and are commonly told they have irritable bowel syndrome, a far less serious condition that is not treated with the gluten-free diet. It's particularly important to get a diagnosis of celiac disease as early as possible, because the more delayed the diagnosis of the disease, the more risky it can be. Researchers did a survey in the mid-1990s, looking at when celiac disease patients had their first symptoms, versus when they were diagnosed with the disease. They found that the typical gap was twelve years. Screening is routine in Europe but not in the United States, where many physicians are not even familiar with the condition.

Practitioners

Gastroenterologists may generally be more likely to recognize celiac disease, but some endocrinologists, physicians who have a nutritional perspective, nutritionists, dietitians, and metabolic and holistic physicians may be more aware of the prevalence of undiagnosed celiac disease and on the lookout for symptoms of this frequently overlooked condition.

Treatment

People with celiac disease must stay on a gluten-free diet for the rest of their lives or risk damaging their small intestine and further losing the ability to absorb nutrients. The gluten-free diet means total avoidance of all wheat, rye, and barley and products made from them. There is some disagreement as to whether oats are also to be avoided. Be careful to avoid hidden glutens, such as "vegetable protein" and malt, modified food starch, some soy sauces, and distilled vinegars, among other food items. A good support group can help you learn how to eat gluten-free among today's variety of food options. It's essential to stay on this diet, and one Italian study found that the death rate for those who failed to stick to it was six times higher than for those who followed it.

A small percentage of celiac disease patients don't respond to a gluten-free diet, and in those cases, corticosteroid drugs such as prednisone are sometimes used.

Things to Know

The incidence of celiac disease in various autoimmune disorders is ten to thirty times more common compared to the general population. In some of these cases, however, the celiac disease symptoms may not be evident.

Type I diabetes is more common at an early age in patients with celiac disease compared to those without celiac disease. Some researchers have found that a gluten-free diet can actually prevent or delay the onset of Type I diabetes in people who are genetically predisposed.

■ Pernicious Anemia

Pernicious anemia occurs after long-term autoimmune gastritis (inflammation of the mucosal lining of the stomach). The destruction of the gastric mucosal cells makes you unable to make intrinsic factor, a substance that enables vitamin B12 to be absorbed from the intestine, resulting in a B12 deficiency.

Pernicious anemia is most common in people of Celtic (i.e., English, Irish, Scottish) and Scandinavian descent and estimated to affect less than 100,000 people. Men and woman are affected somewhat equally, with some studies showing a skew toward women. It usually occurs in people ages 40 to 70. Among Caucasians, the mean age of onset is 60 years, but it shows up at an average age of 50 in African-Americans. The concentration of pernicious anemia in families suggests a hereditary component. An association with *Helicobacter pylori* infections has been suggested but not definitively proven.

Symptoms

The symptoms of pernicious anemia are usually slow and vague, making diagnosis difficult. The most common symptoms include weakness, sore tongue, and paresthesias (numbness, tingling, burning sensations). Other symptoms include

- Lack of appetite, weight loss of 10 to 15 pounds in about 50 percent of patients, due to lack of appetite
- Low-grade fever
- Anemia
- Smooth tongue in 50 percent of patients that may be painful and red; may be accompanied by changes in taste and loss of appetite
- Constipation or several semisolid bowel movements daily
- Numbness and tingling in hands and feet
- Nausea, vomiting, heartburn
- Flatulence, diarrhea
- Sense of fullness, abdominal pain
- Fatigue, weakness
- Pale skin, pallor, lemon-yellow waxy appearance to the skin

- Impaired smell
- Bleeding gums
- Shortness of breath
- Headache
- Ringing in the ears (tinnitus)
- Loss of bladder control
- Impotence
- Clumsiness and unsteady gait (worse in the dark)
- Irritability, personality changes, memory loss
- Delusions, hallucinations
- Premature whitening of the hair
- Rapid heartbeat

Diagnosis

Pernicious anemia can frequently be diagnosed through various tests, including

- Bloodwork to assess iron levels, typically a complete blood count (CBC), which can measure various iron levels
- Blood tests for vitamin B12 and folic acid deficiencies
- Measurement of methylmalonic acid and homocysteine, which can be elevated in pernicious anemia
- Testing for antibodies to intrinsic factor
- Indirect bilirubin may be elevated
- Other red blood cells, enzymes, and serum iron saturation may be elevated
- Serum potassium, cholesterol, and alkaline phosphatase may be decreased
- Other disorders that interfere with the absorption and metabolism of vitamin B12 can produce cobalamine (Cbl) deficiency, so many of the tests to rule out and diagnose pernicious anemia focus on identifying the cause of Cbl deficiency. Some of these results include low serum Cbl levels.

- Schilling test to measure Cbl absorption, which shows that anemia is not secondary to other causes of Cbl deficiency

Practitioners

Gastroenterologists, internists, or hematologists may be best able to recognize and diagnose pernicious anemia.

Treatment

Iron replacement can treat general anemia but not pernicious anemia. For pernicious anemia, injections of vitamin B12 (called cyanocobalamin or hydroxyocobalamin), oral folic acid therapy, or both, can reverse the production of abnormal blood cells. To deal with acute situations, B12 injections are given daily for several weeks, then twice a week for a month, and monthly thereafter. Usually, the B12 shots must be taken for life, although some patients can be maintained on an orally administered form. It's difficult to get people to take monthly injections, so other forms are being investigated. In Europe, a nasal spray form of hydroxocobalamin is showing promise and is expected to reach the United States soon.

In the uncommon circumstance where there are many neurological symptoms, a neurologist may need to be consulted.

Things to Know

Because an increased familial incidence of pernicious anemia is occurring, family members should be aware that they are at greater risk of developing this disease and should seek medical attention promptly if they develop anemia or mental and neurological symptoms. Sometimes there is a risk of potassium deficiency during treatment, so patients should ask their physicians about supplementation.

Pernicious anemia is connected with autoimmune endocrine conditions, including Hashimoto's thyroiditis, diabetes, Addison's, primary ovarian failure, and thyrotoxicosis. Patient advocate Dr. Marie Savard cautions about the thyroid connection and the potential difficulty in diagnosis:

I treat a lot of elderly retired nuns. I have found that the combination of hypothyroid and pernicious anemia is not that unusual. As the elderly sometimes begin to get confused, tired, etc., their doctors write it off to old age. Every senior who is developing some confusion, etc., should get a B12 level and a TSH test. Doctors sometimes think that if the patient is not anemic, they can't have pernicious anemia. Not true. Dementia can begin from low B12 before the patient gets anemic. It is treatable with monthly shots. This is an important autoimmune disease that people need to ask about when they are taking a family history from family members. I reviewed a legal case of a man who had dementia, was falling a lot, and was finally diagnosed almost too late with pernicious anemia. His daughter had hypothyroidism and his son had testicular failure. Of course, the doctor didn't think of taking a family history of his children—the family history goes both ways!

9

Joint and Muscle-Related Conditions

Among the autoimmune diseases that affect joints and muscles, rheumatoid arthritis is one of the most widespread and debilitating autoimmune diseases. With its ability to cause permanent disability to joints and bones, it's an autoimmune condition that is particularly important to diagnose and treat early, because early treatment can help ward off the worst progression of the disease in some people.

■ Rheumatoid Arthritis

Rheumatoid arthritis (RA) is an autoimmune disease that affects the joints, and most frequently, the free-moving joints, especially the small joints of the hands, as well as the knees, ankles, hips, elbows, wrists, and shoulders. As the tissue lining the joints—the synovium—becomes more inflamed and thickened, pain and swelling increase, and ultimately can cause destruction of the bones, along with deformity. The bone and joint damage can also lead to disability. Inflammation of the synovium usually occurs on both sides of the body, which distinguishes RA from the more common osteoarthritis, which is age- and usage-related "wear-and-tear" arthritis.

RA can range from mild to crippling severity. A small proportion of patients—from 5 to 20 percent—will have mild symptoms that resolve within a year or two and require only pain relief as treatment. Another 5 to 20 percent of patients have slow progression and will respond to disease-modifying antirheumatic drugs (DMARDs). For the majority of patients, however, the disease is progressive despite treatment, and one-fourth of all RA patients can expect to have a major joint replacement. An estimated 50 percent of patients suffer a decrease in their functional status within the first two years, and 75 percent will have joint damage. As many as half may be work disabled after ten years, and up to 75 percent after twenty years.

The condition generally starts between ages 25 and 50, although it can begin at any age. RA affects females two to four times more frequently than males. Prevalence in the United States is 1 percent, which means that as many as 2.5 to 3 million people may have this condition. RA is more common in some Native American populations. Some experts have suggested that overall RA has become less common over the past 40 years; however, the survival rate has not improved substantially. Approximately 65,000 to 70,000 children have a juvenile form of rheumatoid arthritis (JRA), which has similar symptoms to RA found in adults.

There is no single cause for RA. The likelihood is that several factors—both bacterial and viral—are triggering the disease in susceptible people. It appears that exposure to some pathogen sets the RA process in motion, but even eliminating the initial pathogen does not necessarily slow or halt the progression of disease. Some of the suspected triggers include viruses such as rubella, cytomegalovirus, Epstein-Barr virus, and parvovirus, which have all been found in the fluid surrounding the affected joints.

Other bacteria implicated include *Mycobacterium tuberculosis* and *Helicobacter pylori*—the bacteria known to cause ulcers. In one study of patients with RA, more than half had *H. pylori* infection, and elimination of the bacteria resulted in improvement of symptoms.

In early 2001, Israeli researchers were able to demonstrate that *Mycoplasma fermentans* is found in the fluid of joints inflamed by rheumatoid arthritis. In their test group of RA patients, *M. fermentans* was found in 20 percent of the joints examined but was not detected in any patients who had other forms of arthritis. Half of the RA patients studied, even those who had no detectable *M. fermentans* in their joints, had high levels of antibodies against the mycoplasma, showing exposure to *M. fermentans*.

A lack of intestinal bacteria in the Bacteriodes, Prevotella, and Porphyromonas families has also been shown to be more common in RA patients.

Another possible trigger or contributory factor is the use of hair dye. It was found that women who use hair dyes for more than twenty years may be nearly doubling their risk of developing rheumatoid arthritis. Interestingly, researchers also found that decaffeinated coffee may raise the risk of developing rheumatoid arthritis. They followed more than 31,000 women between ages 55 and 69, using the Iowa Women's Health Study from 1986 through 1997. Among the 158 women who developed rheumatoid arthritis, women drinking four or more cups of decaffeinated coffee a day faced more than twice the risk of developing rheumatoid arthritis. Women who drank regular coffee had no increased risk, and those drinking more than three cups of tea had a 60 percent reduced risk. Some of the experts speculated that the use of industrial solvents to decaffeinate the coffee may play a role in triggering RA. The study's lead author, Dr. Ted R. Mikuls, at the University of Alabama at Birmingham, said, "We concluded that decaffeinated coffee consumption was an important yet modifiable risk factor in the development of rheumatoid arthritis. Given the global popularity of coffee, our findings have potential public health implications."

Smoking is also a risk factor, particularly for severe RA, though the mechanism isn't entirely understood.

Symptoms

In about half of RA patients, symptoms start slowly, and there are months or even years of on-and-off fatigue, joint pain, and arthritic symptoms. Eventually, the symptoms become more continuous. In about 25 percent of patients, the symptoms begin rapidly and develop immediately. Relapsing and remitting RA occurs in 75 percent of patients; 10 percent have symptoms less than a year, followed by remission, and 10 percent have an aggressive form of RA that rapidly progresses to deformed joints and disability.

Because rheumatoid arthritis can come on fairly slowly, it can be more difficult to diagnose. Already diagnosed with hypothyroidism, 42-year-old Mari, busy raising two teenage boys and under stress from helping her husband through a major operation and a new job, began having joint pain. Says Mari:

The joint pain was all over, particularly in the fingers, wrists, feet, knees, and shoulders. First my primary doctor thought it was a virus. But after three months of the pain getting worse and no relief with prescriptions, they put me on prednisone for five days, and I was pain-free! After that, the pain came back, but not as bad. It's mainly in the fingers and wrists and occasionally elsewhere if I get off Celebrex, which I'm on now. My primary doctor referred me to a rheumatologist, and he has diagnosed me with rheumatoid arthritis.

The primary symptom is joint pain and aches. This can begin with morning stiffness, or severe stiffness after sitting for a long period, and progress to frequent or near-constant pain and stiffness. Other symptoms include

- Swollen lymph glands
- Low-grade fever
- Eye problems, including dry eyes, burning, itching, mucus discharge
- Dry mouth
- Nerve-ending pain in hands and feet
- Weakness
- Weight loss
- Tendinitis, swelling and warmth in joints
- Joints tender to the touch
- Reduced range of motion
- Skin bumps called rheumatoid nodules, located near joints

Diagnosis

To diagnose RA, the American Rheumatism Association looks for four of seven criteria:

- Morning stiffness that lasts at least an hour before improving; even stiffness that persists for thirty minutes or longer can be a strong suggestion of some sort of inflammatory disease; stiffness that goes away with morning activity but returns later with continued activity, or after sitting for a long period
- Arthritic swelling involving three or more joints
- Arthritis of the hand, particularly the proximal interphalangeal (PIP) joints, metacarpophalangeal (MCP) joints, or wrist joints
- Bilateral (both-sided) involvement of joint areas (e.g., both wrists, not just one)
- Positive serum rheumatoid factor (RF) via blood test: positive in approximately 70 percent of patients, but negative RF does not exclude diagnosis of RA
- Rheumatoid nodules, small nodules in joint area, under the skin
- X-ray evidence of RA, including erosions or decalcifications

Some other diagnostic signs include

- Slight anemia, present in approximately 80 percent of patients
- Erythrocyte sedimentation rate (ESR) elevated in approximately 90 percent of patients, showing inflammation
- Positive antinuclear antibodies (ANAs) present in around 30 percent of patients
- Specific genetic marker, HLA-DR4, found in about 65 percent of RA patients but not required for a diagnosis
- Synovial fluid from an inflamed joint to show elevated white blood count, evidence of infection
- Magnetic resonance imaging (MRI) and computed tomography (CT scan or CAT scan) to show other damage to soft tissue, muscle, cartilage, and joints

But it's important to note that during early-stage RA all laboratory tests may be normal and may lead practitioners to believe that treatment is not needed. The earliest stage, however, is when treatment can be most effective, so if your symptoms qualify you for an RA diagnosis, it is important to consult with a rheumatologist as quickly as possible.

Practitioners

Rheumatologists are essential, because the stakes are high in RA. As noted, if not properly treated, RA can permanently damage joints in just one year.

Traditionally, general practitioners have not referred patients with RA symptoms to a rheumatologist unless the symptoms weren't responding to pain relievers and nonsteroidal anti-inflammatory drugs (NSAIDs). But rapid referral in the case of suspected RA is essential, and experts are now saying that doctors should refer RA patients to a specialist within twelve weeks after the first onset of symptoms, in order to initiate disease-suppressing therapies and prevent damage.

Carol Eustice, who has lived with RA for more than twenty-five years and is now an RA educator and patient advocate, believes someone newly diagnosed with RA should first consult with a well-respected rheumatologist:

> *The newly diagnosed patient needs to become educated about the disease too. In so doing, patients can more easily communicate with their rheumatologists and became partners in their own health care, helping to make decisions about the best course of treatment. Though fear naturally accompanies a new diagnosis of RA, the patient should realize that the future cannot be predicted. It is imperative that an aggressive treatment plan begin soon after diagnosis, for the best chance of controlling the disease.*

In a study from UCLA, it was confirmed that seeing a rheumatologist is the gold-standard strategy in treatment. Half of the more than 1,300 study participants were not under the care of a rheumatologist, even though they had health insurance that would have covered their treatment. About 75 percent of the time, rheumatologists were providing the level of care as recommended by the American College of Rheumatology, but only 50 percent of the people without a rheumatologist were getting that level of care.

Katia, a nurse who has worked in the orthopedics/arthritis field for almost twenty years, emphasizes the importance of early consultation with a rheumatologist:

> *Our hospital treats many patients with rheumatoid arthritis, lupus, fibromyalgia, etc. So when I suspected I had developed rheumatoid arthritis last fall, I didn't waste any time. I went*

straight to a rheumatologist I've worked with two decades and trusted completely. Unfortunately, I was right, but because it was caught so early, I have a better chance of avoiding major deformities of my joints. It took us a while to get the meds balanced, but I can still work full-time and lead an active life. I've worked with rheumatoids for so long that some are like extended family. This is not a disease for sissies. It hurts . . . every single day. But I have a great doctor, supportive family and co-workers. I've decided to control the disease instead of letting it control me. I intend to make the best of it.

Treatment

The objective of treatment for RA is primarily to control inflammation, prevent or slow joint damage, and ultimately to put the condition into remission.

Nonsteroidal Anti-inflammatory Drugs

The first level of treatment starts with nonsteroidal anti-inflammatory drugs (NSAIDs), such as ibuprofen, ketoprofen, or prescription NSAIDs. Although these drugs can help with pain and swelling symptomatically, they don't slow or stop the progression of the disease, or prevent long-term joint damage. General guidelines say that if joint symptoms, stiffness, and fatigue continue for three months, more aggressive treatment with disease-modifying antirheumatic drugs (DMARDs) should begin. Other experts are now suggesting that RA patients should consult with a specialist right away, who may begin DMARD therapy even more quickly to reduce damage.

Corticosteroids

Some patients who are in the early stages of rheumatoid arthritis are prescribed corticosteroids such as oral prednisone to help prevent joint damage. While it can offer symptomatic relief, a study conducted in the Netherlands found that long-term use of prednisone, even at low doses, increases the risk of bone fracture. The dose considered "low" was 10 milligrams per day; however, some physicians disagree and find this to be an intermediate or high dose, claiming that prednisone in doses of 5 milligrams or less per day has minimal side effects.

DISEASE-MODIFYING ANTIRHEUMATIC DRUGS (DMARDs)

There are a variety of DMARDs that offer some hope in slowing the progress of RA and have the potential to prevent joint damage.

- **Methotrexate (Rheumatrex):** Originally a cancer treatment, methotrexate is an immunosuppressant drug that is one of the most commonly used DMARDs for RA. It is frequently used alone in active RA, or given with infliximab (Remicade) or etanercept (Enbrel) when there is insufficient response to methotrexate alone. Results are typically seen within four to eight weeks. A key benefit of methotrexate is that it substantially reduces an RA patient's cardiovascular risk and is therefore associated with longer survival. Most common adverse effects include elevated liver function tests, nausea, vomiting, diarrhea, low white and red blood cell counts, rash, hair loss, and dizziness. More serious side effects can include liver fibrosis, cirrhosis, lung inflammation, and lymphoma. Patients on methotrexate need to have regular bloodwork, including a full blood count, platelets, liver function tests, albumin, and serum creatinine levels. About 30 percent of patients discontinue methotrexate treatment early due to liver toxicity, but researchers have found that patients who took folic acid or folinic acid supplements with methotrexate were less likely to have a malfunctioning liver.
- **Leflunomide (Arava):** This is a newer immunomodulator used for early RA therapy. Developed specifically for RA, in recent studies leflunomide appears to be at least as effective as methotrexate and more effective than sulfasalazine (Azulfidine). It had faster

onset of action—four weeks—than methotrexate or sulfasalazine. The most common adverse effects include diarrhea, respiratory infections, nausea, headache, rash, elevated liver function tests, and hair loss. Serious side effects include skin and liver reactions. Patients should be monitored by periodic liver function tests. According to some experts, these side effects are reported six times more often to the FDA with Arava, versus methotrexate. Some consumer groups are even calling for a ban on this drug.

• **Penicillamine (Cuprimine):** This drug is typically used for chelation (removing metals from the bloodstream) but has anti-inflammatory effects. It can take two to three months to take effect in RA patients. Common side effects include altered taste, nausea, vomiting, diarrhea, loss of appetite, rashes, hair loss, and many other symptoms. Some potentially serious side effects include toxic hepatitis, lupus syndrome, and kidney damage.

• **Sulfasalazine:** This sulfa drug was used as an antibiotic. The main side effects can include loss of appetite, headache, nausea, vomiting, itching, rashes, and fever.

• **Antimalarials:** Chloroquine and hydroxychloroquine (Plaquenil) can have some positive results in RA. One key side effect is the possibility of worsening psoriasis. Misty vision and visual halos are serious side effects that need to be reported to the doctor immediately.

• **Oral or intramuscular gold (Aurolate, Myochrysine):** Gold acts as an anti-inflammatory. Some side effects can include itching, rash, diarrhea, and abdominal pain. Potentially serious side effects include difficulty breathing, swelling throat, face, tongue, and lips, hives, and other indications of severe or life-threatening allergy.

• **Azathioprine (Imuran):** This immunosuppressant is used with patients who have severe, active, and erosive RA that is not responding to other therapies. Side effects include low white and red blood cell counts, anemia, nausea, vomiting, diarrhea, abdominal pain, skin rashes, alopecia, fever, and malaise. Serious side effects include increased risk of cancer, severe infections, and liver toxicity.

• **Cyclosporine (Sandimmune):** Originally used to prevent organ rejection in people who had undergone transplants, cyclosporine is an immunosuppressant. Common side effects include nausea, vomiting, diarrhea, hiccoughs, abdominal discomfort, and other symptoms. More severe and less common side effects include serious anaphylactic allergic reactions, heart attack, infections, pneumonia, and increased risk of cancer.

• **Infliximab (Remicade):** This anti-TNF drug is given along with methotrexate when there is insufficient response to methotrexate alone. Results are generally seen within one to two weeks. Most common negative side effects include upper respiratory tract infections, headache, reactions at the injection site, and nausea. Serious side effects can include pneumonia, shortness of breath, lupus-like syndrome, and malignancies. (One important note about infliximab: The drug was found to have triggered seventy reported cases of tuberculosis (TB)—four of them fatal—among U.S. patients who received the medication between 1998 and May 2001, and who had prior, latent TB. Since as many as 15 million Americans are thought to have latent TB infections, patients should be tested and treated for inactive or latent TB prior to infliximab therapy.)

• **Etanercept (Enbrel):** This anti-TNF drug can be given alone in moderate to severely active RA, or is combined with methotrexate when there is insufficient response to methotrexate alone. The drug was approved in 1998 for the reduction of the signs and symptoms of the disease. Since then, the drug gained FDA approval for inhibiting the progression of joint damage in patients with moderately to severely active rheumatoid arthritis, and was also approved by the FDA to treat patients with early-stage RA, to help prevent disease progression.

Etanercept interrupts the inflammation process and may be used in early RA. There is evidence that it can slow joint damage, and etanercept was found to be generally superior to methotrexate in reducing RA disease activity and inhibiting its progression over a two-year period. Results typically are observed within one to two weeks. Most common adverse effects include reactions at the injection site, upper respiratory tract infections, headache, and rhinitis. Serious side effects include infection and malignancies.

Leslie Garrison, a physician and senior vice president of clinical development at Immunex, one of the manufacturers of Enbrel, noted a recent study of early-stage RA patients, all of whom were experiencing a rapid progression of the disease. Approximately 600 people were split into three test groups. The first group took 20 mg of oral methotrexate once a week; the second, a twice-weekly injectable 10 mg dose of Enbrel; and the third, a 25 mg dose of Enbrel, injected two times a week. Researchers studied the subjects' x-rays, looking for changes in bone erosion and joint-space narrowing, and found that the patients who received the 25 mg dose of Enbrel fared far better than the group taking methotrexate. Among patients who received the 25 mg dose of Enbrel, 72 percent showed no change in erosion scores, as compared with 60 percent of patients in the methotrexate group. According to Garrison, in this same patient population the results are still holding. The people in the early-stage Enbrel study will be followed for five years.

• **Anakinra (Kineret):** The recently approved injectable drug Kineret will likely be used with arthritis patients who have failed other treatments. Kineret works differently from other rheumatoid arthritis drugs, by blocking an inflammatory chemical in the body called interleukin-1, which is a cause of joint swelling.

Researchers studied x-rays noting bone erosion and joint-space narrowing, and found the patients who took Kineret, especially those who were on it for a full year, experienced less bone and joint destruction. After six months, Kineret-treated patients experienced nearly twice the rate of reduction in joint destruction than a placebo group.

Dr. Barry Bresnihan, professor of rheumatology at University College Dublin, said in a press statement: "Not only did patients on anakinra see benefits as early as six months on treatment, but the longer they were on therapy, the more improvement they experienced. This suggests that anakinra may have a cumulative effect on joint destruction."

• **Combination therapy:** For patients who don't respond to a single DMARD, combination therapies may be more effective. Methotrexate is most commonly used as a base drug, with other DMARDs added to it. One study showed that patients with RA who were treated with a combination of leflunomide and methotrexate were more than twice as likely to experience significant symptomatic improvement compared with patients receiving placebo plus methotrexate. In a study of patients taking anakinra in combination with methotrexate, compared with those taking methotrexate alone and those given a placebo, the patients taking anakinra and methotrexate experienced at least a 20 percent improvement in five measures. A majority (55 percent) of the anakinra plus methotrexate patients reported a capability to perform functions with some or no difficulty, compared with 7 percent of placebo patients.

Antibiotic Therapy

Tetracycline compounds have some therapeutic effect in some RA patients, pointing toward a possible bacterial relationship in RA. Daily oral minocycline (Minocin) therapy offered significant improvement in RA disease activity in some patients. Note, however, that there have been some reports linking exposure to minocycline to development of lupus-like syndromes and symptoms that cause arthritis, pneumonitis, and hepatitis, which have been fatal on rare occasions.

TREATMENT FOR CHILDREN

Treatment for children does not necessarily follow the same program as adults. The FDA has approved a formulation of the drug sulfasalazine for the treatment of JRA in children ages 6 to 16. Etanercept has also been approved for children. Other drugs used in JRA include

- Naproxen (Naprosyn)
- Diclofenac sodium (Voltaren)
- Ibuprofen (Motrin/Advil)
- Methotrexate (Rheumatrex)

OTHER TREATMENTS

Because rheumatoid arthritis is so debilitating, it is an area for extensive research of new drugs.

- **D2E7:** Abbott Labs is likely to introduce a new product, currently with the working name of D2E7, which is similar to Enbrel. According to Abbott researchers, however, the drug is superior to Enbrel and another popular RA drug, Remicade, because it requires fewer doses, making it more convenient for patients. Studies have been encouraging so far; the drug has been found to improve joint condition and slow the disease's progression.
- **Disease simulation computer model:** In something that only a few years ago would have come solely out of a science fiction novel, two companies have jointly developed a disease simulation computer program. Entelos, in partnership with the European pharmaceutical company Organon, has created a simulated model of RA. Using the program, researchers can simulate experiments and clinical trials that would otherwise take months or years. This allows them to explore their drug development ideas more quickly, safely, and at less cost, enabling them to determine which drugs have the best potential, focus on those, run the most informative clinical tri-

als and experiments, and get these new drugs to patients faster. Entelos and Organon have also created a "virtual patient," which allows researchers to test new treatments on different types of patients.

• **AGIX-4207 IV:** Trials are under way for a drug with the working title AGIX-4207 IV, an intravenous treatment. Unlike the currently available tumor necrosis factor alpha inhibitors, AGIX-4207 targets a specific subset of TNF-alpha activity and may decrease chronic inflammation in RA without impairing the body's ability to respond to infection. AGIX-4207 IV was designed for RA patients who need to quickly reach target drug levels in the blood, including people in active serious flares, those who aren't tolerating other drugs, or those who are undergoing surgery with its accompanying risk of flare.

• **Vitaxin:** The biotech company MedImmune is testing this drug. Vitaxin is an antibody that has the potential to inhibit the progression of a variety of diseases, including RA, psoriasis, psoriatic arthritis, and certain forms of cancer and eye disease. In a statement issued by MedImmune, Dr. Ronald Wilder, director of clinical development, said, "We believe that Vitaxin may have the ability to impede the advancement of this disease by exerting both antiangiogenic and antiosteolytic effects." Testing will also look at the safety and tolerability of escalating single and multiple doses of Vitaxin in patients with active RA who are currently treated with methotrexate with or without additional antirheumatic drugs.

• **Gene therapy:** In animal studies, Japanese researchers have found a way to reduce the severity of rheumatoid arthritis symptoms using gene therapy. Attaching two different genes to an adenovirus, which they then injected into the mice, the researchers found that one of the genes, CIS3, had a dramatic effect on reducing the severity of the symptoms. Researchers are looking to determine ways that this technology can be applied to human treatment of rheumatoid arthritis.

• **IL-10:** Other biologic agents that target different chemicals are in development. One agent in the late stages of clinical testing is IL-10, which is similar to an anti-inflammatory chemical made naturally by the body.

• **B-lymphocyte depletion therapy:** In some studies this treatment reduced RA symptoms by 70 percent and kept patients feeling nearly symptom-free for more than a year. It combines intravenous and oral medications that remove B-lymphocyte cells from the bloodstream. These cells produce the antibodies believed to cause RA.

Things to Know

Many nonmedication therapies are available for RA, including exercise, massage, counseling, stress reduction, physical therapy, and surgery such as joint replacement. Although some of the newer TNF-inhibiting DMARDs such as infliximab and etanercept show greater promise in RA, insurance companies favor some of the older, traditional DMARDs that can slow joint damage because they are far less expensive. Some insurance companies are requiring that patients must fail to respond to as many as three traditional DMARDs before they will pay for treatment with a TNF-alpha inhibitor.

Many approaches have been suggested to prevent or minimize recurrences or flares. These include proper nutrition, relaxation, low-impact exercise, flexibility exercises, yoga, tai chi, counseling, meditation, hydrotherapy, and stress reduction.

RA decreases in about 70 percent of women during pregnancy but then flares after pregnancy. Richard Eustice, an RA sufferer for more than thirteen years, explains that some men may take RA particularly hard: "As RA imposes more limitations, men can be devastated by how it diminishes their physical ability. The disease takes as much of a psychological toll on its sufferer as it does a physical toll. The impact on both mind and body need to be addressed with your rheumatologist."

If you have rheumatoid arthritis, you should make sure to get your thyroid function evaluated. According to researchers, people with rheumatoid arthritis have a higher incidence of hypothyroidism, and proper and early treatment of the underlying hypothyroidism may help with the course of the rheumatoid arthritis.

Women with RA are at high risk of developing osteoporosis, but researchers have found that muscle-building exercise can help protect bones in RA patients.

People who suffer from RA may be prone to developing chronic gum disease, which can lead to tooth and bone loss. One study found that RA patients were twice as likely as others to develop periodontitis—a chronic infection of the gums and tissues supporting the teeth.

In children with JRA, there is a higher risk of developing chronic uveitis, an infection of the eyes, and vision should be checked every three months for several years.

■ Spondyloarthropathies: Reiter's Syndrome and Ankylosing Spondylitis

Reiter's syndrome and ankylosing spondylitis are chronic, progressive autoimmune diseases known as spondyloarthropathies, which typically involve inflammation and arthritic reactions of the joints, the skeleton, and sometimes the spine. The cause is unknown, but as with other autoimmune diseases, it's assumed that genetic and environmental factors are involved.

Reiter's syndrome is also known as reactive arthritis because joint and tendon inflammation appears to be in reaction to an infection. In addition to the arthritic symptoms, problems include inflammation of the urethra, conjunctivitis of the eyes and other mucous membranes such as the mouth and genitourinary area, and a rash. Bouts of Reiter's syndrome typically last from several weeks to up to six months, and as many as half of all Reiter's sufferers will have recurring arthritis or chronic arthritic symptoms. One form of Reiter's occurs with sexually transmitted infections and is most common in sexually active men; the other occurs after an intestinal infection and diarrheal illness with foodborne bacteria. Everyone who has these infections does not develop Reiter's. There appears to be some genetic factor that makes some people more susceptible to developing Reiter's after these types of infections. It's not clear how many people have the condition, but it's estimated to occur in about 3 to 4 out of every 100,000 people. Some experts have suggested that there may be many more undiagnosed cases of Reiter's syndrome, given that symptoms can be difficult to pinpoint. Reiter's syndrome is generally considered more common in men than women, and the age of onset is most typically between 20 and 40.

Ankylosing spondylitis may also be referred to as Marie-Strümpell disease, Strümpell-Marie disease, spondyloarthritis, and von Bechterew's disease. In ankylosing spondylitis, the spine becomes stiff, and eventually the vertebrae—the bones in the spine—may grow or fuse together. Ankylosing spondylitis can also cause arthritis in other joints and bones. It usually begins between the ages of 15 and 35. The disease affects young white males three times more frequently than women. Symptoms are generally milder in females. This disorder is seen rarely among non-Caucasians. In the United States, the incidence is approximately 0.1 to 0.2 percent of the general population, or around a quarter- to half-million people. The cause is unknown, but it is assumed to be a combination of genetic susceptibility and environmental factors or triggers.

Symptoms

Symptoms of Reiter's syndrome typically begin one to two weeks after the initial infection, and the first symptom is frequently inflammation of the urethra. This shows up as pain and discharge from the penis in men and an inflamed and painful prostate, and in women, slight vaginal discharge or uncomfortable urination. In addition to these genitourinary symptoms, other symptoms include

- Itchy, burning, tearing, swollen, or light-sensitive eyes
- Joint pain, inflammation (especially knees, toes, and areas where tendons are attached to bones, such as the heel)
- Joint stiffness, especially affecting knees, ankles, and feet
- Pain in the spine, back pain, lower back pain
- Painless sores on tongue and mouth
- A rash of hard, thickened spots on palms and soles
- Fever
- Malaise
- Plantar's fasciitis (pain in the bottom of the foot)
- Achilles tendinitis (pain in Achilles tendon in foot)

Symptoms of ankylosing spondylitis include

- Stiffness and pain in lower back, the buttocks and hips upon waking or after periods of inactivity, radiation of pain into the buttocks from the back, pain in hips, difficulty bending the spine
- Back pain relieved by movement or exercise
- Difficulty walking, bent-over posture, poor spinal range of motion
- Pain in heels, pain in soles of feet
- Fever
- Loss of appetite, weight loss
- Fatigue
- Swollen, red, painful, or light-sensitive eyes
- Difficulty taking a deep breath

Diagnosis

There are no simple tests to confirm Reiter's syndrome. Instead, Reiter's is typically diagnosed over time, after observing joint, genital, urinary, skin, and eye problems. For an official diagnosis of Reiter's, two or more of the following criteria must be observed, and one must affect the musculoskeletal system:

- Diarrhea
- Conjunctivitis or iritis (inflammation of the iris of the eye), swollen eyelids
- Genital ulceration or urethritis
- Tenderness in prostate area
- Inflammation in vulva or vaginal area
- Painless ulcers on the penis
- Papules and nodules on feet, toes, palms, scrotum, trunk, and scalp
- Nail thickening and ridging
- Mouth sores
- Joint stiffness, especially affecting knees, ankles, and feet (musculoskeletal symptom), toe or heel pain, inflammation of fingers

There are no specific laboratory tests to diagnose ankylosing spondylitis. Primarily, doctors look at x-rays for evidence of inflammation in the joint between the sacrum (the pelvic bone between hipbones) and the ilium (the flat pelvic bone on either side of the sacrum). Other signs include

- Inflammatory back pain
- Pain and stiffness that is worse in the morning
- Reduced mobility of the spine
- Reduced ability to expand the chest

Bloodwork findings that can help to confirm a diagnosis include

- Elevated erythrocyte sedimentation rate
- Elevated C-reactive protein, a sign of inflammation
- Anemia
- Absence of rheumatoid factor and antinuclear antibodies

Practitioners

Rheumatologists or orthopedists are best able to diagnose Reiter's syndrome, ankylosing spondylitis, and the spondylo-arthropathies.

Treatment

For joint pain and other arthritic symptoms, nonsteroidal anti-inflammatory drugs (NSAIDs) such as ibuprofen (Advil, Motrin) are the best treatment for both conditions. Corticosteroid injections may be given directly into particularly inflamed joints, and short-term oral corticosteroids may occasionally be used. In more debilitating cases of Reiter's, immunosuppressive drugs used in RA, such as sulfasalazine or methotrexate, may be used.

For Reiter's syndrome, antibiotics may be given to treat the underlying sexually transmitted or intestinal infection. Reiter's syndrome usually goes into remission within six months of a flare-up, but as many as half of all patients will have relapses with recurrent arthritis, and up to a third may develop chronic arthritis.

Some researchers suggest that the anti-TNF-alpha drugs used for RA—etanercept and infliximab—may be useful in ankylosing spondylitis. For ankylosing spondylitis patients, surgery is occasionally needed to correct spinal deformities or repair damaged joints, particularly hips and shoulders. For both conditions, physical therapy, including exercise, deep breathing, and postural training, is important.

Things to Know

Frequently, Reiter's syndrome begins one to three weeks after sexual contact or an episode of infectious diarrhea. If there's a chance that your Reiter's syndrome was due to chlamydia infection, you and your sexual partner will need a three-month course of tetracycline antibiotics in order to prevent recurrence of the underlying infection.

Water therapy and swimming are frequently recommended to maintain maximum mobility for ankylosing spondylitis patients.

10

Neuromuscular Conditions

Both the nerves and the connections between muscles are targets for some of the most debilitating autoimmune conditions.

■ Multiple Sclerosis

Multiple sclerosis (MS) is a chronic inflammatory autoimmune disease of the central nervous system that affects the brain and the spinal cord. In MS, the autoimmune reaction is the body's attack on the covering of nerves, known as the myelin sheath. The process of destruction of the myelin is known as demyelination. The myelin sheath can be compared to the insulation covering an electrical wire. Much like when insulation is damaged, a wire cannot conduct electricity, and when demyelination occurs, the nerves cannot transmit impulses quickly or properly. As demyelination occurs in the nerves of the eye, brain, and spinal cord, a variety of neurological disturbances can appear, including psychological and cognitive changes, weakness or paralysis of limbs, numbness, vision problems, speech difficulties, problems with walking or motor skills, bladder problems, and sexual dysfunction.

Commonly, damage to the central nervous system occurs intermittently, which creates a remitting/relapsing condition, allowing for periods of fairly normal functioning. In its most severe form, however, MS symptoms can become constant and progress to blindness, paralysis, and even premature death.

Symptoms of MS are very diverse, and the condition is usually quite hard to diagnose in its early stages. Symptoms can appear slowly over time and may disappear for long periods. In some people, symptoms may appear only two to three times per year, then not appear for months, years, or even decades.

- Overall, some 60 percent of MS sufferers will experience intermittent symptoms, interspersed with periods of normal health.
- Around 20 percent have essentially no impact and few symptoms.
- Approximately 15 percent of sufferers will have intermittent periods of symptoms that grow progressively worse.
- An estimated 5 percent will see their symptoms rapidly worsen, sometimes in just a few days.
- Approximately 15 percent of all MS patients end up needing substantial care and may end up in a wheelchair.

MS is estimated to affect up to 350,000 people in the United States and is the most common acquired neurological disease in young adults. According to the National Institutes of Neurological Disorders and Strokes, about 200 new cases are diagnosed each week. According to the Centers for Disease Control, the numbers are also on the rise. Among women, the numbert of MS cases increased 50 percent between 1982 and the mid 1990s.

The disease can strike at any age but is most commonly diagnosed between ages 20 and 40. MS strikes women twice as often as men, and is more common in Caucasians, particularly those of northern European descent. African-Americans and Asian-Americans have half the risk of Caucasians. MS has a hereditary factor; approximately 5 percent of MS sufferers have an affected brother or sister, and 15 percent have a close relative also affected. It's not a purely genetic transmission, however, as even if an identical twin has MS, there is only a 30 to 50 percent chance that the other twin will get it.

Where you spend your first decade of life seems to have more influence than current geographic location. MS is far more common in those who grew up in temperate climates; it's rare in people who grow up near the equator or in tropical climates.

As with most autoimmune diseases, the exact cause is not known. It is currently thought that exposure to a virus, chemicals, or a trauma may be launching the autoimmune process in susceptible individuals, who then begin to produce antibodies against their own myelin. Other suspected trigger factors include poor diet, viral infections, and stress.

Research is currently examining whether the Epstein-Barr virus (EBV) may be a cause of MS. According to Harvard University researchers, women with significant levels of Epstein-Barr virus antibodies were four times more likely to develop multiple sclerosis than women without high levels. It has been noted that both MS and EBV sufferers have low levels of essential fatty acids. This may help to explain why MS is more common in the United States and northern Europe, where high-fatty-acid diets—diets based on fruits, oily fish, olive and seed oils—are far less common than in other parts of the world.

It's estimated that the yearly economic, social, and medical costs of MS exceed $2.5 billion.

Symptoms

Symptoms of MS depend on what part of the nerves have experienced demyelination. The most common symptoms include

- Increased reflexes
- Problems with balance and coordination

- General weakness
- Eye problems, with jerky eye movements

Other symptoms frequently seen in MS include

- Sensation of warmth, burning and prickling, itching, tingling, numbness
- Frequency or difficulty urinating, bowel- and bladder-control problems, constipation
- Fatigue
- Loss of arm, hand, leg strength
- Clumsiness in arms, hands, and legs, difficulty walking
- Tremor
- Stiffness
- Impotence in men, lack of sensation in the vagina, difficulty reaching orgasm
- Dizziness, vertigo
- Double vision, partial blindness, pain in one eye, color distortion, dim vision, blurred vision, depth perception problems, pain when eyes move, flashes of light when the eyes move, loss of central vision
- Emotional changes
- Body pain
- Problems with thinking, concentration, memory, and judgment
- Paralysis
- Difficulty speaking

Since for many people MS goes into remission, then flares up, it's important to note that some of the most common triggers for flares include

- Very hot weather
- Hot bath or shower

- Fever
- Infection

For one patient, Michelle, her odyssey went on for thirty years. On-and-off symptoms included dropping things, bladder problems, interstitial cystitis, anxiety attacks, and what she called "shaky days"—days when she dropped things and felt uncoordinated. Says Michelle:

While I am far from the athletic type, I used to be a dancer, so acute uncoordination was noticeable to me. At this point, the symptoms started to interfere with my life, but I attributed them to other physical conditions, and my dropping of objects had reached the point where members of my family and I considered it normal. Around that same time, I became extremely tired all the time. I fell asleep driving . . . I fought sleepiness constantly. Finally, a doctor ordered an MRI, and it revealed lesions that were indicative of multiple sclerosis.

Diagnosis

There is no single test for MS, but a variety of tests can help to confirm or rule out a clinical diagnosis. Doctors will look closely at the symptoms and clinical signs, and MS is suspected particularly when there is the characteristic pattern of remission and relapse. A thorough neurological evaluation includes muscle strength, numbness, inflammation of the optic nerve, and other evident symptoms. Specific tests that can be of help include

- Magnetic resonance imaging (MRI), which can sometimes show areas of the brain that have lost myelin; over 90 percent of those with MS have abnormal brain scans that show evidence of tissue destruction

- A spinal tap, which can show elevated white blood cell counts, protein and certain antibodies in spinal fluid
- Nerve stimulation tests, which can reveal slower responses that may point to demyelination
- Electroencephalogram (EEG), looking at the speed of brain waves and electrical activity in the nervous system
- CT scan of the brain
- General bloodwork, to rule out other conditions

If you suspect MS, it's particularly important to keep a detailed, descriptive log of your symptoms on a daily basis. This log can help your physician in reaching a diagnosis. Patient advocate Dr. Marie Savard tells this story of the difficulty one woman had in getting diagnosed:

One 46-year-old woman loved to walk. She had noticed over about five to seven years that she was developing a foot drop or weakness of her left leg whenever she walked greater than a few blocks . . . she also started to fall on occasion . . . always thinking she simply tripped, but never really thinking why. She never thought to tell her family doctor. An orthopedic surgeon said it was a probable slipped disk pinching on a lumbar nerve to her leg. She could get an MRI of the back to be sure, but unless she wanted surgery, why bother! She chose to do nothing. Three years earlier, she had developed uveitis of her eyes, an autoimmune condition . . . again she saw a specialist, who didn't know about her chronic leg problem. After a particularly serious fall, she finally went to a neurologist. After an MRI of the spine and brain, she was diagnosed with MS. She later learned from a specialist that there is a connection between the uveitis and MS, yet no doctor took a complete history to learn of the different problems. She is now on daily injections with beta-interferon and is relieved to finally know that she is doing something about her problem.

If this patient had done some research herself, insisted on seeing a neurologist when she had leg weakness and was falling, and told the ophthalmologist about her other problems, she could have been diagnosed sooner.

Practitioners

The best possible diagnosis and treatment for MS typically comes from a neurologist, who is trained to be able to identify the sometimes difficult-to-diagnose symptoms and differentiate them from other conditions. Neurologists are typically up to date on all the latest MS drugs and treatments, which are frequently changing as new drugs are introduced.

Treatment

Treatment of MS can focus on symptoms and on the underlying disease itself. To work with the disease itself, the drugs include interferons, steroids, and immunosuppressant medications.

INTERFERONS: BETA-1B (BETASERON) AND BETA-1A (AVONEX OR REBIF)

Interferons stop inflammation in the brain, reducing the relapse rate of attacks. Interferons can reduce the severity of attacks and generally show evidence of an ability to prevent myelin damage. Betaseron is taken in an every-other-day self-administered subcutaneous (under the skin) injection. Avonex and Rebif are administered by a weekly intramuscular injection. Occasionally, Betaseron can have negative side effects, including serious depression, with more common side effects including flu-like symptoms, shortness of breath, menstrual disorders, and injection site reactions.

GLATIRAMER ACETATE (COPAXONE)

This drug is similar to myelin and can help suppress the immune system's attack on its own myelin. Several studies have found that long-term use of Copaxone reduces the relapse rate and delayed disability in those with a relapse-remitting form of MS. Copaxone is taken daily by subcutaneous injection and has fewer side effects than interferons.

CORTICOSTEROIDS

Corticosteroids such as methyl prednisolone and prednisone may help shorten the length of MS flares but come with side effects, including lowered resistance to infection, risk of diabetes, weight gain, fatigue, bone thinning, and ulcers.

OTHER TREATMENTS

Intravenous immunoglobulins (IVIG)—chemicals the body uses to fight infections—can be beneficial, but these are costly and must come from human blood, which poses its own set of risks.

Recent research has indicated that a new treatment, antigen-specific immunotherapy, may offer protection from MS and other autoimmune diseases. The treatment uses proteins from myelin itself. In MS, these myelin proteins are attacked by the immune system's T cells. But when the T cells were exposed to an "overdose" of the myelin protein, they self-destructed.

On the alternative front, preliminary research has indicated that bee venom injections may provide patients with significant benefits. Injections have allowed some patients to regain some muscle control and to feel more energetic.

Many cutting-edge treatments are also being researched and tested for MS.

• **Oral versus injectable versions of drugs:** Oral agents are one of the cutting-edge areas of research, which would eliminate the need for painful injections. Four drug companies, Teva Pharmaceutical Industries Ltd, Schering AG, Biogen Inc., and Genzyme Corp, are working on oral MS treatments. Teva has an oral version of its current Copaxone that releases protein-blocking cells in order to suppress inflammation. The drug is undergoing testing in 1,650 relapsing-remitting MS patients worldwide. Schering is working on three different pills that would be at least as effective, if not more, than current treatments. It aims to reduce the frequency and severity of MS attacks by at least 30 percent. Biogen is working on an inhalable version of its Avonex treatment for relapsing-remitting MS sufferers. Genzyme is also looking at oral agents and is studying how these protein-blocking compounds work individually or in combination.

• **The antibiotic minocycline:** Researchers are currently testing whether the common tetracycline antibiotic minocycline, sometimes known by its brand name, Minocin, may be able to significantly decrease the severity of disease attacks or even block relapses.

• **New "old" drugs:** Some of the "new" drugs for multiple sclerosis aren't new at all; in fact, they've been prescribed for years to patients with other disorders. But now scientists and researchers are studying their usage in people with MS. One company, Viragen, was given approval by the Medicines Control Agency (the British version of the FDA) to begin testing natural alpha interferon (Omniferon) on MS patients. A natural alpha-interferon derived from human white blood cells, Omniferon was undergoing clinical trials for patients with hepatitis C. According to Viragen's chief operating officer, Dr. Magnus Nicolson, current drug therapies to treat MS are genetically engineed beta-interferons, and the fact that Omniferon is a naturally derived substance may be key to its success:

> There is a growing body of evidence showing that a significant percentage of patients develop antibodies to recombinant beta-interferon. This may limit their efficacy and potentially cause adverse side effects. Since our natural alpha-interferon is derived from human white blood cells, we

believe that it should be less immunogenic and possibly better tolerated. Omniferon may represent a potent alternative in the treatment of multiple sclerosis patients, particularly those with antibody responses to recombinant type 1 interferons.

The drug Provigil has been used to treat people with narcolepsy—a disease characterized by sudden episodes of unconsciousness—but more recent studies show that the drug can alleviate some of the fatigue in MS patients. A team of researchers at Ohio State University reported that a moderate dose, 200 milligrams each day, of modafinil (which is sold as Provigil by the manufacturer, Cephalon) improved patients' scores on three separate fatigue tests.

• **Early Pregnancy Factor (EPF):** A modified version of a hormone that prevents the immune system of a pregnant woman from attacking the developing fetus is currently being studied as a possible MS treatment. The drug could potentially halt the progress of MS.

• **Gene Trust Project:** One company is aiming to explore how to treat disease, including MS, by collecting genetic information from a large pool of volunteers. DNA Sciences is focused on discovering the genetic basis of treatment response, disease susceptibility, and disease progression. More than 10,000 people have registered for the DNA Sciences Gene Trust Project, an Internet-based research initiative designed to discover the links between genetics and common diseases. DNA Sciences researchers say the project will help identify the genetic basis of common diseases such as MS—a crucial step toward developing new diagnostics and treatments. DNA Sciences' current research focus includes autoimmune diseases such as psoriasis, multiple sclerosis, and Type II diabetes, as well as cardiac arrhythmias, breast cancer, and colon cancer.

You can register for the Gene Trust by completing a brief health questionnaire on the company's website at www.dna.com. If your health history matches a current DNA Sciences research project, you may be asked to volunteer a small blood sample. A qualified health professional collects the blood sample at the participant's convenience anywhere in the United States.

• **Stem Cell Transplants:** Severe MS is now being selectively considered for stem cell transplant, and results are encouraging for patients with severe cases of primary progressive MS.

Things to Know

In one study of multiple sclerosis patients conducted at the University of California–San Francisco/Mount Zion Medical Center, researchers found that stress caused new brain lesions to form in the study participants. Stress reduction is, therefore, an important component of living with MS. Regular exercise is also recommended, as it can help reduce the spasticity of muscles and maintain muscle health and strength. Be careful about raising body temperature, however, as that can trigger a flare. Swimming is a good choice because the water both supports your body and keeps your temperature down. Physical therapy can be useful to help with balance and range of motion and to counteract weakness.

Animal research has shown that diets high in curcumin, a compound found in the curry spice turmeric, may block the progress of MS. This may explain why MS is relatively rare in Asian countries with higher turmeric consumption.

■ Raynaud's Phenomenon

Raynaud's phenomenon (RP) is a common autoimmune condition in which small arteries in fingers and toes spasm, usually in response to exposure to cold or a rapid change in temperature. This spasming causes the skin to change colors and leads to sensations of tingling, pain, and numbness in the extremities.

RP can exist on its own, but more often it's found alongside other autoimmune diseases. It occurs in as many as 10 percent of the general population and 25 percent of younger women.

In RP, blood flow is reduced to the arteries and capillaries of the fingers and toes in response to cold or temperature change. Incidence of RP is high among autoimmune disease patients. For example, approximately 40 percent of people with lupus have RP, and 90 percent of patients with scleroderma have RP.

From 60 to 90 percent of RP sufferers are women, and onset is most commonly during the teenage years. RP is common among postmenopausal women, however; among that age group, only 3 to 8 percent go on to develop connective tissue autoimmune diseases such as lupus or scleroderma.

Symptoms

Symptoms of RP include

- Cold fingers and toes
- Numbness, tingling or throbbing in fingers and toes
- Pins and needles or burning sensation in fingers and toes
- Skin color changes to white, blue, or red
- Feeling of clumsiness in hands and fingers

Diagnosis

Diagnosis of RP is usually made by observation and report of symptoms; however, blood-flow studies may also be used to diagnose the condition.

Practitioners

Most types of practitioners should be able to recognize, diagnose, and treat RP. In the rare case of severe RP, where blood flow becomes permanently decreased and ulceration or gangrene becomes a risk, a neurologist or vascular expert should be consulted.

Treatment

Some treatments for RP are essentially lifestyle approaches, including

- Avoiding cold exposure for arms and legs
- Stopping smoking, because it constricts blood vessels
- Practicing relaxation techniques
- Practicing biofeedback

In some cases, medication to relax the walls of blood vessels may be prescribed, but treatment for the underlying autoimmune dysfunction is the most important factor.

Things to Know

Smoking can aggravate RP and should be avoided, as it can also increase the risk of severe RP. Some RP patients have found help in paraffin baths. Says Corinne:

I have hypothyroidism, and when my hands were really cold, white, and numb, I thought maybe my meds needed updating. It turned out to be Raynaud's phenomenon. I was a bit disheartened to hear my doctor suggest warm mittens—and if it gets unbearable, to get a prescription for a heart medication. Anyway, the list of potential side effects included dizziness to the point of passing out! I decided to hold off on any prescription drugs and see what I can do about it. My solution was really a gift from my husband—a home paraffin bath. They used them where he works to help people with repetitive motion injuries, and he thought it would help. A parabath is a tank filled with a pure medical grade of paraffin pellets, melted and held at a constant yet safe temperature. You simply dip (don't soak) your hands (or fingers or elbows or feet) into the warm paraffin about five times and the wax builds up. Then let the heat soak in for about ten to fifteen minutes, and it feels soooo good. And the only side effect is the paraffin moistens your skin to protect it from chapping in these cold northern winters!

■ Guillain-Barré Syndrome

Guillain-Barré (pronounced "ghee-yan-bah-ray") syndrome (GBS) is also known as acute ascending polyneuritis. The body's immune system attacks myelin sheath around the nerves, or even the actual nerves. As with multiple sclerosis, in GBS the damage to the myelin sheath leaves muscles unable to properly respond to brain signals. But the acute nature and onset of GBS makes it a dangerous condition; unlike many of the long-term, chronic autoimmune diseases, the fatality rate of GBS is 5 to 10 percent.

GBS can strike at any age, although it is most likely to occur from ages 15 to 35 and 50 to 75. GBS affects both men and women but is more likely to strike men. It affects only about 1 person in every 100,000.

In about 80 percent of people, symptoms start from five days to three weeks after a mild infection, surgery, or immunization. As many as 20 percent of cases are associated with *Campylobacter jejuni* infection, 10 percent follow cytomegalovirus, 5 percent follow Epstein-Barr virus, and 5 percent follow *Mycoplasma pneumoniae*. Other suspected triggers are some vaccinations (such as the flu vaccine, rabies, and strep), lymphomas, surgery, pregnancy, and some drugs, such as heroin, penicillamine, and gold, among others.

Symptoms

Symptoms of GBS include

- Weakness, tingling, and loss of sensation in the legs that progresses up to the arms

- Muscle weakness
- Numbness and tingling
- Pain in the buttocks and lower back
- Facial weakness
- Difficulty speaking or putting words in order (dysphasia)
- Fluctuations of heart rate, blood pressure, and temperature
- Urinary difficulties
- Reduced or absent reflexes

In as many as 25 percent of cases, the muscles that support breathing become too weak, and ventilatory assistance (i.e., a respirator) is needed for a time. Up to 10 percent of people need support with food (IV or tube feeding) because facial and swallowing muscles become too weak to eat by mouth.

Diagnosis

Diagnosis is mainly by clinical observation. There are no formal tests to diagnose GBS. A variety of tests can be done to rule out other conditions—for example, spinal taps, nerve conduction tests, blood tests, pregnancy test, liver function tests, analysis of spinal fluid, nerve conduction tests, and an electrocardiogram.

Practitioners

A neurologist may be the likeliest practitioner to diagnose GBS.

Treatment

It's important that if GBS is suspected, medical treatment be sought as soon as possible, because the earlier a diagnosis can be made, the greater likelihood there is that a more serious course of the condition can be avoided.

GBS usually requires hospitalization, as the condition needs to be closely monitored. Plasmapheresis, a process by which toxic substances are filtered from the blood, can be a help in some cases, as can intravenous gamma globulin. Both treatments have been found to shorten recovery time by as much as 50 percent.

With early diagnosis and treatment, recovery may be just days or weeks. Typically, however, recovery can take several months. But most people will enjoy almost complete recovery from GBS and will be left with only some residual weakness.

Among the small percentage of GBS patients with a chronic recurring form of the disease, gamma globulins, corticosteroids, plasmapheresis, and immunosuppressive drugs may be effective treatments.

Things to Know

Some patients believe that GBS may be triggered by a chemical exposure. One patient, Nancy, who has chronic inflammatory demyelinating polyneuropathy (CIDP), a chronic form of GBS, said, "I have this disorder due to formaldehyde in a mobile home we lived in for two years."

Guillain-Barré comes on quickly, can be more debilitating, and subsides with treatment. CIDP is slower to appear, more difficult to control, and may never actually go away.

■ Myasthenia Gravis

Myasthenia gravis (MG) is a rare, chronic autoimmune disease in which the skeletal muscles are affected. There are a variety of types of MG, including

- Restricted ocular MG (ROMG), which weakens the eye muscles, causing the eyes to droop and giving the appearance that eyes are sleepy
- Generalized MG (GMG), which can affect any skeletal muscles

- Drug-induced MG, which is caused by the prescription drug D-penicillamine

Muscle weakness results from an immune attack on the muscle's acetylcholine receptors. Acetylcholine acts as a neurotransmitter. The cause of MG is unknown, but it is suspected that some sort of abnormality or dysfunction in the thymus may cause the formation of antibodies against acetylcholine receptors.

MG can be either early onset or late onset. Early-onset GMG typically strikes women before age 40. Late-onset GMG affects men and women equally and occurs after age 40, and is usually related to a mass in the thymus, known as a thymoma.

Symptoms
Symptoms include

- Drooping or weak eyelids
- Weak eye muscles, causing double vision
- Excessive muscle fatigue and weakness after exercise
- Difficulty speaking or swallowing in more advanced cases

In almost half of all patients, the eye muscles are the first ones affected, and eventually almost everyone with this condition has some eye involvement.

Diagnosis
Diagnosis is by clinical observation, particularly when the MG is manifesting itself in eye or facial muscle weakness, common symptoms. Some tests that can help pinpoint an MG diagnosis include

- Acetylcholine testing; a temporary improvement on muscle strength after testing is a sign of MG.
- Nerve and muscle function testing with an electromyogram

- Acetylcholine receptor antibody blood testing
- Computed tomography (CT) scan or MRI of the chest to identify a tumor of the thymus gland
- Single-fiber electromyography (SFEMG)
- X-ray looking for pneumonia, because pneumonia is a common side effect of MG

Practitioners

Because an MG diagnosis means a patient will need to follow lifelong medical treatment and possibly even surgery, diagnosis has to be done extremely carefully by a trained neurologist.

Treatment

Drugs known as chlorinesterase inhibitors are given to increase the level of acetylcholine, including pyridostigmine and neostigmine. Side effects include abdominal cramps and diarrhea, so doctors may prescribe other drugs to help alleviate those symptoms.

In some cases, corticosteroids such as prednisone or the immunosuppressant drug azathioprine (Imuran) can help. When a patient doesn't respond to drugs, plasmapheresis may be performed to remove the actual antibodies from the blood.

Surgery is done more frequently in MG than in many other autoimmune diseases, because even in patients without thymomas, as many as 80 percent who have their thymus surgically removed (thymectomy) seem to show improvement.

Things to Know

Thyroid disorders are found in up to 4 percent of MG patients, and related symptoms may be found, so it's important for MG patients to be aware of and proactive about any seemingly thyroid-related symptoms. MG can be transmitted from the mother to the fetus but will normally disappear in the newborn a few weeks after birth.

11

The Intersection of Autoimmune Disease: Prognosis and Treatment

In the course of my autoimmune disease, Hashimoto's thyroiditis, I've had the classic symptoms of this condition, including fatigue, weight gain, hair loss, depression, difficulty concentrating, and longer/heavier periods. But in the seven years since I was diagnosed, I've gone through very distinct periods when I've had clusters of symptoms that have made me strongly suspect I was developing another autoimmune disorder.

For example, I went through a year-long period where I awoke with morning stiffness that lasted several hours, I had tendinitis in my forearms and calves, my joints were excruciatingly tender, I ran a low-grade fever, and I had numbness and tingling in my hands and feet. Was I developing rheumatoid arthritis, or did I have fibromyalgia? No specific tests were run, but my physician decided to try a short course of the antibiotic doxycycline, and within a few days, all the muscle, joint, and neurological symptoms disappeared. I remained on the antibiotics for a year, and after slowly weaning off of them, in conjunction with a rigorous holistic herbal program, I have been able to avoid a return of these symptoms.

Then there was the summer I spent several weeks in Florida. Every time I came in from the sunny pool to the air-conditioned indoors, I had numbness and tingling in my arms and legs. For about ten minutes, it was as if I was taking a powerful shower of tiny needles. A sign of Raynaud's phenomenon? And if so, since Raynaud's is far more common in people with lupus or scleroderma, could it be a warning of future autoimmune diseases in progress?

Then there was a recent episode of severe eye pain and blurry vision. A trip to the eye doctor revealed that I was having an acute episode of dry eyes—so bad that my cornea had a small abrasion in it. Due to frequent thirst and dry mouth, I also walk around with a water bottle constantly. Am I developing Sjögren's syndrome perhaps?

What becomes clear in my own story and in the thousands of stories of autoimmune disease patients that I've heard in researching this book is that very few of us are textbook patients, with symptoms limited to just those that go along with our diagnosed condition. Most of us suffer from a variety of symptoms that are more common in other autoimmune diseases—symptoms that wax and wane. They may even represent periodic flare-ups of actual subclinical forms of autoimmune diseases.

So, is it possible that I have another autoimmune disease? Certainly having one autoimmune disease increases my risk of developing other diseases. But I would need to dedicate months and many thousands of dollars to the various tests necessary to diagnose or rule out all the possible conditions these symptoms could represent. What I find more effective is to concentrate on my overall health and some of the holistic approaches—outlined later in this book— to help deal with the underlying issue of autoimmunity in general.

I call these various constellations of sporadic symptoms the *autoimmune syndrome*. On a more formal basis, some specific autoimmune diseases are actually grouped together and named as formal syndromes. For example, the polyglandular syndromes present crossover symptoms that affect a number of organs or glands. Autoimmune Addison's disease, along with an underactive parathyroid gland and candidiasis (chronic yeast overgrowth), is polyglandular autoimmune syndrome type I, also known as autoimmune polyendocrinopathy–candidiasis–ectodermal dystrophy (APECED). When Addison's is found with Type I diabetes and the thyroid conditions Hashimoto's thyroiditis or Graves' disease, the syndrome is known as polyglandular autoimmune syndrome type II. And Addison's disease and Hashimoto's thyroiditis together are known as Schmidt's syndrome.

■ Subclinical Autoimmune Disease

In addition to the idea of an autoimmune syndrome featuring multiple symptoms or the crossover syndromes, it's likely that some people have one or more autoimmune diseases in a subclinical form. A subclinical autoimmune disease would mean that laboratory tests might be slightly abnormal—but still within a normal range—or many but not all of the required symptoms for diagnosis are present. So, laboratory tests and clinical signs cannot support an official diagnosis. But the signs are there that the autoimmune attack is already under way, and some signs and symptoms of a condition are already present. This is a phenomenon seen commonly in Hashimoto's disease, for example, where the presence of antithyroid antibodies, even with normal thyroid function tests, may indicate subclinical autoimmune thyroid disease, and its sufferers can experience the full range of hypothyroidism symptoms. Those same symptoms frequently will improve after treatment with low-dose thyroid hormone replacement.

Subclinical disease is also the mechanism behind prediabetes, when diabetic-like changes are in progress, but blood sugar has not become sufficiently abnormal for an official diagnosis. Researchers have even discovered that autoreactive T cells from both diabetic patients and multiple sclerosis (MS) patients target autoantigens in islet cells and the central nervous system. Reporting in the *Journal of Immunology*, the authors stated, "what (usually) protects diabetics from MS, and MS patients from diabetes . . . could have therapeutic ramifications."

In an interview with Reuters Health, Dr. H.-Michael Dosch from the Hospital for Sick Children in Toronto, Ontario, Canada, said:

> *Our work implies that there is a lengthy, clinically silent pre-MS phase analogous to prediabetes. That's good news: there is strong consensus that we will stop diabetes within a reasonable time frame through intervention therapies that are targeted to early prediabetes. We hope (and have some reason) that the same will turn out to be true for MS.*

Autoimmune expert Dr. Noel Rose acknowledges the likelihood of subclinical autoimmune diseases:

> *I wouldn't be surprised that there are people who have autoimmune processes, but don't quite reach the point where the disease is clinically relevant. We do have situations where we see, as in the thyroid, for example, extensive lymphocytic infiltration and antibodies, although thyroid tests are perfectly normal. This suggests that other autoimmune processes may well be going on in many of us.*

■ 100 Autoimmune Diseases?

How many autoimmune diseases are there? Recently, some well-known diseases have actually been reclassified as autoimmune. For example, experts have stated that there is overwhelming evidence that there is an autoimmune component to the condition endometriosis, which affects as many as 15 percent of all women in their reproductive years. It's likely that autoimmune components will be discovered in even more diseases and conditions as more is understood about the nature of autoimmunity.

The diseases covered in this book are just some of the estimated 80 to 100 different conditions currently considered autoimmune in origin. Also included as autoimmune diseases are the following:

Antiphospholipid syndrome: body attacks various fats that can affect blood clotting, among other effects

Autoimmune hemolytic anemia: red blood cells destroyed prematurely

Autoimmune hepatitis: immune system targets the liver

Behçet's disease: inflammation of the blood vessels, can lead to blindness

Bullous pemphigoid: a skin disorder, similar to pemphigus

Chronic inflammatory demyelinating polyneuropathy: where nerve roots swell, destroying the myelin sheath covering the nerves, leading to weakness, paralysis, and/or impairment

Churg-Strauss syndrome: where antibodies accumulate, blood vessels become inflamed, and white blood cells cluster abnormally, leading to kidney, lung, and other organ damage

Cicatricial pemphigoid: an autoimmune disease of the mucous membranes, including the lining of the mouth and eyes

Cold agglutinin disease: a form of autoimmune hemolytic anemia

Eosinophilia-myalgia syndrome: affecting the skin, fascia, muscle, nerve, blood vessels, lung, and heart

Essential mixed cryoglobulinemia: in which the immune system attacks the blood and other tissues and organs

Idiopathic pulmonary fibrosis: inflammation resulting in scarring, or fibrosis, of the lungs

Idiopathic thrombocytopenia purpura (ITP): an autoimmune attack on the platelets

IgA nephropathy: an autoimmune kidney disease

Lichen planus: an inflammatory skin disease that targets eyes, skin, and the mucous membranes

Meniere's disease: ringing in the ears, dizziness, and a sensation of fullness or pressure in the ears, even deafness

Polyarteritis nodosa: an autoimmune attack on the vascular system that creates narrowing vessels and increases the risk of clots and aneurysms

Polychondritis: causing recurrent inflammation of the cartilage

Polymyalgia rheumatica: inflammation of connective tissues

Polymyositis and dermatomyositis: autoimmune neuromuscular/connective tissue diseases that cause limb and neck weakness

Primary agammaglobulinemia: where an antibody deficiency compromises the immune system

Primary biliary cirrhosis: where the autoimmune attack is against the bile ducts of the liver

Rheumatic fever: in which the body overreacts to a strep infection and attacks the heart

Stiff-man syndrome: a neurologic disease where an attack on the central nervous system causes stiffness and spasms

Takayasu arteritis: an autoimmune disorder involving inflammation of the vascular system

Temporal arteritis/giant cell arteritis: inflammatory autoimmune disease with vascular inflammation

Uveitis: inflammation of the uvea, the area of the eye where many blood vessels become inflamed

Vasculitis: inflammation of blood vessels, including veins, arteries, and capillaries

Wegener's granulomatosis: vascular and kidney inflammation disease

■ Autoimmune-like Conditions

There are other conditions or syndromes that are thought—but not known—to be autoimmune, particularly because they are so commonly seen in autoimmune patients. One such condition is dysautonomia, an imbalance in the autonomic nervous system, which controls "unconscious" functions such as heart rate, digestion, and breathing. Within the autonomic nervous system, there's the sympathetic system, which controls the body's fight-or-flight reactions, and the parasympathetic nervous system, which controls the quieter body functions such as digestion. Usually, the sympathetic and parasympathetic systems are in balance, but in dysautonomia, they are not.

Patient advocate and cardiologist Dr. Richard Fogoros has found that some patients inherit the propensity to develop dysautonomia syndromes. There are also theories that viruses can trigger dysautonomia syndrome, as can chemical exposures and head and chest trauma. According to Dr. Fogoros, recent research confirms that some cases of acute dysautonomia may represent a milder form of Guillain-Barré syndrome. But what's clear is that many autoimmune disease patients complain of dysautonomia symptoms. Says Dr. Fogoros:

> In dysautonomia, the autonomic nervous system loses its balance, and at various times the parasympathetic or sympathetic systems become inappropriately predominant. Symptoms can include frequent, vague but disturbing aches and pains, faintness (or even actual fainting spells), fatigue and inertia, severe anxiety attacks, rapid heartbeat (tachycardia), hypotension (low blood pressure), poor exercise tolerance, gastrointestinal symptoms such as irritable bowel syndrome, sweating, dizziness, blurred vision, numbness and tingling, anxiety, and (quite understandably) depression.

According to Dr. Fogoros, all of these syndromes are real physiologic (as opposed to psychologic) disorders and probably variants of the same general disorder of the autonomic nervous system.

One of the most effective treatments for dysautonomia is regular physical exercise, which helps stabilize the autonomic nervous system. Also, some patients have found that antidepressants have been helpful in rebalancing the autonomic nervous sytem, and antianxiety drugs may help with anxiety or panic disorder. Nonsteroidal anti-inflammatory drugs (NSAIDs) can be a help to some people as well.

■ Broad-Spectrum Treatments of the Future

The future of autoimmune disease prevention and treatments can only be described as exciting! As noted in the previous chapters, there are many promising conventional drugs and treatments in the works for specific conditions. As researchers develop a more unified theory of the interrelationships among autoimmune diseases, even more promising developments are likely to take place. In addition to the disease-specific treatments discussed, there are some broader-spectrum approaches that are applicable to numerous autoimmune conditions.

Bone Marrow Transplants

Although bone marrow transplant is a treatment used most often for cancer, more recently it has been used in rare cases when autoimmune diseases such as scleroderma, multiple sclerosis, or rheumatoid arthritis become life-threatening. Only a small number of people have received bone marrow transplants for autoimmune diseases to date, but the treatment is promising for otherwise untreatable cases.

In a bone marrow transplant, the patient's marrow is removed and frozen to protect it. Then chemotherapy is used to destroy the immune system. The marrow is put back to rebuild a healthy immune system. According to Dr. Noel Rose:

> *For the moment, it's for people who do not respond to any other form of treatment, such as life-threatening lupus, or when they've gone through all the medications available, or for the rare patient with myasthenia gravis or pemphigus that becomes life-threatening. Most people can be controlled with medications, but some don't respond or have run out of medicines to try. For these patients, bone marrow transplantation may be appropriate. There are colleagues who say that this treatment has become sufficiently benign that many other patients who are not at the "end of the road" might prefer this kind of treatment. Someone with lupus or rheumatoid arthritis, where treatments can be horrendous and difficult with many side effects, might prefer bone marrow transplantation. But it is still a risky and difficult experience.*

Stem Cell Therapies

Researchers are looking at stem cells for possible use in autoimmune treatment. Stem cells are primitive cells that have the ability to grow into other cell types. According to Dr. Rose, stem cells could be useful in one of two ways:

> *They can be used instead of external marrow transplantation in some cases, or may play a role in restoring a defective organ, such as pancreatic islet cells, or maybe even a thyroid. When we would see this sort of application for patients depends on national policy. If this research is supported and encouraged by NIH and readily available by NIH, we could be looking at three to five years. If it becomes difficult to get the cells, NIH's support dries up, and the research may have to be done overseas.*

In early 2001, researchers reported that they had the "ultimate adult stem cell"—a cell in the bone marrow that can transform itself into almost any organ in the body. The study, by New York University School of Medicine, Yale University School of Medicine, and Johns Hopkins School of Medicine researchers, said that the discovery of this cell means that theoretically any organ could be repaired using cells generated from the stem cell. Stem cells in the marrow may be recruited to a damaged organ where they will develop into the mature tissue of that organ in response to certain signals. Applications for autoimmune diseases would be huge— with possibilities to heal the damaged pancreas as a diabetes treatment, or to repair a damaged thyroid, for example.

Some stem cell treatments are already in progress. Stem cells taken from the blood of two Crohn's disease patients were used to rebuild their defective immune systems. The same technique has also been successfully applied in patients with multiple sclerosis and lupus. Stem cells are taken from a patient's own blood or bone marrow (which is optimal, because there is no risk of rejection), from the umbilical cord of a newborn, or from embryos (a practice that has sparked a heated national debate). The defective immune system is destroyed with chemotherapy as well as a protein that reduces the number of white blood cells, which leaves the body susceptible to infection. In self-harvesting, a growth factor is given to stimulate the bone marrow to produce stem cells. After harvesting, the stem cells are injected back into the patient via a vein in the neck or arm. The whole process, including recovery, takes about three weeks. As with marrow transplant, this treatment is quite dangerous and is only used as a last resort for patients who are unresponsive to other therapies.

Multiple sclerosis patients who had the treatment stopped developing new lesions, but the treatment did not heal the damage already present. Lupus patients, however, did see some organ repair. In animal studies, researchers found a way to make stem cells grow into islet cells similar to those that produce insulin in the pancreas. When sugar was added to the area surrounding the cells, the cells produced a small amount of insulin. While federal laws prohibit testing these same processes using human embryo cells, animal tests are continuing. If testing becomes possible, it's theoretically conceivable that stem cells could cure diabetes and perhaps other autoimmune diseases as well.

Another promising treatment is cord blood transplant, a variation on stem cell transplants or bone marrow transplants. Healthy white blood cells from umbilical cord blood are used instead of bone marrow cells. The umbilical cord blood offers a healthy immune system. The cord blood also doesn't have to be as close a match and presents less chance of rejection. Unlike bone marrow harvesting, obtaining cord blood is a noninvasive, painless procedure, involving donation of umbilical cords and their stem cell–rich blood by parents of newborns. Researchers believe that this sort of technology that is used for immune deficiencies may also be applied to serious autoimmune diseases in the future.

Antigen-Specific Immunotherapy

Antigen-specific immunotherapy is being tested against MS and other autoimmune diseases in humans. The therapy has already had promising results in animal testing. According to Dr. Michael Lenardo of the National Institute of Allergy and Infectious Diseases (NIAID) Laboratory of Immunology, the current treatments for MS suppress the immune system and can cause toxic side effects. This new treatment can specifically target the immune system's T cells that cause the disease and may not lead to such extensive side effects. Antigen-specific immunotherapy is based on a discovery by Dr. Lenardo and his colleagues that T cells exposed to small amounts of the proteins making up the myelin sheaths are stimulated to attack the sheaths. But T cells exposed to large amounts of the same proteins will undergo a preprogrammed self-destruct sequence. (In fact, T cells exposed to large amounts of any antigen—a substance that provokes them to attack—will self-destruct.) Therefore, introducing large amounts of myelin proteins into the body should remove the problematic T cells and halt the disease. Dr. Lenardo explains:

> *The therapy is counterintuitive; one might think it would be like pouring gasoline on a fire. But the self-destruct sequence actually protects the body from having too many active T cells, which can themselves be toxic. Like any potent weapon, you want to control how much is deployed. The immune system doesn't let your T cells grow uncontrolled and kill you. In this case, adding more antigen smothers the fire.*

Dr. Lenardo and his colleagues are investigating how the therapy works against other autoimmune diseases in lab mice. One disease under investigation is myasthenia gravis.

Intravenous Immunoglobulin G

Intravenous immunoglobulin G (IVIG) is a preparation of human-derived antibodies made from pooled donor blood that is washed and processed. IVIG works by taming responses of the immune system, particularly by cutting back the toxic activities of natural killer (NK) cells. In the last two decades, IVIG has become the treatment of choice for several autoimmune diseases, including Guillain-Barré syndrome, chronic inflammatory demyelinating polyradiculoneuropathy, and Kawasaki's syndrome. While official studies have not been extensively conducted on IVIG in various autoimmune diseases, the list of disorders that have reportedly responded to intravenous immune globulin include

- Guillain-Barré syndrome
- Multiple sclerosis

- Myasthenia gravis
- Idiopathic thrombocytopenic purpura
- Corticosteroid-resistant dermatomyositis
- Kawasaki's disease
- Autoimmune uveitis

IVIG has been found helpful when autoimmunity seems to be interfering with pregnancy. Women with unexplained miscarriages who had the presence of various autoimmune antibodies were able to get pregnant and maintain pregnancy after IVIG treatment. IVIG appears to counteract the immune response, which can reject a woman's fetus and cause repeated pregnancy losses.

Cytoxan Rebooting

Researchers from MCP Hahnemann University in Philadelphia announced in late 2001 that a newly proven cure for severe aplastic anemia, a fatal bone marrow failure disorder, has implications for cures for the entire array of autoimmune diseases. The remedy, which consists primarily of a ten-times higher dosage of what has been considered the standard administration of the nearly fifty-year-old chemotherapy drug cyclophosphamide (Cytoxan), has been proven in clinical studies of patients from MCP Hahnemann University, Johns Hopkins University, and the University of Maryland. The therapy is a four-day treatment and produced "durable treatment-free remission." The remedy, according to the study, had 73 percent of the patients off all medication at two years. At fifty months, 65 percent of the patients were in treatment-free remission. In severe aplastic anemia, the immune system attacks the stem cells, the progenitors of all blood cells produced in the bone marrow, and renders them incapable of making new oxygen-carrying red blood cells, infection-fighting white cells, and clot-inducing platelets.

According to the researchers, the impact of Cytoxan is that the marrow stem cell reconstitutes the bone marrow and "reboots" the patient's immune system, allowing it to function normally without any further therapy. Preliminary trials in treating other autoimmune diseases—such as lupus, Crohn's disease, rheumatoid arthritis, and neurologic disorders—with similar high doses of Cytoxan were previously published. The researchers concluded at that time that the high-dose treatment of cyclophosphamide "can induce complete remission in patients with refractory, severe autoimmune disease. Reemergence of marrow function is similar to that seen after autologous transplantation and does not carry the risk for reinfusion of autoaggressive lymphocytes with the autograft."

PART III

Holistic Approaches

Herbal and Alternative Medicine for Autoimmune Disease

Conventional medicine really offers few cures for autoimmune diseases, and even the treatments that doctors present as simple "cures"—such as thyroid hormone replacement drugs for hypothyroidism, or moisturizers and eye drops for Sjögren's syndrome—leave a substantial percentage of patients condemned to suffer a variety of subclinical syndromes, persistent symptoms, and varying degrees of chronic illness. Many patients struggle with the following questions:

- What could possibly be causing my autoimmune disease, and is there anything I can do about it?
- Can I avoid getting other autoimmune diseases?
- Are there supplements I can take or other things I can do to prevent or minimize flares and help reduce my overall level of symptoms?
- Is there any way to cure—or at least go into remission—with my condition?

I hear from thousands of patients each week, and it's interesting that many who have reported that they've gone into long-term remission have all had one thing in common—they have combined conventional treatments with comprehensive herbalism. Usually, those who report the greatest success are under the care of experts in Ayurvedic or traditional Chinese medicine, or a practitioner who integrates these approaches into a Western herbal approach.

I can't emphasize enough how important it is to add a qualified herbalist to your health care team for autoimmune disease. Autoimmune diseases are complex conditions, and the best conventional medicine can offer is a partial solution. With some conditions, there aren't any effective treatments, only measures to minimize damage. Herbal medicine offers a possibility of remission, healing, or even cure in some cases.

You may be expecting me to provide a standard recipe or formula for each condition—that is, "If you have Graves' disease, take this vitamin, this mineral, and this herb, in this quantity, daily, for three months, and you'll feel better." Or, you may be looking for prescriptions for particular symptoms—that is, "If you're depressed, take St. John's Wort. If you're tired, take ginseng." If you read many of today's popular health magazines, or visit a vitamin store, this is the approach you'll find applied to vitamins, supplements, and herbs. But the reality is that autoimmune diseases are complex, involve multiple dysfunctions, and plague patients with very different symptoms. Therefore, autoimmune diseases are not easily treated by one remedy or one formula. This becomes even more evident when you add in your own genetic predispositions, your diet and nutritional status, your environmental exposures, and your stress levels.

One person with multiple sclerosis may have eye involvement, another may have memory problems, another may have difficulty walking, while a fourth has all of these symptoms and more. One Hashimoto's thyroiditis patient may present with only fatigue, another with weight gain, and another with depression, while a fourth has swollen face, hair loss from the eyebrows, and heavy menstrual periods. While there may be some herbs and supplements applicable to all patients with a particular condition, patients need them in amounts that correlate to symptoms and body weight. Patients might also require additional supplements, herbs, dietary and lifestyle changes that would better address their particular situations.

Is is clear that in order to get effective herbal treatment, you can't just go to the health food store and ask for advice, or read one article in a health magazine or website. For proper herbal treatment, you need a practitioner who will take into account your genetics, your own triggers and exposures, your diet, your lifestyle, your particular disease and symptoms, and then offer customized recommendations. That means you need a trained and experienced herbalist who comes out of a complete herbal tradition, such as India's Ayurvedic system, or traditional Chinese medicine, or Western herbalism. Once you start treatment, a trained herbalist will carefully monitor your response to the treatment, making adjustments along the way based on your results.

It's tempting to try to self-diagnose and self-treat, because so few insurance programs and HMOs today cover the costs of alternative therapies and herbal remedies. But it's important that you have professional guidance, or you may waste your time and money on herbs and treatments that are not a good fit for you and your condition.

The General Herbal Approach

Karta Purkh Singh Khalsa, CN, AHG, and Alan Tillotson, PhD, AHG, DAy, are two of the world's premier herbalists. Both renowned members of the American Herbalists Guild and diagnosticians, practitioners, educators, and authors with decades of experience with medicinal herbs and natural healing, they represent the most astute and innovative experts on herbal medicine in the United States. They both suffered from and overcame serious illnesses using herbal medicine, which has motivated them in their own study and practice.

Khalsa, an accomplished Kundalini yoga master and natural healer, focuses his studies, teaching, and writing on Ayurvedic medicine, Chinese medicine, and North American herbalism. Khalsa is widely known as the co-author of an immensely respected book, *Herbal Defense,* which integrates herbal information from a variety of traditions, including Ayurveda (the medical system of India), Chinese medicine, and Native American herbalism, with information on preventing and treating conditions using herbal medicine, focusing on the immune system and how to support it.

Alan Tillotson is the codirector of Chrysalis Natural Medicine Clinic, along with his wife, Dr. Nai-shing Hu Tillotson, a doctor of Oriental medicine. Tillotson holds a PhD degree in health sciences, a master's degree for his work in Asian medical systems, and is a diplomate in Ayurvedic health sciences. As a master herbalist, he has lectured extensively on herbal medicine and meditation and serves as an executive board member of the American Herbalists Guilds. Tillotson is also known as a gifted formulator, and his CNS (central nervous system) Myelin Sheath Repair, created for Planetary Formulas, is one of the most popular herbal supplements for multiple sclerosis. People travel from all over the country to his Wilmington, Delaware, clinic, and I have had the pleasure of being his patient. I credit him with my own improvements in health. Tillotson's seminal book, *The One Earth Herbal Sourcebook,* covers everything you need to know about Chinese, Western, and Ayurvedic herbal treatments in almost 600 pages.

According to Tillotson, the Western idea of autoimmunity is that immune system cells go haywire and start attacking healthy cells for no reason. So, in the Western mode, the treatment should be to depress the immune system with drugs such as corticosteroids, or with proteins that block specific parts of the immune system such as interferons. Says Tillotson:

> *They're looking to inject specific drugs to block the immune system from being able to do what it wants to do. And the "Holy Grail" of autoimmunity is to induce tolerance, where the immune system no longer tries to attack the tissue. These are all ways to trick the immune system into not attacking. This approach is doomed to fail, however, because it lacks a fundamental understanding. The immune system is attacking the tissue because the tissue itself is unhealthy prior to the attack. And in autoimmunity, once a tissue is targeted, the immune system memorizes it, and then continues to attack it. Under those circumstances, if you suppress the immune system, the attack slows down. But after you go off the drug, like prednisone, that is suppressing the system, the tissue is further degraded and unhealthy, and it still gets attacked.*

Both Tillotson and Khalsa believe the treatment objective should be to create a nourishing, strengthening, healing, and detoxifying herbal formula—plus dietary and lifestyle recommendations—focused on the following key steps:

1. Remove toxins. This may involve removing food allergens such as corn, wheat, milk products, and soy products from the diet, or switching to organic and hormone-free foods, or generally avoiding or removing other toxins such as metals.

2. Nourish and strengthen the tissue under attack. Strengthening the tissues under attack is a complex process, and figuring out what to do first is the hardest part. You may be dealing with weak digestion or intestinal imbalance, food allergies, kidney dysfunction, emotional issues, blood sugar imbalances, or a liver out of balance, and it's critical for your practitioner to identify the various factors and then decide what should be the priority in terms of treatment.

Khalsa lends additional perspective to this issue. He believes you must identify some of the general health triggers that allow for the autoimmune condition to take place:

> As people begin to degenerate and experience imbalance, they begin to develop inflammation in various places. Why does one person get arthritis, another thyroiditis? Because they have a particular familiar tendency, or ate a lot of something that triggers an allergic sensitivity, or for some reason, the immune system didn't have the resources it needed to support appropriate vigilance. Ultimately what works very well is to get healthy. The way to treat this disease and many of these other slipperier, obscure inflammatory and autoimmune diseases is to treat what ails them.

3. Support an underfunctioning immune system. When you have an autoimmune disease, it may seem counterintuitive to try to boost or support the immune system. After all, an autoimmune disease represents an overresponse of the immune system to its own organs and cells, so why would you want to give the immune system even more ammunition? Some people also erroneously believe that because the immune system goes into overdrive with autoimmune disease, they have a properly functioning—just overzealous—immune system. The reality is that autoimmune disease is a sign that the immune system is dysfunctional. Says Tillotson: "Actually, while the immune system is thought of as an attack force, in reality, immune cells also release growth factors, clear away debris, and are part of a repair process taking place that is not truly understood. Using immune system stimulants may benefit some autoimmune patients."

4. Calm an overactive immune system without completely suppressing it. In autoimmunity, since the immune system is inappropriately overreacting, the objective is to minimize or eliminate that overreaction—but not by suppressing the immune system. In autoimmunity, once a tissue is targeted, the immune system memorizes it, then continues to attack it. Under those circumstances, if you suppress the immune system, the attack slows down or stops. But after you go off the drug (e.g., prednisone) that is suppressing the system, the tissue is further degraded, and it still gets attacked.

5. Downregulate the attack process while strengthening the detoxification and clearing process. This is where the customized herbal, dietary, and lifestyle recommendations come in, and where it's critical to have the advice of an expert. Says Khalsa:

> Trying to pick your own herbs and self-treat autoimmune disease is tricky. The most common story is that people are interested in herbal medicine, and enthusiastic, so they go to Walmart and buy a particular remedy, try it, and it doesn't work. Practitioners will suggest things that are more potent, effective, and really do the job. I always encourage people to see a practitioner at least once or twice.

Khalsa believes that there's not a "one-size-fits-all" formula for each condition, and expert advice is needed: "You probably can't really self-treat an autoimmune disease in general, as you have to take a whole body point of view to get better results." He doesn't even feel that an herbal approach focused solely on a particular condition is always called for. In the case of autoimmune thyroid disease, for example, Khalsa says:

> I don't think that the approach always needs to be specially focused on the thyroid. What people almost always have is generalized chaos in the endocrine system, a chronic endocrine

dysregulation. You can see thyroid disease, or adrenal disease, or even female hormone imbalance. It depends on the lens the practitioner is looking through.

6. Make dietary changes. Tillotson recommends that we vary our diets. We're not meant to eat the same foods all the time. In the United States, for example, there are many people who have corn allergies, because so many foods that we eat regularly contain corn syrup, and frequent exposure to the same foods can trigger allergies. But corn allergies are not common in the United Kingdom. Instead, beet sugar allergies are far more common, because beets are typically used more often where corn syrup would be used in the United States.

Holistic practitioners and authors Richard Shames and Karilee Shames, who run a popular holistic health practice in Mill Valley, California, specializing in autoimmune diseases, agree that variety in the diet is essential:

We would certainly recommend that people avoid the same foods on a consistent basis. This is countered to most people's standard habits, but it's a habit worth changing. It would be far better to alternate and pick from a wide variety of items so as to avoid the possibilities that the immune system would start finding one particular thing irritating or sensitive. This particular maneuver is called "rotation."

Tillotson suggests that you also follow some of the seasons in terms of what you eat. In summer, with hot weather, leafy vegetables are best suited for the digestive system. You need lighter, drier foods that are nutritious but not high in fat; they don't produce excess fat and oil. In the cold weather, however, you can tax your immune system by living on salads to lose weight, and you'll feel cold all the time.

While both Khalsa and Tillotson urge autoimmune patients to find an herbal practitioner to develop a customized program, both *Herbal Defense* and *The One Earth Herbal Sourcebook* have detailed sections that cover the variety of herbs, minerals, and supplements that can be useful in particular autoimmune conditions, as well as immune enhancers, immune tonics, and anti-inflammatory herbs, supplements, and foods. Before you set out to find a practitioner, I recommend a thorough reading of both books. Not only will you understand your autoimmune condition much more thoroughly but you'll be prepared to find and work with an herbalist on a program that will be of help specifically to you.

Remember, however, that even in the most expert of hands, herbal treatments can take time. Khalsa counsels patience, as he has found that autoimmune conditions are "some of the slowest responding conditions."

■ The Traditional Chinese Medicine Model

Traditional Chinese medicine (TCM) is the ancient Chinese system of health and wellness that incorporates a variety of tools, including herbal medicine, acupuncture, and energy work such as qigong as part of treatment. Patrick Purdue is a highly respected doctor of Oriental medicine and acupuncture physician, and a graduate of the Florida Institute of Traditional Chinese Medicine. His Seminole, Florida, practice focuses on women's health, gastrointestinal conditions, and autoimmune diseases. According to Purdue, until modern times TCM wouldn't have used the term *autoimmune disease,* because TCM has an entirely different language and viewpoint to describe a patient's symptoms. Says Purdue:

> *In the modern TCM hospitals, Western-style diagnostic techniques are used, such as measuring blood ANA (antinuclear*

antibodies) levels, thyroid antibodies where appropriate, and various blood inflammatory markers such as erythrocyte sedimentation rate, C-reactive protein, and so on. Alongside this, standard, time-tested TCM diagnostic techniques are also done, involving extensive questioning about symptoms, palpation, pulse diagnosis (there are twenty-eight different types, or qualities, of pulse), appearance of the tongue, and so on. From this, a pattern diagnosis is made.

In TCM, a pattern diagnosis is a unique constellation of symptoms that describe one patient. In the TCM model, it's possible, therefore, for ten lupus patients to have ten different patterns, and therefore ten different treatments. This is very different from the Western medical approach to treat everyone with lupus with the same protocol. The TCM approach recognizes that everyone is different and is affected differently by disease processes and treatments. Says Purdue:

I've treated several cases of lupus, as diagnosed by their medical doctors based upon signs and symptoms, ANA levels, and so on. Some of these cases did not want to, for whatever reasons, follow my dietary instructions, or take the formula I made for them as prescribed. Of those who have, the vast majority have had improvement in symptoms, and in two cases, complete remission, as verified by normalized blood lab, absence of symptoms, and so on. One case was a nurse who had terrible reactions to the drugs prescribed by her doctor, and the other was a young, single mom who had been on complete disability with her condition. I was pleased to see her return back to her career. The latter case had had her condition for several years before coming to see me. The nurse had been recently diagnosed. The time for both of them to get to this point was six months. The other cases all had various degrees of reduced symptoms, and three to six months to get to this point seems to be the average.

The basic formula Dr. Purdue starts with in these cases is Lang Chuang Kang Fu Tang, or Lupus Health Returning Decoction, which was shown to have positive effects in an outcome-based study published in China in 1995. But Dr. Purdue cautions that as with all TCM formulas this is only a starting point and must be altered to fit each individual patient by an expert practitioner.

■ Some Condition-Specific Alternatives

While I would urge autoimmune disease patients to specifically consult both *Herbal Defense* and *The One Earth Herbal Sourcebook,* as well as their own alternative practitioner, for specific guidance on the best alternatives for an autoimmune condition, the following are tips regarding a few selected alternative treatments and supplements for some key autoimmune diseases.

Lupus
Some practitioners recommend that lupus patients add a variety of supplements, including

- Essential fatty acids and fish oils
- Grapeseed extract
- Vitamin C
- Bromelain
- Glucosamine sulfate
- L-lysine

There is also some evidence that lupus patients may need sulfur, which is found in garlic, onions, eggs, and asparagus.

Some experts believe that lupus can be exacerbated or triggered by high levels of heavy metals in the body, including mercury, arsenic, cadmium, lead, and aluminum, among others, as well as a buildup of pesticides. These alternative practitioners recommend oral or IV chelation therapy as part of the detoxification process.

Dietary changes can be important in lupus, and some practitioners recommend a diet free of food allergens, a switch to organically raised foods, and use of filtered water. One lupus patient, Joan, had success with a rigorous change in diet:

> I found Dr. Joel Fuhrman, an MD/hygienic physician, who supervised water-only fasts. His book, Fasting and Eating for Health: A Medical Doctor's Program for Conquering Disease, convinced me to call him—one chapter specifically addresses autoimmune conditions. Dr. Fuhrman put me on a very strict vegetarian diet for one month (no animal products, no dairy, no wheat, and no processed foods), supplemented by a multivitamin and essential fatty acids. Then I traveled to his fasting facility in New Jersey, where I did not eat or drink anything but water for twenty-four days. This approach is so drastic that I told only my husband and immediate family what I was doing. Everyone else thought I went for a supervised elimination diet to determine the cause of a skin allergy—my rash was hard to hide! I stayed in New Jersey four more days for "refeeding" and then went back to the eating program described above, probably for the rest of my life, to keep my conditions under control. After five months, I had great results, and time will tell how long-lasting it will be (and if I can stick to my new lifestyle). I have been very disciplined, hanging on to the mantra of "Nothing can possibly taste as good as I feel."

Type II Diabetes

Having one autoimmune disease increases your risk of developing Type I diabetes. But there's also evidence that having an autoimmune disease increases your risk of developing Type II diabetes. You can dramatically lower that risk, however—some experts say nine out of ten cases can actually be prevented—by eating a better diet and getting more exercise, as well as stopping smoking.

The most important risk factor for Type II diabetes is being overweight. Even having a weight at the high end of the normal range can triple the risk of diabetes. Revise your diet, to focus on vegetables, low-fat protein, good fat, fruits, and limit the high-glycemic carbohydrates and flour/sugar-based food products.

Women who exercised for seven or more hours per week were half as likely to develop diabetes than women who exercised for less than half an hour weekly. You should work on building up to at least thirty minutes of exercise a day. It doesn't have to be rigorous; even a brisk walk is fine. The Diabetes Prevention Program, sponsored by the National Institutes of Health, was able to definitively demonstrate this when they found that among those people at risk of developing diabetes, those who ate a low-fat diet and exercised moderately (walking, bike riding) for thirty minutes, five times a week, reduced their risk of diabetes by 58 percent without taking medication. These people also lost an average of 5 to 7 percent of their body weight. (Those who took medication alone—in this case, metformin (Glucophage)—without diet or exercise changes, reduced their risk by 31 percent.) Drug therapy was also found to be far less effective than lifestyle changes in older people and those less overweight.

A study reported in late 2001 found that patients with Type II diabetes who took supplements containing 300 mcg chromium picolinate and 150 mcg biotin, twice daily, had significantly reduced elevations in blood sugar and fatigue.

Thyroid Disease

In the arena of thyroid disease, one promising supplement is the South American medicinal root known as maca. In some animal studies, it was shown that maca can stimulate the hypothalamus and pituitary gland to better balance the entire endocrine system.

Several years ago, Dr. Viana Muller, an anthropologist and expert on South American herbal remedies, began to study the impact that taking maca was having on several women with thyroid disease who had moderate to severe menopausal symptoms. Interestingly, according to Dr. Muller, they had been able to reduce their thyroid medication—or in a few cases stop it entirely—after using maca for two or three months. Says Dr. Muller:

They all reported feeling so much better, much more energetic. What they noticed after a month or two was that they were beginning to feel some of the symptoms of an overactive thyroid, and so they cut back their thyroid medication and the symptoms went away. Some got stabilized at 50 percent of their former dosage of thyroid medication and some were able to stop all thyroid medication. They did this, however, little by little, with frequent testing of thyroid function in order not to shock the thyroid and make their condition worse.

Dr. Stephen Langer refers to thyroiditis as an "arthritis of the thyroid." Just as arthritis attacks the joints with pain and inflammation, thyroiditis can mean pain and inflammation in the thyroid for some sufferers. During a thyroiditis attack, common symptoms include anxiety, panic attacks, heart palpitations, swelling in the thyroid area, problems swallowing, and problems sleeping. Since thyroiditis attacks can classically happen in the middle of the night and interrupt sleep, Dr. Langer suggests taking calcium/magnesium before going to bed, which may have a sedative effect, and a pain reliever to relieve inflammation—for example, buffered aspirin or ibuprofen. He's found that this protocol helps about two-thirds of his patients. Reducing swelling is a key aspect of dealing with thyroiditis attacks, according to Dr. Langer. "Just as with arthritis, an anti-inflammatory pain reliever doesn't cure the problem, but it temporarily ameliorates the symptoms."

Palpitations are a common symptom of thyroiditis, as well as a symptom of autonomic imbalances that commonly result from autoimmune disease. According to Dr. Langer, patients can end up in the emergency room seeing a cardiologist, and if it happens enough times, they may even be labeled as having a psychiatric disorder. Usually, these patients end up with antianxiety medications or antidepressants. Dr. Langer cautions that palpitations can be a sign that too much thyroid medicine is being taken and a person has become hyperthyroid. But if an overactive thyroid or cardiac problem has been ruled out, Dr. Langer has found that nutritional deficiencies may be to blame, particularly deficiencies of calcium, magnesium, or vitamin D. Says Dr. Langer:

> There's compelling evidence coming to the surface that vitamin D is not only a vitamin but a hormone. . . . The recommended daily allowance for vitamin D is 400 IU, but scientists doing studies actually believe that people who do not get regular exposure to sunshine should be getting 2,000 to 4,000 IU of vitamin D. The vitamin D also has profound effects on absorption of calcium and magnesium.

Chronic Fatigue Immune Dysfunction Syndrome

On the alternative front, practitioners offer a variety of treatment options. For example, many practitioners agree that some activity and exercise are essential for recovery from CFIDS. But you have to find the right amount. Too much exercise, and you end up exhausted for several days. But with no exercise, you become stiff, deconditioned, and muscle and joint pain increases. At a minimum, you should begin stretching exercises of some sort under the guidance of a practitioner. Formal physical therapy can help accomplish this, or regular yoga classes can provide sufficient stretching.

Some alternative practitioners strongly recommend that CFIDS patients learn proper breathing techniques. Specialized breath instruction can be sought, or classes in pranayam (yoga breathing) can teach deep breathing techniques that can help with fatigue. Acupuncture is another recommended pain treatment for CFIDS patients.

Some practitioners recommend that you avoid or limit all foods with sugar, caffeine, alcohol, the artificial sweetener aspartame, and tobacco. Those who are sensitive to dairy and wheat, or have bloating and diarrhea, should try an elimination diet, with particular emphasis on identifying dairy and wheat allergies. Some experts suggest that high-dose vitamin B12 (usually provided by injection or intravenously) may help relieve symptoms.

Fatty acids such as omega 3 (evening primrose oil) and omega 6 (fish oil), as well as flaxseed oil and borage oil, are known to fight inflammation. You can ask your practitioner about an optimum combination of these essential fatty acids in oil or supplement form, or consider taking a product such as Udo's Oil, which combines them in a predetermined, optimal balance and ratio for many people.

A substantial percentage of patients report some improvement with dehydroepiandrosterone (DHEA). For women, the dosage is 25 to 50 milligrams a day, and for men, 50 to 100 milligrams a day, taken in the morning. One controversial alternative treatment for both CFIDS and fibromyalgia is a drug called Kutapressin, an extract of pig liver that works as an antiviral and immune modulator. Kutapressin quickly gets costly, as therapy requires a shot in the hip every day for a month, then every other day for five months, and each shot can cost $10. But some practitioners believe that Kutapressin can put these conditions into remission fairly quickly.

Fibromyalgia

Relaxation therapies are frequently recommended as part of the treatment for fibromyalgia. These could include breath work, meditation, yoga, or even biofeedback—some sort of therapy that allows you to start the body's relaxation response.

Alternative practitioners such as Dr. Andrew Weil recommend cognitive behavioral therapy, which offers specific tools to help you cope with particularly troublesome symptoms or stresses that tend to worsen fibromyalgia. For fibromyalgia sufferers, Dr. Weil also recommends acupuncture for pain relief and better sleep, and has found that it reduces morning stiffness in some of his patients. He also advocates massage—but gentle massage, not deep tissue—for relief of insomnia, pain, and stiffness.

Water therapy, known as hydrotherapy, is frequently recommended for fibromyalgia patients. Water should be warm—but not hot—for maximum benefit.

A controversial treatment that some practitioners and patients find useful is injections into fibromyalgia trigger points, either by dry needling (nothing injected) or needling with infiltration (injecting the anesthetics lidocaine or procaine.)

Some practitioners recommend that fibromyalgia patients take magnesium and calcium supplements: with 750 milligrams of magnesium and 1,500 milligrams of calcium daily. Other recommended supplements include melatonin, general antioxidant formulas, amino acid combinations, and various herbal formulas.

Some alternative practitioners believe that the optimal diet for fibromyalgia is a low-glycemic diet that avoids simple carbohydrates as much as possible. One of the most popular alternative recommendations for fibromyalgia and chronic fatigue syndrome is outlined by Dr. R. Paul St. Amand, an assistant clinical professor of medicine in endocrinology at UCLA. Dr. St. Amand, who wrote the best-seller *What Your Doctor May Not Tell You About Fibromyalgia,* believes that a genetic flaw leads to an inability to form ATP, the source of power that energizes most cell functions. He has found that the expectorant guaifenesin—a common cough syrup ingredient—can reverse fibromyalgia, and for most patients, complete reversal is seen within a year. Thousands of fibromyalgia patients who are following the "guai" protocol have claimed success with Dr. St. Amand's regimen, which also includes special dietary considerations and other wellness components.

Finally, according to a study reported in late 2001, some people with fibromyalgia have reduced symptoms when they eliminate allergenic foods from their diet. Dr. Joel S. Edman of the Center for Integrative Medicine at Thomas Jefferson University Hospital in Philadelphia, Pennsylvania, reported on research among fibromyalgia patients who eliminated common allergens from their diet, including corn, wheat, dairy, citrus, soy, and nuts. After two weeks without eating any of the potential food allergens, nearly half of the patients reported "significant reduction of pain." More than 75 percent of patients reported a reduction in other symptoms such as headache, fatigue, bloating, heartburn, and breathing difficulties.

Vitiligo

Some alternative experts believe that vitiligo is the result of nutritional deficiencies, especially folic acid and vitamin B12. One study looked at 100 patients given 10 mg per day of folic acid and 2,000 mcg per day of B12. Among that group, who were also told to avoid exposure to the sun, more than half had repigmentation of the skin, and six had total repigmentation. Other suspected deficiencies include para-amino-benzoic acid (PABA), tyrosine, and copper.

There is a clear link between vitiligo and low stomach acid, and some patients have benefited by supplementing with hydrochloric acid plus pepsin.

Inflammatory Bowel Disease

According to patient advocate Amber Tresca, who runs a popular website on irritable bowel syndrome and Crohn's disease, there have been significant research findings for ulcerative colitis:

> *Cognitive behavior therapy (CBT) has proven to be very effective, with one study resulting in 75 to 80 percent of patients seeing improvement. A study on boswellia (also known as frankincense) for ulcerative colitis also had dramatic results. Complete remission was achieved by 82 percent of those taking boswellia, 350 mg three times a day (compared to 75 percent with conventional therapy). Complementary therapies are finally seeing the light of day, but traditional medicine continues to dominate the treatment of these conditions.*

Tresca suggests caution when looking for dietary therapies for Crohn's, irritable bowel syndrome, and ulcerative colitis:

> *I have talked to many patients who swear by this diet or that diet to treat their symptoms. But there are several factors to take into consideration. So little is known about these conditions, and misdiagnosis is frequent. It is also possible that a proper diet could be treating other underlying conditions that were previously attributed to IBD. However, as I often tell the people who write to me in email and my forum—if it works, do it! I also talk to many people who have tried nutritional approaches and get no relief whatsoever (myself included). Therefore, it is really a case-by-case situation, and as in so many things, one size does not fit all.*

Rheumatoid Arthritis

In an article in *Arthritis Today*, one integrative rheumatologist, Dr. James McKoy, of Honolulu, Hawaii, described his treatment of

246 Living Well with Autoimmune Disease

a patient who was so debilitated by RA that she was unable to walk after just two years. Dr. McKoy drained her knees, injected them with cortisone, and began disease-modifying drugs. But he also recommended other treatments, including vitamins, minerals, aromatherapy, breathing exercises, and omega-3 fish oil capsules with each meal. Two or three times a day, her aching joints were massaged with essential oils from ginger, lemon, nutmeg, black pepper, and peppermint; and he prescribed self-help classes and guided visual imagery. The patient described her response as near miraculous, and reported, "I was out of my wheelchair the day he drained my knees," and within several months she had substantial improvement in pain and other symptoms.

Exercise is particularly important for RA patients, and low-impact forms are frequently recommended, including water aerobics, swimming, yoga, and tai chi, with instructors specially trained to help those with musculoskeletal problems. Generally, even conventional physicians feel that some alternatives can be safely recommended for most RA patients, including

- Use of "natural anti-inflammatories" such as omega-3 fish and flaxseed oils
- Gentle exercise, such as yoga, tai chi, and qigong
- Acupuncture
- Massage and physical therapy
- Glucosamine and/or chondroitin, which may relieve osteoarthritis pain and stiffness and possibly stop further cartilage loss

In a Chinese study, the supplement Wobenzym was found to reduce morning stiffness, SED rate, rheumatoid factor, and proved to be a good basic treatment of RA.

Multiple Sclerosis

In his book *Dr. Atkins' Vita-Nutrient Solution: Nature's Answers to Drugs,* Dr. Robert Atkins discusses the use of the supplement calcium AEP—also known as colamine phosphate, or calcium 2 amino ethanol phosphate—for autoimmune disease. Although it isn't always easy to get in the United States, Dr. Atkins finds calcium AEP "ideally suited to treat any autoimmune disorder—including rheumatoid arthritis, lupus, scleroderma, Crohn's disease." He feels that the greatest results are seen in multiple sclerosis and early Type I diabetes.

According to Dr. Atkins, his results parallel those of research conducted by Dr. Hans Nieper in Germany, finding that more than 60 percent of those trying calcium AEP for MS noted stabilization of symptoms, with reduced fatigue, steadier walking gait, and better balance. Some research suggests that a natural, healthy diet can result in improvement in MS. The assumption is that MS has its roots in moving away from natural healthy foods. This means that alcohol, salt, sugar, nicotine, white flour, condiments, spices, preserved foods, coffee, and tea should be banished from the diet. Researchers have also suggested that those suffering from MS should eat less than 15 grams of saturated fat per day.

13

Dietary and Health Approaches

In researching cutting-edge conventional and alternative ways to prevent, minimize, or treat autoimmune diseases, diet comes up again and again. One of the most important ways you can have the potential to change your immune system is through your diet and nutrition, as well as identifying allergens, pathogens, and other factors that can tax your immune system. The following are some dietary recommendations that apply to all autoimmune diseases. *Note:* Remember that if you have a gastrointestinal autoimmune condition, you should consult with your practitioner before making any dietary changes.

■ Food and Environmental Sensitivities and Allergies

Identifying and Treating Sensitivities and Allergies

The most common allergenic foods include

- Wheat
- Dairy foods
- Corn
- Soy
- Fish (especially shellfish)

- Nuts
- Fruits

Dr. Larrian Gillespie, an expert on hormones and diet, is a firm believer that unsuspected and unidentified allergenic reactions may be causing inflammation and contributing to the autoimmune process:

> *Many people are allergic to food products. This causes the gut to "leak" highly charged by-products of metabolism into the lymphatic system. In turn, the by-products alter the protective surface layer, called glycosaminoglycans, which act as the first barrier between the joint/muscle tendons and the fluid bathing them. Think of this as a giant bug zapper trying to prevent the bugs from getting through. When the membrane is damaged by altering the charge on the surface of the membrane, it allows larger molecules to pass in, causing inflammation. By using a diet that avoids allergens, you can help prevent attacks of inflammation.*

Food allergies are high on Dr. Donna Hurlock's list of possible triggers and culprits in some autoimmune reactions. Hurlock, a women's health and hormonal medicine expert, gynecologist, and surgeon, urges her autoimmune disease patients to find out whether they have food allergies:

> *But don't waste a lot of money doing food allergy testing. You can spend $500 to $800 to do food allergy testing, and you'll find out you're allergic to wheat, or dairy, or another common allergen. Instead, a simple elimination diet—where you remove foods from your diet, and then reintroduce them, noting symptomatic reactions—will tell you all you need to know.*

Dr. Hurlock found that her own allergy to citrus juices caused her to have joint pain with rheumatoid arthritis–like symptoms. After an elimination diet showed that she was allergic to orange juice, she got rid of the pain by removing it from her diet. Dr. Hurlock believes that while conventional medicine can solve some problems, autoimmune disease patients should go on an elimination diet to assess food allergies.

You need to remove an item completely from your diet for two weeks, then eat a large amount of the food you're testing, to see if you have any noticeable reaction over the next three days. You're looking for diarrhea, nausea, gas, headache, rashes, skin eruptions, itching, fatigue, irritability, and other strong reactions or symptoms.

According to registered dietitian and nutrition educator Rick Hall, insensitivity to foods may be more prevalent than we know: "The most known food sensitivities are to dairy, corn, and wheat. There's additional evidence that soy may also be problematic. A food challenge test can be conducted to isolate which foods cause adverse reactions."

Functional medicine practitioner Dr. John Dommisse is a believer in more formal testing: "I like the IgG4 and IgG1 (delayed) food allergy testing in the blood, by the ELISA method. This test is not popular with allergists, but I have found it to be very useful in my practice. For one thing, it reveals those food sensitivities that are virtually impossible for patients to discover themselves, because the reactions are delayed."

The Gluten-Free Diet

Gluten is one of the most common food sensitivities linked to autoimmune disease. It is a protein found in the grains of wheat, rye, and barley. In its full expression, it can cause celiac disease, which is a complete intolerance to gluten products. But even a sensitivity to gluten may contribute to autoimmune disease. Dr. James

Braly, an author, lecturer, and researcher, argues that human beings have strayed far from the diet we originally subsisted on of animal proteins, fruits, and vegetables. It was only relatively recently on the human timeline that grains were introduced. Yet gluten is now one of our most common foods, and even the newly revised food pyramid advises people to eat six to eleven servings of grains each day. Says Dr. Braly:

We've gone from being hunter-gatherers to being canaries. Yet our society's dependence on gluten may not at all be healthy. From 20 to 30 percent of the population actually has undiagnosed, untreated gluten sensitivity, which manifests itself in a variety of health problems, including autoimmune conditions like insulin-dependent diabetes and other disorders.

Certain foods—such as gluten, soy, and casein, a protein found in cow's milk—tend to be diabetogenic, or linked to the development of diabetes. British researchers recently reported that celiac disease is common in Type 1 diabetes and recommended that screening for celiac disease should be part of the routine examinations offered to all patients. In a diabetic with celiac disease, the benefits of a gluten-free diet include control of symptoms, better stabilization of diabetes, and prevention of celiac complications.

Dr. Braly says the gluten sensitivity and celiac disease linkage needs to be ruled out in a number of autoimmune diseases, including diabetes, multiple sclerosis, lupus, Crohn's disease, sarcoidosis, alopecia, rheumatoid arthritis, fibromyalgia, Sjögren's, and thyroid disease. He feels that it's worth evaluating, especially in high-risk individuals, such as those with autoimmune conditions or a family history of diabetes, because there's hope to lessen the symptoms, possibly eliminate the need for medication, and prevent other autoimmune diseases.

Despite numerous studies suggesting that gluten-free diets can help a variety of health problems, Dr. Braly finds that most doctors are still unaware of the research. He urges patients to serve as their own health advocates and "surround yourself with a cadre of knowledgeable health professionals. If your doctor completely dismisses your concerns about food sensitivities, then find one who will listen."

A gastroenterologist or nutritionally oriented practitioner can perform the various antibody tests, including antigliadin antibodies, to help diagnose gluten insensitivity. Laura Dolson, a writer who runs a popular patient-oriented website on gynecological cancers, has been on the gluten-free diet for more than three years. She describes what it's like to follow the diet:

> It was very difficult at first. European and North American diets are very wheat based, and there is a steep learning curve as you realize everything in your pantry that has wheat in it! Also, you can make alternative pizza dough and breads, but until you forget how the "real" stuff tasted, it's pretty disappointing! But after a while, you learn new ways to cook!

Identifying and Clearing Allergies with NAET, JMT, and BRT

Dr. Eric Berg is the first person to admit that what he does can seem a little unusual. But when it comes to his patients, they say that results speak for themselves. And the results they speak of can be surprising, including a patient who claims that her lifelong allergy to dairy products, which manifested itself as full-body hives, disappeared practically overnight, and now she enjoys a bowl of ice cream, or cheese, anytime she wishes. Or a patient who said that her joint pain and aches were significantly improved after a series of treatments to clear her sensitivities to various toxins, allergens, and other pathogens.

Dr. Berg, a certified doctor of chiropractic, practices several relatively unknown but increasingly popular therapies known as

NAET, JMT, and BRT (body restoration technique), which was developed by Dr. Berg himself. NAET stands for Nambudripad allergy elimination technique, which allows for diagnosis and treatment of allergies, combining muscle response testing of kinesiology with chiropractic and Chinese medicine techniques to clear allergic reactions by reprogramming the brain's response to allergens. Recipients of NAET treatment claim dramatic reduction or elimination of allergy symptoms after a series of ten to twenty sessions. NAET uses concepts from Chinese medicine, which recognize that symptoms can result when allergic responses disrupt energy flows and pathways. The aim of NAET is to desensitize the response to allergens. Small vials filled with various allergens are placed in the patient's hand, and muscle response testing is used to determine sensitivities. Once the various allergens are identified, treatment involves holding a vial of the allergen while particular acupuncture points are stimulated. This technique is supposed to clear the sensitivity, and if the allergen is avoided for twenty-four hours, the system claims that the sensitivity will be gone.

A related therapy is the Jaffe-Mellor technique (JMT), which is performed similarly to NAET. JMT focuses on the symptoms, including joint and muscle pain and inflammation, which result from various forms of arthritis and degenerative joint disease. JMT was developed by two practitioners, Carolyn Jaffe, DAc, Dipl NCCA, PhD, and Judy M. Mellor, RN, PhD, directors of the Health and Wellness Alternative Medical Center near Reading, Pennsylvania, who identified microorganisms in all of their patients with arthritis and "autoimmune" diseases, and developed a therapy to neutralize the body's reaction to the organisms.

Jaffe and Mellor believe that the microorganisms stress the body's immune system and establish themselves in muscles, joints, cartilage, and bone tissue. Eventually, they believe that the microorganisms and resulting response will destroy healthy tissue and organs, and can lead to pain, as well as what appears to be autoimmune disease but actually is not. Speaking to *Alternative Medicine* magazine, Dr. Jaffe clarified this point: "This 'autoimmune' response is in actuality a normal, pathogen-induced immune defense reaction that occurs in arthritis and in many diseases besides arthritis . . . they are in fact the immune system's attempt to spew out the pathogen."

Dr. Berg practices NAET and JMT but uses BRT for hormone and endocrine problems. According to Dr. Berg, estrogens and toxic substances that resemble estrogens found in the food supply may be a reason behind chronic symptoms of endocrine imbalance and autoimmune disease in some people: "With BRT, we're focusing on bringing the hormone system into balance naturally—without giving hormones or medication. Using the body's acupuncture points, BRT may rejuvenate and revitalize the hormonal and endocrine system."

Berg describes the way these therapies work:

It's similar to an opera singer reaching a high note that can shatter glass. The singer reaches a frequency that is the same as the wine glass . . . the wavelength is duplicated, and in physics, when this happens, the wave vibration gets canceled out. The same thing happens in BRT. By energetically exposing patients to substances that they are sensitive to, and using noninvasive treatments that incorporate acupressure and breathing, we can retrain the body's sensitivity.

One of Dr. Berg's patients, Veronica, a retired two-star admiral with the Navy, said that she had chronic food allergies and sinusitis for thirty years, which were exacerbated by the discovery of a thyroid problem in her 40s. Suffering from profound fatigue and worsening allergy symptoms, she felt at the end of her rope when she went to see Dr. Berg. But she was skeptical at first:

I couldn't talk about it with my friends, they would think I was off my rocker. I promised myself I would only go for a couple months and then see. But I saw immediate results. Right from the start, I had dramatic results in energy. That's what kept me going back. I can't explain how it worked, but it did. All I can do is talk about results. My allergies are gone. I'm feeling great, my energy is off the charts, and now, when I get a cold, it doesn't go into a sinus infection.

Veronica also reported that she had gone off her thyroid medicine, under the supervision of her regular physician, and now had a normal TSH level, with no thyroid-related symptoms whatsoever.

Another patient, Dorie, reported her daughter's success with NAET: "She was allergic to practically everything by the time we took her there and the traditional doctors couldn't even figure out what was wrong, much less know how to treat it. In about four months, she was a completely different person—practically normal, free from pain and fatigue."

■ Other Dietary Considerations

There are a variety of other dietary factors to consider in relationship to autoimmune disease.

Consider a Low-Fat Diet

Dr. Shari Lieberman from the University of Bridgeport School of Human Nutrition in Connecticut advocates very low-fat diets, with 20 grams a day or less of fat, to help people with lupus, multiple sclerosis, scleroderma, and rheumatoid arthritis. In a thirty-four-year study of MS patients following a very low-fat diet, 95 percent of patients survived and remained physically active, which was substantially higher than usual rates. Deviating from the diet, even after five to ten years of strict adherence, triggered symptoms again.

Consider a Diet Higher in Protein

Since weight gain is a problem for many patients with autoimmune disease, it may be worth considering a switch to a diet somewhat higher in protein. Recent research has suggested that a diet higher in protein and lower in carbohydrates than is currently recommended may help people maintain desirable body weight and overall health. Donald Layman, professor of nutritional sciences at the University of Illinois, did a study of two groups of middle-aged women. One group ate a classic diet of 55 percent carbohydrates, 15 percent protein, and 30 percent fat, and a total of 1,700 calories. Another group ate 40 percent carbohydrates, 30 percent protein, and 30 percent fat, and 1,700 calories total. Both groups lost approximately 16 pounds, but the high-protein group lost mostly body fat and just a small amount of muscle mass, and women eating the higher-protein diet showed the ability to burn more calories at the end of the study. Higher levels of thyroid hormone were documented among women who ate the higher-protein diet, suggesting a higher rate of metabolism. Triglycerides also declined significantly, and an increase in HDL, the "good" cholesterol, was seen.

Consider a Low-Glycemic Diet

Sugar in the diet is thought by many practitioners to be an immune irritant and trigger for inflammation. Many alternative practitioners recommend a low-glycemic diet for autoimmune disease patients. The glycemic index (GI) assigns a number to carbohydrate-based foods, based on how they affect your blood sugar. Foods with a lower GI cause only a slight increase in blood sugar, foods with a medium-range GI cause a higher increase in blood sugar, and high-glycemic foods cause blood sugar to raise significantly.

A low-GI diet has been shown to help with diabetes by helping control blood sugar and promoting weight loss—two factors that alone can actually reverse Type II diabetes. A 1999 study in Sweden showed that Type II diabetics could lower blood glucose and insulin by 30 percent after only four weeks on a low-GI diet. And in a study of men over six years, those on the lowest-GI diets were 25 percent less likely to develop diabetes.

The low-glycemic diet flies in the face of some current nutritional guidelines, which encourage heavy consumption of grains. Rick Hall, dietitian and nutritional educator, says:

A low-fat, high-carbohydrate diet, can—here it goes—make you fat. Eat too much refined carbohydrate, your body will reconstruct it to fat for long-term storage. In most cases, we eat too much. A small portion of pasta is healthy. A large bowl of spaghetti with unlimited bread sticks and soda is not. Much research supports a lower glycemic index diet for reduced weight and, potentially, diabetes prevention. Starchy foods, including corn and potatoes, should be eaten in moderation.

When it comes to GI ratings, particularly with grains, it's a safe bet to look for higher fiber. Higher-fiber breads, for example, have a lower GI than lower-fiber breads. A variety of resources can help you choose healthy low-glycemic foods, and some suggested books are listed in Appendix A.

Consider Eating Smaller Meals More Frequently

Another way to maintain a more consistent blood sugar and avoid stress on the immune system is to eat smaller meals more frequently. Author and diet expert Dr. Larrian Gillespie recommends that most people construct small meals of around 250 calories per meal, and spread them out throughout the day, based on total calorie requirements:

Stress is reduced, as frequent feedings stimulate the key CP450 enzymes in the liver, which revs up your metabolism. These enzymes are a key to aging, as their ability to convert foods into available energy diminishes with age. By frequently challenging the system, you keep them in a higher state of energy utilization.

The immune system benefits from smaller, more frequent meals, according to holistic practitioners and authors Richard Shames and Karilee Shames, who run a popular holistic health practice that specializes in autoimmune diseases in Mill Valley, California:

A good approach is to present to the immune system at any one moment of intake a multiplicity of foods. This maneuver is called the "eight mini-food meals" and the "five mini-food snacks," meaning that whenever you eat, you eat from a variety of food choices, perhaps in smaller amounts than if that individual food were eaten alone. This is another method of avoiding the immune system's tendency to zero in on any one particular substance that it confronts frequently.

Maximize Your Digestion

Ensuring proper digestion is an important part of dealing with autoimmune disease. According to metabolic experts Drs. John Lowe and Gina Honeyman-Lowe, in the 1970s, researchers found evidence for "intestinal toxemia," an age-old notion much maligned in mainstream medicine:

Researchers found that when they introduced undigested, whole, radioactively labeled proteins into the small intestine and colon, some of the protein molecules passed into the lymph and blood circulation. Like all proteins foreign to the body, these food proteins are capable of setting off antigen-

antibody reactions. The antibodies that form are capable of crossreacting with body proteins. This, of course, is the basis of some autoimmune disease.

According to Dr. Lowe, people must be careful to thoroughly digest food proteins before they reach the colon. For some patients, this means taking the time to chew food thoroughly. This disrupts the collagen in meat, allowing digestive enzymes to more effectively reach the proteins encased in the collagen. It may also mean that patients take supplemental protein-digestive enzymes with meals. The supplements should contain pepsin, which breaks down collagen, betaine hydrochloride to lower GI pH and activate the digestive enzymes, and bromelain. Studies show that bromelain is an effective treatment for the virus herpes zoster, and it is an effective anti-inflammatory in conditions such as sinusitis, rheumatoid arthritis, and lupus.

Consider Losing Weight

If you are overweight, losing weight can be a tremendous help in almost any autoimmune disease. Reducing body weight reduces excess stress on joints and muscles. Weight loss has a positive effect on the endocrine system and can benefit patients with diabetes, thyroid disease, and premature ovarian decline. In general, a healthy weight enables the immune system to function better.

For many people, the process of simply identifying and removing food allergens allows them to lose weight naturally. The gut inflammation and dysfunction of the digestive system caused by food sensitivities can help contribute to malnutrition and weight gain.

Many autoimmune disease patients—myself included—have found that some variation on the low-glycemic diet is the best way to safely lose weight. In my case, after trying numerous diets, I was able to lose weight by going to a limited (but not low) calorie diet of smaller, more frequent meals, and an emphasis on vegetables, low-fat protein sources, some fruit, and limited starches.

Some people consider the diet drugs, and that's a decision you need to make with your practitioner. Research shows, however, that most people who use diet drugs do not keep off the weight once they stop the drugs. Dr. Stephen Langer, who wrote the best-selling book *Solved: The Riddle of Weight Loss,* doesn't believe in diet drugs such as Xenical or Meridia for most autoimmune disease patients, and he typically does not prescribe them. Says Dr. Langer: "I don't think an overweight condition is due to a Meridia deficiency."

■ Other Key Dietary Changes

There are a variety of other dietary changes you may want to make to help your immune system.

Add Probiotics

Probiotics are supplements that contain live bacteria that we are meant to have in sufficient quantities in our intestinal system—the "good" bacteria found in fermented foods such as miso and dairy products such as yogurt and some cheeses. One of the more well-known bacteria in this category is acidophilus, the live cultures found in yogurt.

According to a report in the *European Journal of Clinical Nutrition,* the probiotic bacteria bifidobacterium lactis HN019 boosts the activity of various disease-killing immune system cells in healthy adults. A Finnish study found that giving probiotic supplements to pregnant women close to delivery, and to their newborns, could help prevent childhood allergies in the babies. Allergy experts say this is evidence that probiotic bacteria can train an infant's immune system to resist allergic reactions. The bacteria used in this study was lactobacillus rhamnosus. Among the babies, all at high risk of developing allergies because of family history, those who themselves took the probiotic therapy and whose mothers did prior to their birth halved their risk of developing eczema by age 2.

Avoid Bad Fats and Get Enough Good Fats

Generally, many experts believe that the type of fat you eat has more of an impact on your overall health than the total fat intake. Saturated fats—found in meats, butter, and tropical oils—can contribute to inflammation and increased cholesterol, while the protective fats—found in olive oil, avocados, fish, and nuts—can help protect against heart disease and reduce inflammation.

You should avoid trans-monounsaturated fatty acids and hydrogenated fats. They are found in shortening, margarine, snacks such as crackers and cookies, and in the oils used by fast-food restaurants. If the label says "partially hydrogenated," the product contains a trans-fatty acid.

Omega 3 Supplementation

In his book *Dr. Atkins' Vita-Nutrient Solution: Nature's Answers to Drugs,* the author talks about how essential omega-3 fatty acids are in helping with autoimmune disease. Addition of omega-3 fatty acids, including via the supplements EPA and DHA, can help reduce inflammation. Dr. Atkins supports the use of fish oils in helping to suppress inflammation such as that found in rheumatoid arthritis, and as a potential alternative to nonsteroidal anti-inflammatory drugs.

Dr. Atkins recommends as much as 3 grams a day of eicosapentaenoic acid (EPA) and dehydroepiandrosterone (DHA) for three weeks, to help slow down the self-destructive process of autoimmune diseases, including lupus, scleroderma, MS, and other conditions. According to Dr. Atkins, every Crohn's and colitis patient he counsels is recommended to take the omega-3 fatty acids. Because it can take time and you need to take a sufficient amount, such as 3 to 4 grams, it may take several months before you really see an impact on your symptoms.

Eat More Fish . . . Carefully

According to some experts, we are meant to have some amount of fish-derived fats. Professor Michael Crawford of the Institute of Brain Chemistry and Human Nutrition at the University of North London says that DHA is one of the important fish fats, but there is no alternative source for it other than fish, or by supplements. The optimal sources of these fats are oily fish such as salmon, tuna, herring, sardines, mackerel, and anchovies. Even mussels, prawns, and oysters have some omega-3s.

Some experts say you need to be somewhat careful about the type of fish you eat, however. Dr. Ronald Hoffman, a popular radio host and nutritional and holistic physician who runs New York City's Hoffman Center, says to be careful about fish that are on the EPA's (Environmental Protection Agency) list as high in toxins. These fish include swordfish, shark, and mackerel. Dr. Hoffman suggests eating tuna in moderation, but that generally the other fish highest in omega-3 oils, such as salmon, usually are fairly safe.

When it comes to fish, Dr. Joseph Mercola, who runs a holistic clinic in Schaumburg, Illinois, urges even greater caution, as he feels most fish have mercury contamination. His list of the only "safe" fish to eat includes summer flounder, wild Pacific salmon, croaker, sardines, haddock, and tilapia.

Eat More Vegetables

With vitamins, nutrients, fiber, and other health benefits, as well as many immune-enhancing properties, there is no question that more vegetables should be incorporated into our diets. While the typical recommendations urge us to eat five fruits and vegetables each day, many practitioners encourage seven to nine fruits and vegetables a day. Practitioners with expertise in autoimmune disease suggest that among these servings, the majority should be vegetables, rather than fruit, because fruit has more allergenic potential and is typically higher-glycemic.

Try to Eat an Immune-Enhancing Food Every Day

Certain foods are known to be immune enhancers, so one dietary improvement you can make is to try to eat an immune-enhancing food every day. These include garlic, medicinal mushrooms such as maitake, broccoli, sea greens (dulse, chlorella, and spirulina), and fruits such as blueberries and elderberries. (*Note:* Be careful with too much raw broccoli or uncooked sea greens, as they can promote goiters and thyroid disease. Cooking, however, removes most of the antithyroid properties.)

Reduce Sodium and Table Salt Intake

Because of its overall impact on cardiovascular health, it's usually a good idea to consider reducing your overall sodium intake. Typically, practitioners recommend you reduce sodium intake to less than 2,400 milligrams a day—that's about 1 teaspoon total of table salt. To cut salt intake, remove your salt shaker, limit the amount of fast food and processed food in your diet, and study food labels to find foods with high hidden sodium levels, such as breads and canned soups.

Since most Americans get enough iodine from the iodized salt in processed foods, if you do use table salt, consider switching from iodized, processed salt to sea salt, which also offers healthy trace minerals. Excess intake of iodine is a known trigger of thyroid disease in some susceptible individuals.

Increase Dietary Fiber

Dietary fiber (i.e., plant materials that are not easily digested) is an essential part of a healthy diet. Fiber helps to normalize bowel func-

264 Living Well with Autoimmune Disease

tion and can help prevent toxins from spending too much time in the intestines, potentially being absorbed into the bloodstream. Fiber also helps to limit the spike in blood sugar that typically occurs after eating and may help prevent or minimize diabetes. A high-fiber intake has been associated with a reduced risk of hormonal cancers such as breast and ovarian cancers. Most of us eat only 14 to 15 grams a day of fiber, but almost everyone should be eating 25 to 30 grams per day. (In some people with gastrointestinal conditions such as Crohn's disease and ulcerative colitis, high fiber can aggravate their condition, so always follow your practitioner's guidelines.)

To add fiber, choose higher-fiber versions of foods over lower-fiber versions—for example, the actual fruits versus juices, whole grains over refined grains, and so on. If you still can't get enough fiber, consider a supplement. When you switch to a high-fiber diet or supplements, add them slowly over time, in order to minimize temporary side effects, which could include gas, cramps, and diarrhea. Double-check with your practitioner or pharmacist regarding any medications you are taking and their absorption. A high-fiber diet can change intestinal absorption rates of some medicines, which can reduce a drug's effectiveness. With thyroid hormone replacement medicine, for example, eating a high-fiber diet can prevent sufficient absorption of the drug, so doctors typically recommend that patients take their thyroid medicine in the morning, an hour before eating, to ensure a sufficient amount is absorbed.

Dr. Joseph Mercola suggests that people with autoimmune disease be cautious about how they eat a high-fiber diet:

> High fiber almost always implies increasing consumption of whole-wheat bread, which will be massively counterproductive, as wheat is one of the major autoimmune triggers. So high-vegetable fiber should be stressed, and I really find most people's health turns around completely once they start vegetable juicing with attention to eating the pulp.

Drink Enough Water

It may sound simplistic, but many people do not drink enough water. The old adage about eight glasses of water a day is often repeated for a reason—it's a basic requirement for good health. Holistic and nutritional physician Dr. David Brownstein believes that dehydration may in fact be the number one health problem affecting Americans today:

> Our bodies are made of over 70 percent water. Without drinking enough water, the immune system cannot function normally, and this will set the stage for infectious problems and autoimmune problems to develop. People (and even children) drink too much nonwater sources such as soda and coffee.
>
> I can't tell you how many patients who complain of joint pain improve when they increase their water intake. In my experience, over 90 percent of those patients suffering from a chronic illness have had a long history of dehydration. The first step to providing the body with the necessary raw materials to heal itself is to hydrate it.

Get Enough Selenium

Selenium has been shown to have cancer-fighting abilities, and many practitioners recommend 200 micrograms a day. Selenium, a trace mineral, is typically found in plant foods, but Brazil nuts, walnuts, beef/calf liver, and canned tuna are very good sources of the mineral. But typically the selenium content of the local soil determines the selenium level of plant foods and the selenium levels of the local population. In places such as China and New Zealand, where the soil is selenium deficient, people are likely to have a higher risk of muscle disease, infertility, heart disease, thyroid problems, and other autoimmune symptoms.

Recent animal studies found that the human flu virus becomes stronger when selenium is deficient, and experts believe that selenium deficiency allows viruses to take hold more strongly in humans as well. Since the 1980s, research has clearly demonstrated selenium's ability to prevent cancer. One ten-year study found selenium takers had 37 percent fewer instances of new cancers and less than half the cancer deaths as placebo takers. Since selenium in high amounts can be toxic, no more than 200 to 400 micrograms a day is considered necessary for beneficial effects.

Eat Organic/Hormone-Free Foods

Pesticides on fruits and vegetables, and hormones and antibiotics found in meat, can contribute to toxic overloads that may trigger or worsen autoimmune disease. Noted herbalist and holistic practitioner Alan Tillotson recommends shifting to organic and hormone-free foods. In particular, with fruits and vegetables, he feels organic is best:

> Carotenoids and bioflavonoids, the pigments found in plants that give them their vibrant, bright, and deep colors, have powerful and now well-known antioxidant actions on the body. For example, the eye depends on carotenoids like lutein, lycopene helps the prostate, bioflavonoids help the immune system, etc. But foods grown in nonorganic conditions have less color/pigment, so choosing brighter, more colorful organic produce is one obvious way to ensure you're getting fruits and vegetables with more powerful antioxidants. Not only are these foods higher in nutrients but organic foods reduce your overall load of exposure to pesticides.

Minimize Chemicals, Artificial Sweeteners, and Processed Foods

Along with eating more organic and hormone/antibiotic-free foods, you can reduce your toxic load by minimizing the amount of chemicals, artificial sweeteners, and processed foods in your diet. Dr. David Brownstein has some thoughts on diet:

> I believe that getting the nutritionally deficient foods—transfatty acids, refined sugars, and flour and others—out of the diet is absolutely necessary for one to allow the healing process to begin. In addition, all artificial sweeteners (especially aspartame) must be removed. I have seen many patients improve their health considerably by removing artificial sweeteners.
>
> People with chronic illnesses must remove all processed foods from their diets. Examples of processed foods include cookies, cakes, donuts, etc. I think that autoimmune problems and infections may begin by ingesting a poor diet. A poor diet leads to nutritional deficiencies and immune system problems, which can set the stage for infections to occur.

Eliminate Toxic Metals

Many holistic practitioners recommend hair or blood tests to assess levels of exposure to toxic metals, such as mercury, found in dental work. Some practitioners then recommend chelation—the process of removing the metals from the bloodstream—via IV treatments or supplements. But some believe that in certain cases it's necessary to replace the mercury fillings to remove the toxic exposure.

Sherrie, who was diagnosed with both lupus and rheumatoid arthritis, ended up having all her mercury fillings removed. Says Sherrie:

> I thought I wouldn't be able to talk or even move my mouth the next day—but it was fine. The next day we were dancing . . . I hadn't danced in a long time! This treatment has totally eliminated fibromyalgia, chronic myofascial pain,

lupus, Sjögren's syndrome, Raynaud's phenomenon, and improved many others.

■ Prevent Infection

Many practitioners believe that overgrowth of bacteria, organisms, and viruses may contribute to the inflammatory process and autoimmune disease. Infection causes inflammation, and inflammation activates the immune system.

Holistic practitioners and authors Richard Shames and Karilee Shames have this to say about infection:

> *Try to avoid as many bacterial and viral infections as possible (i.e., rather than get a bronchitis or strep throat and then take antibiotics for the infection, instead live your life so strong and so carefully as to not get the infection in the first place, or nip it in the bud right away with a homeopathic first-aid kit). Moreover, most people know that they would be healthier and more resistant to infection if they simply got more sleep, and maybe did a little bit more walking.*

There are some other common-sense things you can do to prevent infection.

Take Care of Your Teeth

Researchers have suggested that chronic periodontal disease may contribute to diabetes. Apparently, when gums are seriously inflamed in periodontal disease, bacteria can gain access to the bloodstream, activating immune cells and inducing Type II diabetes. This process can take place even in healthy individuals who have no risk factors for diabetes. This same mechanism is thought to be at play in many other autoimmune diseases. Experts advise that you take excellent care of your teeth and gums to help prevent gum disease. That means regular brushing and flossing, checkups, and professional cleanings.

Wash Your Hands

It may sound ridiculously simple, but many bacterial and viral infections are spread hand to hand, or hand to a surface where a hand touched. There, infectious organisms accumulate under your nails, or remain on the skin. Then, rubbing the hand to the membranes of the eyes, nose, or mouth completes the process of self-infection.

Clean Your Nose

Cleaning the membranes of the nasal passage can eliminate allergens, antigens, and infectious organisms, and prevent infections. A practice that yogis and Ayurvedic medicine practitioners have followed for centuries is neti, a simple daily washing of the nasal passages using warm salt water dispensed by a small pot. But similar benefits can be gained by regular use of a saline nasal spray, or other techniques to rinse out the nasal passages.

■ Eliminate Pathogens and Infection

Frequently, the body is infected in ways that are not immediately obvious. There can be foodborne bacterial overgrowth, or yeast, parasites, and other pathogens that have infected tissue, organs, or the bloodstream and are causing inflammation and activation of the immune system. Under the guidance of an experienced practitioner, one useful process to consider is testing to look for infectious organisms and pathogens.

There are too many linkages between bacteria and autoimmune disease to list them all here, but a notable one is the bacteria that causes ulcers: *Helicobacter pylori.* This bacteria appears to be a possible trigger in rheumatoid arthritis, Raynaud's phenomenon, and Sjögren's syndrome, and treatment to eliminate bacteria has resolved symptoms in some patients.

People with autoimmune thyroid disease have a higher-than-average chance of overgrowth of the foodborne bacteria *Yersinia enterocolitica,* which has been found to be a potentially potent trigger in thyroid conditions. Since many laboratories do not routinely test for *Y. enterocolitica,* it is particularly important for your doctor to notify laboratory personnel when infection with this bacterium is suspected so that special tests can be done. (Great Smokies Diagnostic Laboratory in Asheville, North Carolina, can do this testing. Specifically, your doctor would need to order the comprehensive digestive stool analysis and request the test for *Y. enterocolitica* be added.)

Typically, for this sort of testing, you would need to consult with a practitioner who specializes in functional medicine. Functional medicine practitioners may be MDs, chiropractors, nutritionists, naturopaths, or other types of practitioners, but their emphasis is on uncovering the causes of symptoms using laboratory assessment, with the purpose of early intervention to improve health. The nutritional status, metabolism, presence of bacteria and pathogens are all looked at, in order to identify deficiencies and imbalances so that they can be corrected. Functional medicine looks at six key areas: the digestion/gastrointestinal system; nutritional status; detoxification/oxidative stress; immunology/allergies; hormonal status; and heart and blood vessels (cardiovascular).

Great Smokies Diagnostic Laboratory is truly a pioneer in these tests. Just a few of the many tests Great Smokies offers that are of use in assessing factors that affect immune function and autoimmune disease include the following:

- Comprehensive digestive stool analysis (CDSA), which can identify bacteria, yeast, malabsorption, and other key digestive issues
- Comprehensive parasitology, which identifies parasites, both pathogenic and "good" bacteria, and yeast overgrowth
- Intestinal permeability assessment, which identifies leaky gut and malabsorption
- *Helicobacter pylori* antibody assay, which identifies antibodies to H. *pylori*
- Vaginosis profile, which identifies candida, gardnerella, and trichomonas, good bacteria, yeast, and other immune measures
- Comprehensive antibody assessment, which identifies allergies to 120 of the most commonly encountered food and environmental allergens
- Elemental analysis, which looks for toxic levels of nutrients and elements in the hair, blood, and urine

Antibiotic Treatment

When particular bacteria or pathogens are identified, many practitioners treat with antibiotics. Even when infection may be suspected but can't be demonstrated by laboratory tests, some practitioners are using antibiotic therapy to treat a variety of autoimmune conditions, including rheumatoid arthritis, lupus, scleroderma and ankylosing spondylitis, among others. Some physicians have been using tetracycline antibiotic therapy for several decades, preferring either straight tetracycline, doxycycline, or minocycline (Minocin).

There's substantial evidence for use of antibiotic treatment in rheumatoid arthritis, and in some studies, more than half of the patients had significant improvement on antibiotic therapy. According to Dr. Joseph Mercola, Minocin is the preferred antibiotic because it is the most effective against the organisms that may be causing rheumatoid arthritis, and it is least likely to cause yeast infections in long-term therapy. For those taking Minocin therapy, Dr. Mercola also recommends the addition of probiotics, such as *Lactobacillus acidophilus,* to help maintain normal bowel flora and decrease the risk of fungal overgrowth. He believes that sugar in foods should be aggressively avoided. Dr. Mercola, who has provided antibiotic therapy to more than 1,500 autoimmune patients, claims that nearly "80 percent of the patients do remarkably better with this program." But Dr. Mercola cautions patience: "The length of therapy can vary widely. In severe cases, it may take up to thirty months for the patients to gain sustained improvement. One requires patience because remissions may take up to three to five years."

Dr. David Brownstein, a family physician who integrates conventional and alternative therapies in his practice, is the author of *Overcoming Arthritis.* He has found that many individuals suffering from autoimmune illnesses often have an underlying infectious component. According to Brownstein, experts have long known that some forms of arthritis can be caused by bacteria. One rheumatologist, Dr. Thomas Brown, isolated *Mycoplasma bacterium* from the joints of people suffering from rheumatoid arthritis and had success treating these patients with antibiotics. Says Dr. Brownstein:

> *When I read Dr. Thomas Brown's research on mycoplasma, I immediately began thinking about my patients who were suffering from autoimmune illnesses, including thyroid patients. I began testing my patients for bacterial infections eight years ago, and I discovered a significant portion of these patients with autoimmune arthritic disorders and autoimmune thyroid disorders have signs of an infection. Perhaps these individuals had a bacterial infection (e.g., mycoplasma) that the body was not able to clear.*

Dr. Brownstein uses nutritional support, plus low-dose antibiotics taken only two to three days per week, as his primary therapy. He believes patients can stay on this therapy indefinitely, and particularly recommends that patients on antibiotic therapy also take probiotic supplements to help prevent side effects.

■ Antiviral Therapy

Viruses are implicated as triggers in many autoimmune diseases. But there are few means to protect yourself against viruses and almost no treatments for active viruses. One promising area is in South American herbal medicine, which offers some potent antiviral herbs.

According to Dr. Viana Muller, an ethnobotanist and expert on South American herbal medicine, since antibiotics only kill bacteria and have no effect whatsoever on viruses, one of the great "holes" in Western medicine has been the lack of good antiviral medications—whether the virus be the common cold, the flu, the hepatitis virus, or the polio virus. Practically the only effective response has been the development of vaccines, which have proved to be dangerous in some cases. Says Muller:

> You can imagine my surprise when I came across two different South American herbs in my investigation which have highly effective antiviral properties. One is the "break-stone" herb (in Spanish, chanca piedra) whose botanical name is Phyllanthus niruri. This is a rainforest plant whose leaves, stems, and roots are made into a tea by native people to combat hepatitis B. It is highly effective in getting rid of jaundice and normalizing liver enzyme levels, and has been shown experimentally in published research to have antiviral properties. Chanca piedra also helps detoxify the liver. Since it is

*improving lipid (fat) metabolism, it is not surprising to learn
that in some cases it has been shown to be helpful in losing
weight.*

Another rainforest herb, actually a fruit, which has powerful
antiviral properties is camu-camu. Camu-camu is most notable for
its high vitamin C content, 8 to 10 percent by weight once it has been
spray dried. According to Dr. Muller, anecdotally camu-camu has
been shown to be effective against cold sores (herpes simplex), genital herpes, herpes zoster (shingles), and even the Epstein-Barr virus.

One particularly powerful antiviral from South America is cat's
claw, also known as *uña de gato,* or by its scientific name, *Uncaria
tomentosa.* The key strengths of cat's claw appear to be the following:

- Reducing inflammation
- Lowering allergic response
- Combating viruses
- Detoxifying the liver and kidneys
- Treating gastrointestinal disorders, such as constipation, nau-
  sea, diarrhea, Crohn's disease, hemorrhoids, leaky bowel syn-
  drome, ulcers, gastritis, and diverticulitis

Dr. Ronald Hoffman of New York City's Hoffman Center
believes that dealing with viruses is important in preventing and
treating autoimmunity:

*Nutritional support is the armament that helps you prevent
getting the initial virus, but you also need to normalize the
response to viruses. You want to try to prevent the initial
onslaught, but if infected, ensure that you have a normal
course with a virus, i.e., ten days of mononucleosis, but not
followed by a lifetime of chronic fatigue syndrome.*

For antiviral and immune support, Dr. Hoffman recommends

- Transfer factor, a colostrum-based product, but only under the guidance of a practitioner
- Olive leaf extract, which has broad-spectrum antimicrobial and antiviral properties
- Fluogen, a sublingual flu vaccine, used almost homeopathically, as it can sometimes affect the course of a virus

When it comes to fighting viruses, Richard Shames and Karilee Shames believe that the task is to assist the genetically controlled constitutional factors and help make cells resistant to viral takeover. This involves increasing antibody levels, increasing the number and aggressiveness of the macrophage white blood cells, increasing the amounts and quick reactivity of the complement system, and ramping up the body's ability to rapidly produce interferon. They explain:

What seems to help people accomplish this incredibly complex laudatory goal is to have increased levels of vitamin C compared to what's normal in the population, and to cover as many of the other nutritional bases as possible (which generally means adequate amounts of high-quality foods/avoidance of junk food, avoidance of the metabolic monkey wrenches—caffeine, alcohol, tobacco, sugar), and a good high-quality multivitamin with multiminerals, as well as a decrease in the typical excessive levels of mucus in the mucous membranes (the excess acts as a breeding ground and way station for viral or bacterial invaders), and also a general decrease in toxic load (chemical pollutants in the air, food, and water generally lead to decreased immune functions).

■ Hormonal Treatment

Two leading experts on women's hormones feel that hormones have a critical role in autoimmune disease. Sherrill Sellman, a natural hormonal expert, health researcher, and author of *Hormone Heresy: What Women Must Know About Their Hormones*, believes that hormones are reflecting the other issues in the body, and ensuring hormonal balance is essential to dealing with autoimmune disease. When the estrogen/progesterone balance is altered, Sellman feels that the problem is usually estrogen excess and/or progesterone deficiency:

> There may be overload of estrogen from hormones, meat, pesticides, environmental estrogens, or sometimes it's due to poorly functioning organs like the liver that aren't properly metabolizing estrogen out of the body, allowing it to get reabsorbed. High levels of sugar can also increase estrogen levels.

Sellman feels the other key component is low progesterone. A woman may not make progesterone because she's not ovulating, she has poor nutrition, or she was exposed to toxins in the environment. Another key issue about progesterone deficiency is the relationship to stress, according to Sellman. Since progesterone is a precursor to stress hormones, when women are under emotional or physical stress, the body uses more progesterone because it's needed to make more stress hormones.

Sellman believes that conventional medicine acts as if hormones exist separately from everything else in the body, but proper hormonal balance is directly related to the healthy functioning of all the systems of the body. Before resorting to hormone replacement, Sellman urges a functional medicine approach to identify and correct hormonal imbalances that may be contributing to immune dysfunction:

If you were healthy, had good digestion, were detoxifying your body, didn't have an overload of toxins, weren't stressed out, you wouldn't have hormonal imbalances and you wouldn't have autoimmune diseases. The myopic view of traditional allopathic medicine is to manipulate hormones when there are hormonal imbalances. But a holistic view is to correct the underlying imbalances.

Hormonal expert and educator Gillian Ford, best-selling author of *Listening to Your Hormones*, also feels that there is a very close reciprocal relationship between the hormonal and immune systems. According to Ford, you can theoretically separate the two systems or physically describe them as separate systems, but in practice they work together with other systems such as the nervous system and the sympathetic nervous system. Their joint interaction is complex and as yet poorly understood.

Medical research has concentrated mainly on hormones such as estrogen, thyroid, cortisol, and, of course, insulin in connection with autoimmune diabetes. They are important hormones, but, according to Ford, the body produces hundreds of different hormones. Some may be more fundamental in their impact on the body in terms of overall importance. Although there's not much public understanding about these other hormones—such as the vitamin Ds, parathyroid, angiotensin II, aldosterone, and prolactin—Ford believes they are where some of the most promising findings may be found:

And as far as the autoimmune system is concerned, my understanding is that treatments mainly suppress the immune system and put the disease into remission. They are not considered cures. Better solutions for those autoimmune problems will almost certainly involve hormone solutions in the future.

Attitude, Lifestyle, Mind, Body, and Spirit

Attitude, lifestyle, mind, and body have a tremendous impact on your ability to live well with autoimmune disease. Here are some of the best suggestions to help you move forward productively.

■ Start with a Positive Attitude

In sixteen studies, it was shown that patients who have positive expectations about recovery usually do recover well and are likely to have a better outcome than negative people. Michelle, who has multiple sclerosis, is a strong believer in positive thinking:

I think the best medicine is positive thinking. My mother constantly tells me I am sick and that I don't know how sick I am, and when I politely ask her to not do this, she chalks it up to a personality change (obviously for the worse!) and that I am cranky because I have MS. I am sometimes cranky because she is a pain in my neck. I am cranky when people sprinkle me with gloom and doom. I am not exactly naive or

Pollyanna, but I think maintaining a healthy attitude is the best thing anyone can do, and that includes family and friends of those who have MS.

Research published in 2001 found that a positive emotional state at an early age can actually help ward off disease and even prolong life. The experts behind the research theorize that the more optimistic a person is, the less stress that person puts on his or her body over time. When there is little stress, the body thrives, is better able to ward off infection, and has more resources to devote to healing.

Patient advocate and writer Kim Carmichael Cox says that when she first started treatment for her illness, she thought she would take a pill and everything would be okay:

I have since come to understand that there is a complex interplay within the body and all the hormonal systems. I have realized that there is no pill that can precisely alleviate every symptom of a disease process. While my health has improved from when I first became ill, there are many days when I still struggle with fatigue and a feeling of depression or brain fog. The biggest challenges for anyone dealing with a chronic illness are managing lingering symptoms and trying to live fulfilling, productive lives. What has kept me going physically, mentally, and spiritually is the belief that no matter how bad things may be, there will be better days ahead.

I think disabilities advocate and writer Gary Presley sums it up well:

Refuse to become your illness or disability. To paraphrase a rabbi who survived the Nazi death camps, our last freedom is how we react to that which happens to us, and that freedom can never be taken away. And then understand that acceptance does not mean defeat. There came a point when I recognized I could be happy or unhappy, and neither would get me out of a wheelchair on my feet. I decided happy was more fun.

■ Empower Yourself

Be Your Own "Conductor"

Patient empowerment expert and best-selling author Dr. Marie Savard feels that autoimmune disease presents the utmost of challenges for practitioners and patients, requiring them to be at their best. Dr. Savard believes that resolving an autoimmune disease requires physicians who take complaints seriously and involve patients in all aspects of their care, taking a thorough medical history and leaving no stone unturned, collecting all medical information, as well as previous tests and findings. The physician then needs to synthesize this information, based on his or her expertise, recognition of patterns of illness, personal experience with similar cases, knowledge of the latest research and technology in the diagnosis and treatment, and his or her well-honed sixth sense about things. Says Dr. Savard:

I liken the diagnosis and treatment of complex illnesses like autoimmune diseases to a symphony orchestra. To get the best, every component needs to be working together, and each member doing their part to the best of their ability. The years of working together also makes a difference in the outcome. Yet how unlikely is it today for a patient to have a longstanding relationship with a practitioner who will give them the detailed time and attention that is necessary to diagnose a challenging and complex condition, collect all the relevant information, and research all aspects of an often frustrating condition. Today the patient often needs to serve as the conductor, seeing that all the specialists have the same complete information (like having the same musical score), assuring that everyone is working together.

Dr. Savard has some rules about how to be your own conductor and get the best possible outcome with autoimmune disease:

1. Trust your instincts. You are the best expert on you!
2. Collect, read, and organize *all* your medical information, making it available to every practitioner you see who needs it.
3. Research your condition/symptoms and do your homework on you so that you truly can learn as much as, if not more than, your practitioner about your condition.
4. Form an active partnership with all your practitioners, which means both sides have obligations to each other and respect each other.
5. Share in all the decisions about your care and treatment.
6. Find the courage to treat yourself right! Once you know the right course for you, stick to it.

Patient advocate and writer Kim Carmichael Cox echoes Dr. Savard's perspectives:

I have learned that while it is important to have a doctor on whom I can rely and trust and who will work with me, I also have learned no one will ever be a better advocate for me than myself. I believe God gives a person guidance in their life, but I also believe He expects us to help ourselves. Being as informed as possible about an illness helps a person live their best with an illness and make more informed decisions regarding their own health.

Join the American Autoimmune Related Diseases Association

One of the most important things you can do is join the American Autoimmune Related Diseases Association (AARDA). An effort to collectively research and understand autoimmune diseases is one of the most important ways that scientists will be able to better pinpoint the risks, triggers, causes, and mechanisms behind autoimmune disease, and ultimately find ways to prevent it, cure it, or fully treat it, rather than simply manage it, as is the case in many conditions.

AARDA's focus is to bring about collaboration in autoimmune research education and awareness. In this effort to get researchers to collaborate, as well as to promote education and public awareness about autoimmune diseases, AARDA has led the way. It has also formed a national coalition of autoimmune patient groups, with eighteen groups to date belonging to a coordinated, national advocacy effort.

AARDA founder, president, and executive Virginia Ladd, a lupus patient herself, was president of the Lupus Foundation of America and was involved with the Lupus Foundation for twenty years. Ladd says that while she understood lupus was an autoimmune disease, as she researched she found multiple autoimmune diseases in her family, not just lupus:

I began to ask myself, why don't we look at autoimmune diseases like cancer, as conditions with a common thread? I realized we should, but no one was carrying that flag. How could we get a neurologist and rheumatologist to speak with each other? Some people were taking the same medications, but they didn't try the same drugs in different conditions. . . . Basically, the research wasn't coordinated. I knew I had to take my experience in nonprofit management and start this organization to bring a more concentrated focus on the underlying cause. I went to Dr. Noel Rose. We made a concerted effort that collaboration would be our main focus. We wanted to bring people together to understand and focus on autoimmune disease, and when people wanted information on particular conditions, we would refer them to the specific organization.

AARDA is making tremendous strides in its efforts to advance the understanding and treatment of autoimmune disease. It publishes a helpful quarterly newsletter, and sponsors various research efforts and functions. Annual membership for an individual is very affordable, and your support and research dollars help the only national organization dedicated to autoimmune disease. To join, contact

American Autoimmune Related Diseases Association
National Office
22100 Gratiot Ave. E.
Detroit, MI 48021
(810) 776-3900
http://www.aarda.org
Email: aarda@aol.com

Find Education and Support

Part of being an empowered patient is educating yourself and finding support. We are fortunate that there has never been a better time than now to find information about autoimmune diseases. In Appendix A of this book, you'll find numerous websites and books that provide in-depth information and the latest news about various autoimmune diseases. Many conditions also have organizations that can provide local or national support groups, hotlines, patient newsletters, and online support communities. A detailed list of many of these organizations is in Appendix A.

You can start your online research with the website for this book: http://www.autoimmunebook.com. Ongoing education and news are provided in the new *Autoimmune Report,* a patient-oriented newsletter that covers both conventional and alternative news, developments, and practical information about autoimmune conditions. For more information on the newsletter, send a self-addressed stamped envelope to *Autoimmune Report,* P.O. Box 0385, Palm Harbor, FL 34682.

Mary Kugler, MSN, RN, C, an expert in patient education on rare diseases who runs a popular website on the topic, feels that patients should consider adopting the two key patient empowerment approaches, self-education and support:

> *I have seen patients take two different routes. Some study everything they can find on their disorder, and could almost earn a medical degree given how much they know. They can talk "doctor talk" and ask medical questions. Not everyone, though, has the time or ability to do this, so there's another group of patients who connect with other patients having the same disorder. These ask each other for referrals to doctors, discuss what treatments did and didn't work for them, and share tips for coping with everyday living.*
>
> *The Internet has allowed people with rare diseases to find each other, both in their own countries and around the world. Many people email me or post on the forum the question, "Am I the only one with this problem?" Actually meeting someone, either online or in person in a local support group, who is experiencing what you are going through, makes a*

tremendous difference. People tell me they cry out of happiness at finding someone else with whom they can talk.

Diabetes patient Michael Phillips counsels, however, that information not be provided in a vacuum, particularly to younger patients. He found that one of the most frightening parts of being diagnosed with Type I diabetes at age 12 was being hit almost immediately with too much information and not enough support:

The literature was replete with all the possible devastating side effects of diabetes—kidney disease requiring dialysis, paralysis, blindness, painful, persistent skin problems, and impotence. I think the literature was meant to scare us into religiously following our medical routines, but it had the opposite impact on me. The cumulative weight of all those possible complications really shaped my attitudes toward relationships, sex, and the amount of energy I wanted to invest in good health. I was led to believe that all the bad side effects were inevitable, that even diabetics who became bores obsessed with the details of their disease became hapless cripples. So I lived accordingly.

It took years before Phillips revised his approach to health. He is now following a healthy diet and managing his diabetes more effectively.

■ Exercise

Exercise has so many positive benefits that it should be included in everyone's wellness efforts. Unless you are trying to lose weight, the type of exercise is not as important as simply incorporating some daily activity into your life. Even a little bit of exercise can be a help. Says rheumatoid arthritis sufferer Lina:

> *Exercise is a very difficult part when the disease affects your energy levels and causes a lot of pain in your muscles and joints. Very gentle exercise daily, even if it's just isometrics from your bed, will help ease the chronic pain in the long run. I do very light gardening, walking to the mailbox, yoga, and tai chi to help keep the joints oiled. It's not much at all, but by far, this has been the most effective in pain management.*

While experts have urged us to get exercise, even in short five- to ten-minute bursts, if you need to lose weight, you'll need to pick up the pace a bit and schedule more time. According to research reported in *Medicine & Science in Sports & Exercise,* a study of thirty middle-aged women found that those who walked briskly for half an hour burned more calories than those who took three ten-minute walks throughout the day. The calorie difference could equal the loss of approximately 5 pounds per year.

■ Get Enough Sleep/Manage Your Energy "Budget"

Insufficient sleep wreaks havoc on your immune system. Being chronically tired reduces your resistance to infection and leaves your body with insufficient levels of critical hormones and brain chemicals needed to maintain good health.

Fatigue is a common complaint in autoimmune disease, but all too frequently patients are actually not getting enough sleep. Sleep experts suggest that most adults need eight hours of sleep a night, so if you are feeling particularly tired, start by making sure you are regularly getting enough sleep.

Sandy, a college student who lives with autoimmune hepatitis, says that it has been difficult to manage this chronic illness, but the most important advice she can give is listen to your body:

I know that is a phrase that is tossed around quite frequently, but it truly is helpful. If I was ever feeling tired or overwhelmed, I took a nap or called in sick to work. Just a day or two of rest, reflection, and rejuvenation did tons for my health. I have found that my diagnosis has been both a challenge and a blessing, and it has taught me never to take health for granted.

Eunice, a nurse with CFIDS and fibromyalgia, believes in "managing her energy budget":

My fatigue level definitely affects my other symptoms. The more tired I am, the more the other symptoms bother me. I don't know if they are actually worse, or if I simply tolerate them less well. So I manage my energy budget.

Eunice's system involves getting as much rest as possible to "bank" energy so that she has extra in reserve for those inevitable times when work, family members' illness, or other stressors make it difficult to cope. Periodically, she's found herself with so much stress, anxiety, anger, and fear that she has to go into reserves, or "use her energy credit card":

Then the energy credit card gets maxed! Finally, my body forces the issue. It says, "No more credit. You must stop pushing yourself and rest/sleep more." I frequently sleep for twelve hours a night, of course interrupted by bathroom breaks and some wakeful periods. If I know I have an activity that will involve most of a day, even if I am just sitting, I rest for two or three days before, sleeping as much as possible, and not expending the energy to go out unless I absolutely have to. And I know I will be exhausted for several days afterward, even if I am able to rest at home during those days. I simply have to plan my life and activities around my energy/fatigue level. When I do that, I am able to participate in some social activities.

■ Laugh

You may remember Norman Cousins, famous as the patient who "laughed away" a near-fatal illness. But what Cousins discovered is definitely a factor in good immune health. In one Japanese study, reported in the *Journal of the American Medical Association,* a significant reduction in allergic response was seen in patients who had their allergy triggered and then watched a comedy film. The researchers concluded that laughter may play some role in helping the immune system alleviate the allergic response.

■ Manage Stress

We can't get rid of all stress, and some stress is good. We just need to manage the stress we do face and do our best to avoid unmanageable stress.

The inability to manage stress can make us more susceptible to illness. The body's response is to produce epinephrine and norepinephrine, the "adrenaline rush" hormones that produce the fight-or-flight response. When adrenaline is flooding into the body, the heart races, blood is redirected away from organs and toward muscles, the liver releases sugar, and the abdomen releases fat cells to provide quick energy. All this is useful if your house is on fire, but it's not appropriate when you get cut off in traffic, are frustrated by a boss, or are rushing from one appointment to the next trying not to be late. All that excess sugar and fat can end up harming organs.

This adrenal system is meant to step in and provide energy during short periods of high stress, but it's not meant to sustain you for long periods of time. Ultimately, the body is cheated. The increased levels of cortisol can lower white blood cell levels, and chronically elevated glucose levels can damage arteries. If you always get sick when you go through a period of great stress, you probably have a susceptible adrenal system and are subject to "adrenal burnout."

Stress can have numerous bad effects on the body:

- The redirection of blood away from the digestive system inhibits peristalsis, the squeezing motion that moves food along the gastrointestinal tract. This can cause poor absorption and inability to get nutrients.
- Reduced or increased stomach acid can damage the digestive tract or set the stage for ulcers.
- High cortisol can lead to leaky gut syndrome, which allows antigens into the bloodstream and increases the risk of food sensitivities.
- Stress imbalances blood sugar, and the resulting insulin imbalance can not only increase the risk of Type II diabetes but can cause weight gain.

Stress may even trigger damage to the body's DNA, which would explain how chronic stress could contribute to a long-term risk of cancer. In a study of medical students, researchers found that during exam time, nervous test-takers had an increase in activity in the DNA repair systems that fix cellular damage. This suggests that during the period of stress, there was an increase in damaged DNA, and damaged DNA is one factor implicated in cancer.

One recent study dispelled any doubt that mental stress can

translate to high levels of harmful hormones. The study of patients with rheumatoid arthritis found that the levels of stress hormones were significantly elevated when patients were under mental stress. But under general anesthesia, the levels dropped substantially. This study illustrated that excessive mental stress had a very specific impact on stress hormone levels, which can then affect the control and course of the disease.

New research has just shown that stress that is imposed on you passively, such as watching violence on television, may weaken your immune system. But intellectual tasks and work deadlines may actually strengthen your immune system.

Consider implementing some of the various techniques reviewed in this chapter regarding the relaxation response. Here are just a few good ways to manage stress:

- Try to eat breakfast and lunch daily.
- Plan to meditate or listen to a relaxation tape for a few minutes each day.
- Instead of drinking coffee all day, switch to herbal tea or water.
- Stop multitasking and instead concentrate on doing one thing at a time.
- Get regular exercise.
- Avoid people who are "stress carriers" or "energy vampires."
- Take a news fast and avoid watching news for a day or a week.
- Don't watch the 11 P.M. news.
- Learn how to assertively turn down requests for your time.
- Learn how to properly breathe when you are feeling stressed.
- Adopt a pet.
- Drive less aggressively.
- Resist the temptation to judge or criticize others.

- Be flexible and recognize that things don't always go as you plan.
- Pray, speak to God, your higher power, nature, or your inner guide.

■ Find a Healing/Mind-Body/Relaxation Approach

Healing refers to the overall balance of the body, mind, and spirit, so healing approaches typically fall into the same category as stress reduction and mind-body techniques. Some of the objectives of healing include

- Calming the mind, achieving a peaceful state
- Coping with stress
- Relaxing the body and mind, generating the relaxation response
- Expressing and clearing emotions
- Changing negative thoughts
- Controlling physical functions such as breathing

According to Harvard physician Dr. Herbert Benson, the nation's foremost mind-body expert, the objective of mind-body medicine is the relaxation response, where body functions become more balanced and actual physiological changes can be observed. In a radio interview with public radio host Diane Rehm, Dr. Benson articulated his thoughts:

We have found that when people regularly go into a quiet state, a large percentage of them feel the presence of a power, a force, an energy, God if you will, and they feel that presence is close to them, within them, then these people have fewer medical symptoms. Now, whether or not this is a physiological reaction independent of an external belief system, or whether or not there is indeed something out there, we cannot answer, but from the patient's point of view, they feel better.

There are so many different ways to achieve these objectives, from guided imagery to meditation to writing therapy to yoga, so how do you choose? Dr. Benson has found that meditation is particularly effective. Tai chi, breathing, prayer, and many other techniques also generate this response in different individuals. Holistic healer and educator Phylameana lila Desy has these thoughts:

Today there are so many treatment choices. I recommend my clients try a variety of methods. I suggest they pay attention not only to how their physical body reacts to these methods but to how their emotional, mental, and spiritual bodies align with the treatment. If a person feels a treatment is bizarre or silly, they may be willing to give it a try, but, in reality, they are not truly trusting that it will result in a cure. This untrusting "thought-form" may actually create a barrier between sickness and wellness. Healing touch, reiki, massage therapy, acupuncture, meditation, herbology, aromatherapy, visualization, and homeopathy are a few of the healing options that are more frequently sought out by chronic sufferers.

Physician and stress management expert Dr. Melissa Stöppler counsels that there are thousands of stress management programs, books, methods, and philosophies. Some are based on spiritual or emotional wellness, others combine mind-body relaxation techniques, and others focus entirely on physical training. The key is to find a program that works best for you and your lifestyle, and this may take some experimentation. Says Dr. Stöppler:

While techniques such as the relaxation response offer proven medical benefits in conjunction with standard therapies, many meditative and relaxation techniques must be learned and practiced before they can be beneficial. Therefore, someone who has little patience and dislikes adhering to a regular schedule may find these techniques of little use. Trying to master a time-intensive or proven stress management technique can become yet another unattainable goal and source of further stress. It is critical to find the technique, practice, or activity that works for you.

According to Dr. Stöppler, many people find that participation in a hobby or other pleasurable activity aids in relaxation. Sometimes a distracting or repetitive activity can be soothing, such as kneading bread, knitting, or even stroking a pet. "Participation in enjoyable activities and contact with close friends and loved ones are some of the best stress management measures that I have seen," says Dr. Stöppler.

Meditation

One effective healing/mind-body technique is meditation. According to the Center for Integrative Medicine at Thomas Jefferson University Hospital in Philadelphia, meditation training helped patients with chronic illnesses reduce symptoms and improve quality of life. Meditation training also helped patients cope with stress, have an improved sense of well-being, reduce body tension, and increase their clearness of thinking—all effects that benefit the immune system. Meditation has been able to lower blood pressure, help clear up skin problems, and increase melatonin levels. Researchers have also established by using magnetic resonance imaging (MRI) that meditation actually activates certain structures in the brain that control the autonomic nervous system.

Meditation has proven to be a helpful tool to Lina, a rheumatoid arthritis sufferer:

I recommend for all to learn meditation, for there have been times that has been my only saving grace from the extreme stress of being sick and disabled, especially in those first few months when I lost my job, my health, and my way of life. It's tough when you have to build your life again from scratch and spend most of your time taking care of your body when you should be out enjoying life. I often spend long hours in blissful meditation while I tend my garden, my mind quietly turned off and my feelings open to the beauty, warmth, and quiet of the world. I can happily say my life is getting back on track, and despite the illness, I am mostly a content and happy person because I take good care of my mind and my feelings.

Guided Imagery

Guided imagery can be an effective technique for healing. You can use your own imagery, or follow a book, audiotape, or practitioner. If you are feeling stress, you might envision progressively relaxing each part of your body as you relax on a warm, sunny beach, or you might envision the body's healing capabilities focusing on a damaged organ.

To try a simple guided imagery exercise, close your eyes, take several deep, full abdominal breaths, and then focus on the symptom that is bothering you. Allow an image—whatever image—to appear that represents your symptom. Don't judge the vision that appears, just accept it and observe it. What feelings do you have about it? Tell the image how you feel about it, silently or out loud. Then visualize that it is answering you, to tell you why it's there, what it wants, what it's trying to tell you to do. Ask the image if it is willing to have your symptom abate. Then decide if you're willing to give it what it wants. Continue the exchange until you feel that you've come to some sort of deal with the vision.

According to therapist and mental health educator Dr. Leonard Holmes, for an autoimmune disorder the goal is to take advantage of the connections between the nervous system and the immune system:

> *A person with rheumatoid arthritis or lupus may think about their immune system as soldiers who are at war with the person's own body. Guided imagery could be used to get them to imagine the soldiers laying down their arms or changing sides and fighting an outside enemy. They might even imagine that the soldiers get new leadership and that the new general is much more intelligent than the old one.*

Dr. O. Carl Simonton, author of the best-selling and highly recommended book *Getting Well Again*, talks about effective mental imagery for illness:

1. Create a mental picture of any ailment or pain that you have now, visualizing it in a form that makes sense to you.
2. Picture any treatment you are receiving and see it either eliminating the source of the ailment or pain or strengthening your body's ability to heal itself.
3. Picture your body's natural defenses and natural processes eliminating the source of the ailment or pain.
4. Imagine yourself healthy and free of the ailment or pain.
5. See yourself proceeding successfully toward meeting your goals in life.
6. Give yourself a mental pat on the back for participating in your recovery.

Self-Hypnosis

Another effective technique to generate the relaxation response is self-hypnosis. Research reported in the *Journal of Consulting and Clinical Psychology* found that students who received "hypnotic-relaxation training" did not have a reduction in key immune system components compared to those who did not practice the relaxation techniques. Interestingly, the more often students practiced the relaxation techniques, the stronger their immune response.

Dr. Leonard Holmes, a clinical psychologist in Virginia, believes that hypnosis can be an excellent relaxation technique for almost anyone:

> *All hypnosis is really self-hypnosis—meaning that the person is putting him or herself into a trance. For most of us, a trance is just a light relaxing state similar to daydreaming. Entering this state on a regular basis calms the sympathetic nervous system and reduces the levels of stress hormones in the bloodstream. Some people have even greater hypnotic ability. These are the people that you see on television acting silly with a stage hypnotist. People with high hypnotic ability can use hypnosis as a way to change things about their mind and body.*

Journaling

Have you ever written an email, bulletin board post, diary entry, or letter about something bothering you, and after you were finished, you felt better about the situation? You weren't imagining it—the act of writing about stressful events and situations can actually have a positive impact on your health. In a 1999 study published in the *Journal of the American Medical Association,* researchers reported that some patients with chronic diseases had improvements in their health after writing about major life stresses, such as car accidents or the death of a close friend or relative. The study looked at 112 patients. Each patient spent an hour each day writing, and four months after the study began, almost half of those who wrote about their stresses had experienced significant improvement in their health. The benefits of downloading your concerns and stresses, whether by writing in a journal or sharing your personal experiences with others who can relate via an online support group, is a natural stress reduction activity. What scientists call "expressive writing" not only gives your mind a place to unload stressful concerns or worries but can be a relaxing or peaceful activity that also helps to reduce stress by calming down your system and allowing you to focus better.

Besides straight journaling or writing-based support group participation, you can use another technique called a worry book, in which you draw a line down the page and list some of your major concerns and stresses on the left, and on the right, what steps you are taking to try to resolve the problems, or solutions you can consider.

Official worry-time writing is another technique that can be helpful. To practice, allow yourself five to fifteen minutes a day of official worry time. Sit down with your journal, and in that time, allow yourself to freely write down all your fears, stresses, and concerns. Then, at the end of the time frame, close your book or computer file, and tell yourself that if you want to worry about something, you will save it up for the next official worry time.

■ Mental Health and Relationships

Deal with Depression

It's clear that the depression associated with various medical conditions is not merely a reaction to the incapacitation, pain, and losses that accompany the physical disease process but may be directly caused by activation of the immune system. While studies have shown that positive emotions can enhance the body's immune response and stress can suppress immune function, researchers have also shown that mood can be lowered when the immune system is activated to fight infection. Patients who received an injection of a toxin that would generate an immune response to fight infection reported a significant increase in depressive symptoms and anxiety—along with a decline in memory function—in the hours after the injection.

The reported prevalence of major depressive episodes in physically ill patients varies from 5 to more than 40 percent, and researchers have discovered that people who are depressed and anxious actually heal more slowly. In one study of adults being treated for leg wounds, delayed wound healing was four times as common in patients who scored in the top half of an anxiety and depression scale. The study found that fifteen out of sixteen patients diagnosed with anxiety experienced delayed healing. Symptoms of depression include

- Persistent sad, anxious, or "empty" mood
- Feelings of hopelessness, pessimism, guilt, worthlessness, helplessness
- Loss of interest or pleasure in hobbies and activities that were once enjoyed, including sex
- Decreased energy, fatigue, being "slowed down"
- Difficulty concentrating, remembering, making decisions
- Insomnia, early morning awakening, or oversleeping
- Loss of appetite and weight loss or overeating and weight gain
- Thoughts of death or suicide; suicide attempts
- Restlessness, irritability
- Persistent physical symptoms that do not respond to treatment, such as headaches, digestive disorders, and chronic pain

If you have these symptoms, you should talk to your doctor about being evaluated for depression. Long-term clinical depression may require antidepressant therapy, in combination with talk therapy. Milder depression can frequently respond to therapy, aerobic exercise, and herbal supplements such as St. John's Wort. Getting help and relief for your depression is an essential part of your overall effort to live well with autoimmune disease.

Holistic practitioner Dr. Gina Honeyman-Lowe counsels, however, not to expect psychotherapy to heal physical conditions:

If people are dealing with the lingering emotional effects of childhood traumas, unhealthy relationships, or any other emotional difficulties, I highly advise competent psychotherapy. Many of my patients, however, before they consult me, have already sought help because a physician told them their fibromyalgia/chronic fatigue syndrome was all in their heads. With open minds and hopeful hearts, they sought help and were physically no better off afterward. Any of us walking this planet may need professional psychological help from time to time, and I advise getting it without delay. But genuine physical problems such as fibromyalgia/chronic fatigue syndrome won't be healed through meditation or psychotherapy.

Manage Family Relationships

Chronic illness can put a tremendous amount of stress on relationships, and sometimes the relationships themselves are contributing to the condition. Therapist, writer, and consultant Andrea Maloney-Schara believes that our mechanism for coping with stress makes us each like a balloon. If subject to enough stress, we will pop. Maloney-Schara says that physical illness can actually become a mechanism for coping with stress, a way to "avoid popping by finding ways to let out the air." She offers this example:

I go to work and my boss yells at me. Feeling anxious and stressed, I stop to get a drink on the way home. I actually start to feel better, so I drink more. Eventually I have to take a taxi home. My husband is waiting for me and he's mad. He says that I got drunk on purpose and begins to yell at me, just like the boss did. I go to bed and wake up with a hangover and cannot go to work. My husband feels sorry for me and begins to take care of me. He asks me what happened and says that I worried him to death.

After being diagnosed with a chronic disease, many people reported that they felt it coming. They knew they could not keep up the workload or could not stand the continual fighting with their husband or mother, and so on. Maloney-Schara explains, "We use to call this a secondary reward, getting out of an intense situation, but I think it's a reflection of the role that stress has in becoming the straw that breaks the camel's back."

Disabilities awareness advocate and writer Gary Presley believes that autoimmune disease and their resulting disabilities can cause the strongest relationships to implode, but they can also bring out a profound expansion of love between two people. Disabilities can reveal character. Says Presley:

I knew a popular local businessman whose wife developed MS. She gradually deteriorated to the point she needed full-time attendant care. He shut the doors on his business, stayed home with her for at least fifteen years (until she died from complications). He left her side only to run errands. He's a personable and outgoing guy who loved the interaction with his customers. I've never heard him complain. I never see him—now or then—that he isn't smiling. Before she died, she had reached the point where he was feeding her puréed food. The only sadness I ever heard him express was for his wife.

On the other hand, a longtime friend sat down and told his wife (a woman who uses a crutch from a bout of polio in her youth) that he couldn't stand to see her deteriorate with post-polio syndrome. He resigned as a church deacon and Sunday school teacher, filed for divorce, and moved out. She suspects an Internet romance and is devastated because he used her condition against her—a condition he knew she had when he married her.

Therapy, says Maloney-Schara, can help work out imbalances in the family that may be contributing to disease, or can help a family that is coping with chronic disease or disability:

I like the idea of a coach. But no matter what, find someone that you are comfortable with. I would advise people to find someone who is trained in systems thinking, as I think that disease and stress and family and work dynamics are an inter-acting part of the issues that one has to deal with, so enjoy your thinking time with someone interesting to you. It is difficult when one is compartmentalized, and this often must happen in medicine as the field requires specialization, but in finding a therapist you're not limited. There are hundreds of different theories that people follow. I would find out how the person decided to enter the profession and what they really think about human behavior.

■ Spirituality and Health

In his book *God, Faith, and Health: Exploring the Spiritual-Healing Connection*, social epidemiologist Jeff Levin said, "The weight of published evidence overwhelmingly confirms that our spiritual life influences our health. This can no longer be ignored."

Some research has shown that people who are considered religious may live as much as seven years longer than others, on average. A study done by California's Human Population Laboratory studied 5,000 people for twenty-eight years and reported that those with frequent church attendance had a 23 percent reduction in the chance of dying. Other studies have found that for each of the three leading causes of death in the United States—heart disease, cancer, and hypertension—people who report a religious affiliation have lower rates of illness. Researchers at Johns Hopkins University have reported that attending religious services at least once a month more than halved the risk of death due to heart disease, emphysema, suicide, and some kinds of cancers.

Dr. Christina Puchalski, director of the George Washington Institute for Spirituality and Health in Washington, DC, believes that it's important to look at things that you're grateful for and look for the positive side:

> *Having an illness can make people self-focused, so on the spiritual side, it's important to look at what you can do with your life in spite of the fact of your illness. Think about volunteerism, your work, church, family, how you can step outside of yourself and look to others to help you and for you to help them.*

Dr. Puchalski advises patients that they are going to be angry and frustrated, but the question is how to move beyond it. What can you find that will give you meaning in your life in the midst of illness? Says Dr. Puchalski:

> *Interestingly, with my younger patients, chronic illness can be a blessing in disguise. Because of their health challenges, they do have to ask those questions a lot sooner than the rest of us. Some people ask those questions, and it causes despair. But if you can move from despair into hope, my patients say they*

find a much deeper, more meaningful life than ever before. Sometimes people are even grateful for their illness.

One patient who found this to be true is long-term Type I diabetic Michael Phillips:

I have lived more intensely in many ways because I've had this sense of mortality from an early age. I've wanted to go more places, sample more cuisines, read more books, learn more, and feel more than anyone else around me because I've felt I had less time. And, ironically, because of the diabetes, and because I am no longer in denial about the disease, I have a much healthier diet than most people. I eat little fast food, very little red meat, lots of fruits and vegetables, etc. If everyone ate a diabetic-prescribed diet, we'd all get birthday greetings from Willard Scott.

Dr. Puchalski believes that although most doctors approach patients with the goal of "fixing" them, a doctor's mission should be to "serve":

Fixing assumes a person is broken. Helping assumes a person is weak. Serving assumes the patient is whole. Most of the things we deal with are not fixable . . . so what I try to tell doctors is that you're not going to be able to fix that person with, for example, lupus, but you will be able to serve them, help them cope with their condition.

While the mind-body connection is important, Dr. Puchalski cautions against the idea that illness is our own fault:

That's been some of the criticism . . . that you can will yourself into healing or remission, and if you don't, "I wasn't meditating hard enough, because I have a recurrence." I've had very religious patients who told me that "I didn't pray hard enough because otherwise my diabetes would have been cured." To say we willed a condition upon ourselves is laying a guilt trip that takes it too far.

One patient, Maddy, was diagnosed with fibromyalgia and has such pain that at times it is difficult to walk. A spiritual/mind-body approach has been an important part of her strategy:

I believe in a spiritual program. When my body won't allow me to do physical things, I have others like sewing, reading, handiwork to fall back on. I also—and I think this is very important—have the total support and encouragement from my husband and family. I have always been able to put pain away; this, of course, does not go away. But I refuse to be negative. I will continue to read, research, rest, take care of myself, and hopefully this will reach a point where I can do more.

■ Energy Work/Reiki

There are many forms of energy work, where practitioners transfer "healing energy" to recipients. One of the most popular and effective methods appears to be reiki (pronounced "ray-key"). Reiki teacher, practitioner, and holistic healer Phylameana lila Desy has described reiki as a vibrational healing modality that consists of an enormous amount of "love energy." Some practitioners may touch recipients; others just pass hands over the body. The practitioner taps into a universal "energy force," then passes on that energy to the recipient, who will receive it where it is most needed—mind or body. Says Desy:

I teach my students that reiki is a "smart energy" because it works at the level of acceptance by each individual client. Reiki will never overwhelm someone who is not accustomed to feeling energy, as it will enter the body slowly. For someone more open to the energy, it will flow more quickly, but only at the level that is needed. Reiki is a balancing remedy. It will flow directly to whatever is in imbalance and nudge it back into a more balanced state. Someone with a chronic problem did not get this condition overnight, so they would be in error to expect reiki to bring about 100 percent alignment of body imbalances following a single session. Reiki will address physical imbalances first before addressing the emotional, mental, and spiritual problems. For this reason alone, I think the benefits someone with a chronic illness could experience from consistent reiki treatments are the receiving of relief from the physical and emotional suffering.

Interestingly, reiki is one of the therapies that autoimmune disease patients frequently mention as being of help to them. One patient, Jeannie, decided to learn reiki herself after experiencing the power of a reiki treatment:

Since being diagnosed with a thyroid problem, I give myself an hour of reiki every day, usually a full-body treatment, as the reiki energy is intelligent enough to know where my body needs it. I often do quite a bit of treatment on my neck and throat area and feel a lot of heat and tingling in this part of the body. I strongly believe that it is reiki that first helped to diagnose the disorder and very definitely has helped to make me better. I had a goiter when I was first diagnosed with hypothyroidism; however, with intense reiki, this has reduced in size and swallowing is now much easier. I also feel ener-

gized following a reiki treatment. I go to regular reiki shares, whereby other reiki practitioners give me a treatment and many of them can detect my thyroid condition without any prior knowledge, just by putting their hands near my throat chakra.

Another autoimmune disease patient, Dena, had an unexpected reiki treatment after a massage:

It just resonated with me and felt so right that I decided to study it myself and became a master. I work on self-healing every day. . . . I would love to see more people become involved and benefit from this totally noninvasive, nonmedical approach to healing, plus the sessions feel just plain wonderful.

PART IV

Autoimmune Repair: Creating Your Plan

Autoimmune Disease Risk Factors and Symptoms Checklist

This checklist will help you to identify your possible risk factors for autoimmune disease and symptoms. Note that risk factors or symptoms common to almost all the key diseases covered in this book are marked as "Super-Risks" or "Super-Symptoms."

It might be helpful to make a copy of this checklist, fill it out, and bring it to your physician to aid in getting a diagnosis. Remember that if you already have an autoimmune disease, you are at risk of developing other conditions. This checklist can be helpful, since you may want to periodically assess your symptoms to see if any new patterns are signaling the onset of additional diseases.

■ Family/Personal History of Autoimmune Disease ■

If in the past you were diagnosed with, or currently have, an autoimmune disease, you have a higher risk of developing other autoimmune diseases. Also, if family members have in the past been diagnosed with, or currently have, an autoimmune disease, you face a higher risk of developing an autoimmune disease. This checklist can help you and your practitioner identify family patterns. For any applicable conditions, mark whether you have presently or in the past been diagnosed with the condition, and identify family members who have currently or in the past been diagnosed:

S for Self   P for Parent
C for Child   S for Sibling
IT for Identical Twin   FT for Fraternal Twin
GP for Grandparent

__ Addison's disease   __ Diabetes
__ Alopecia   __ Type I diabetes
__ Ankylosing spondylitis   __ Type II diabetes
__ Antiphospholipid syndrome   __ Dysautonomia
__ Autoimmune hemolytic   __ Endometriosis
   anemia   __ Eosinophilia myalgia
__ Autoimmune hepatitis   syndrome
__ Autoimmune oophoritis   __ Essential mixed
__ Behçet's disease   cryoglobulinemia
__ Bullous pemphigoid   __ Fibromyalgia
__ Celiac disease   syndrome/fibromyositis
__ Chronic fatigue immune   __ Graves' disease
   dysfunction syndrome   __ Guillain-Barré syndrome
   (CFIDS)   __ Hashimoto's thyroiditis
__ Chronic inflammatory   __ Idiopathic pulmonary
   demyelinating   fibrosis
   polyneuropathy   __ Idiopathic thrombocytopenia
__ Churg-Strauss syndrome   purpura (ITP)
__ Cicatricial pemphigoid   __ Inflammatory bowel disease
__ Cold agglutinin disease   (IBD)
__ CREST syndrome   __ Lichen planus
__ Crohn's disease   __ Lupus

___ Meniere's disease

___ Mixed connective tissue
disease (MCTD)

___ Multiple sclerosis

___ Myasthenia gravis

___ Pemphigus

___ Pernicious anemia

___ Polyarteritis nodosa

___ Polychondritis

___ Polymyalgia rheumatica

___ Polymyositis and
dermatomyositis

___ Primary agammaglobulinemia

___ Primary biliary cirrhosis

___ Psoriasis

___ Raynaud's phenomenon

___ Reiter's syndrome

___ Rheumatic fever

___ Rheumatoid arthritis

___ Sarcoidosis

___ Scleroderma

___ Sjögren's syndrome

___ Spondyloarthropathy

___ Stiff-man syndrome

___ Takayasu arteritis

___ Temporal arteritis/giant cell
arteritis

___ Thyroid disease

___ Ulcerative colitis

___ Uveitis

___ Vasculitis

___ Vitiligo

___ Wegener's granulomatosis

___ Other

___ Other

___ Other

■ Risk Factors Checklist ■

Gender/Hormonal Status

__SUPER-RISK—FEMALE: is a risk factor for most autoimmune diseases

__Currently pregnant: is a risk factor for most autoimmune diseases, particularly the autoimmune thyroid diseases

__Recent pregnancy: is a risk factor for most autoimmune diseases, particularly the autoimmune thyroid diseases, and is a trigger for flares in conditions such as lupus, multiple sclerosis, and rheumatoid arthritis

__Long menstrual cycles of more than 40 days: can be a risk factor for Type II diabetes

Nationality/Ethnicity/Origin

While autoimmune diseases are thought to strike more often in colder, industrialized countries, and generally thought to affect Caucasians and those of European descent more frequently, a few specific associations have been found.

__**Scandinavian descent:** increases your risk of developing diabetes

__**Ashkenazi Jewish descent (Jews from eastern or central Europe):** increases your risk of developing celiac disease and the irritable bowel disease ulcerative colitis

__**Jewish:** increases your risk of developing irritable bowel diseases

__**European descent:** increases your risk of developing celiac disease

__**Native American:** increases your risk of developing rheumatoid arthritis

__**Living in the Southeastern United States:** increases your risk of developing sarcoidosis

__**African-American:** increases your risk of developing sarcoidosis

Work/Chemical/Occupational Exposures

__**Exposure to silica:** occupational exposure to silica; a risk for stone masons, among others; is a risk factor for scleroderma, lupus, and connective tissue disorders

__**Exposure to silicone:** occupationally, or via ruptured breast implants, is considered a risk factor for lupus and scleroderma

__**Exposure to quartz:** is a risk factor for scleroderma and connective tissue disorders

__**Exposure to polyvinyl/vinyl chloride:** is a risk factor for scleroderma

__**Exposure to epoxy resins:** is a risk factor for scleroderma

__Exposure to solvents:__ is a risk factor for scleroderma

__Exposure to benzene:__ is a risk factor for scleroderma

__Exposure to carbon tetrachloride:__ is a risk factor for scleroderma

__Exposure to diesel fuel:__ is a risk factor for scleroderma

__Exposure to epoxy resins:__ is a risk factor for scleroderma

__Exposure to naphtha:__ is a risk factor for scleroderma

__Exposure to perchlorethylenes:__ is a risk factor for scleroderma

__Exposure to toluene:__ is a risk factor for scleroderma

__Exposure to trichloroethylene:__ is a risk factor for scleroderma

__Exposure to perchlorate:__ whether via occupational exposure or in water supply, is a risk factor for autoimmune thyroid disease

__Exposure to dioxins:__ whether via occupational exposure or environmentally, is a risk factor for autoimmune thyroid disease

__Exposure to methyl tertiary butyl (MTBE):__ whether via occupational exposure or in water supply, is a risk factor for autoimmune thyroid disease

__Exposure to fluoride:__ whether via occupational exposure or in water supply, is a risk factor for autoimmune thyroid disease

__Exposure to hair-coloring solutions:__ whether via occupational exposure or via frequent use, is a risk factor for lupus and rheumatoid arthritis

Sun, Heat, Cold Exposures

__Exposure to sunlight:__ can trigger a flare of lupus

__Hot bath or shower:__ can trigger a flare of multiple sclerosis

__Very hot weather:__ can trigger a flare of multiple sclerosis

__Fever:__ can trigger a flare of multiple sclerosis

__Exposure to changes in temperature:__ can trigger an episode of Raynaud's phenomenon

__**Exposure to cold:** can trigger an episode of Raynaud's phenomenon

Nuclear Exposure

__**Exposure to nuclear plant emissions:** is a risk factor for autoimmune thyroid disease

__**Chernobyl exposure, or living in path of the fallout in 1986/1987:** is a risk factor for autoimmune thyroid disease

__**Nevada test bombs/fallout exposure in 1950s/1960s:** living in the area of the Nevada nuclear testing during this time period is a risk factor for autoimmune thyroid disease

__**Radiation treatment to the head, neck, or chest:** is a risk factor for autoimmune thyroid disease

__**Nasal radium therapy, given from the 1940s to 1960s:** is a risk factor for autoimmune thyroid disease

Metals Exposure

__**Overexposure to mercury:** whether occupationally or environmentally, can be a risk factor for all autoimmune diseases

__**Extensive mercury dental fillings:** can be a risk factor and trigger for all autoimmune diseases

__**Overexposure to gold:** whether occupationally or environmentally, can be a risk factor for all autoimmune diseases

__**Overexposure to cadmium:** whether occupationally or environmentally, can be a risk factor for all autoimmune diseases

Dietary Factors

__**SUPER-RISK—GLUTEN/GRAIN SENSITIVITY/ALLERGY:** is a risk factor for all autoimmune diseases, particularly diabetes and autoimmune thyroid disease

__**Food allergies/sensitivities to fish (especially shellfish):** is a risk factor for all autoimmune diseases

__Food allergies/sensitivities to fruits:__ is a risk factor for all autoimmune diseases

__Food allergies/sensitivities to nuts:__ is a risk factor for all autoimmune diseases

__Food allergies/sensitivities to corn:__ is a risk factor for all autoimmune diseases

__Food allergies/sensitivities to milk products:__ is a risk factor for all autoimmune diseases

__Food allergies/sensitivities to soy products:__ is a risk factor for all autoimmune diseases

__Overconsumption of processed foods:__ is a risk factor for all autoimmune diseases

__Little to no fish or fish oils in diet:__ is a risk factor for all autoimmune diseases

__Overconsumption of the same foods:__ is a risk factor for all autoimmune diseases

__Low-protein diet:__ is a risk factor for all autoimmune diseases

__Overconsumption of sugar and simple carbohydrates:__ is a risk factor for all autoimmune diseases, particularly Type II diabetes

__Overconsumption of decaffeinated coffee:__ more than four cups a day doubles risk for rheumatoid arthritis

__Overconsumption of cow's milk:__ is a risk factor for Type I diabetes

__Not being breastfed as an infant:__ is a risk factor for Type I diabetes

__Overconsumption of animal fats:__ is a risk factor for lupus

__Overconsumption of alfalfa sprouts:__ is a risk factor for lupus

__Overconsumption of soy and "goitrogenic" food:__ is a risk factor for autoimmune thyroid disease (Goitrogenic foods include raw brussels sprouts, rutabaga, turnips, kohlrabi, radishes, cauliflower, cassava, millet, babassu, cabbage, and kale.)

__Overconsumption of coffee (i.e., 10+ cups):__ is a risk factor for rheumatoid arthritis

__Denatured rapeseed oil:__ can be a risk factor or trigger for toxic oil syndrome and scleroderma

__*Yersinia enterocolitica* infection:__ can be a risk factor for autoimmune thyroid disease

Drugs/Supplements

__Taking tainted L-tryptophan in the 1980s:__ is a risk factor for eosinophilia myalgia syndrome (EMS)

__Interferon drugs (alpha-, beta-, and gamma-interferon) and interleukin-2:__ are risk factors for lupus

__D-penicillamine:__ can be a risk factor or trigger for myasthenia gravis, scleroderma, drug-induced lupus, and Guillain-Barré syndrome

__Quinidine:__ can be a risk factor or trigger for myasthenia gravis

__Propanolol:__ can be a risk factor or trigger for myasthenia gravis

__Trimethadone:__ can be a risk factor or trigger for myasthenia gravis

__Lithium:__ can be a risk factor or trigger for myasthenia gravis, autoimmune hypothyroidism, and psoriasis

__Iodine/iodine supplements (kelp, bladder wrack, or bugleweed):__ can be a risk factor or trigger for autoimmune thyroid disease

__Hydralazine (Apresoline):__ can be a risk factor or trigger for lupus

__Isoniazid (Laniazid):__ can be a risk factor or trigger for lupus

__Procainamide (Pronestyl, Procanbid):__ can be a risk factor or trigger for lupus

__Methyldopa (Aldomet):__ can be a risk factor or trigger for lupus

__Thorazine (Chlorpromazine):__ can be a risk factor or trigger for lupus

__Medicinal gold:__ can be a risk factor or trigger for Guillain-Barré syndrome

__Beta-blockers:__ can be a risk factor or trigger for psoriasis

__Fenfluramine use:__ can be a risk factor or trigger for scleroderma

__Cocaine use:__ can be a risk factor or trigger for scleroderma

__Heroin use:__ can be a risk factor or trigger for Guillain-Barré syndrome

Bacterial and Viral Infections and Illnesses

__SUPER-RISK—RECENT INFECTION (GENERAL):__ Having had a recent infection in general can increase your risk of developing an autoimmune disease, particularly Guillain-Barré syndrome and multiple sclerosis.

__Epstein-Barr virus/mononucleosis:__ Having had a recent bout of mononucleosis, or a flare-up of Epstein-Barr, the virus that causes mononucleosis, is a risk factor for all autoimmune diseases, but particularly rheumatoid arthritis, Sjögren's syndrome, and Guillain-Barré syndrome

__Coxsackie groups A and B viruses:__ Having one of these viruses is a risk factor for Type I diabetes but may be a risk factor for other autoimmune diseases as well.

__*Mycoplasma pneumoniae* infection:__ is a risk factor for rheumatoid arthritis and Guillain-Barré syndrome

__*Mycoplasma fermentans* infection:__ is a risk factor for rheumatoid arthritis, chronic fatigue, and fibromyalgia

__*Mycobacterium tuberculosis* infection:__ is a risk factor for rheumatoid arthritis

__Cytomegalovirus (CMV) infection:__ is a risk factor for Sjögren's syndrome, rheumatoid arthritis, and Guillain-Barré syndrome

__Parvovirus infection: is a risk factor for rheumatoid arthritis

__Rubella infection: is a risk factor for rheumatoid arthritis

__*Yersinia enterocolitica* infection: is a risk factor for autoimmune thyroid disease

__Human herpes virus type 6 (HHV-6) infection: is a risk factor for Sjögren's syndrome

__Herpes infection: is a risk factor for Sjögren's syndrome

__Hepatitis C infection: is a risk factor for Sjögren's syndrome

__Infection with *Helicobacter pylori:* is a risk factor for rheumatoid arthritis and pernicious anemia

__Sexually transmitted infection (i.e., chlamydia): is a risk factor for Reiter's syndrome

__*Campylobacter jejuni* infection: is a risk factor for Guillain-Barré syndrome

__Polio infection: is a risk factor for Type I diabetes

Other Factors

__Obesity: can be a risk factor for Type II diabetes

__Periodontal disease: is a risk factor for all autoimmune diseases

__Not drinking enough water: is a general risk factor for all autoimmune diseases

__Not enough sleep: is a general risk factor for low immune function, which adds to risk of developing autoimmune diseases

__Not washing hands regularly: is a general risk factor for infection, which adds to risk of developing autoimmune diseases

__Frequent use of or exposure to hair dye: may contribute to the risk of rheumatoid arthritis and lupus

__Lack of exercise: is a risk factor for Type II diabetes

__Recent surgery: is a risk factor for Guillain-Barré syndrome

Smoking
__Current or past smoking: can in general reduce immune function, but a history of smoking is a particular risk factor for autoimmune thyroid disease, lupus, psoriasis, and autoimmune oophoritis/premature ovarian failure.

Vaccinations/Immunizations
__Anthrax vaccine: is a risk factor for lupus, inflammatory demyelinating diseases, and Guillain-Barré syndrome
__Hepatitis B vaccine: is a risk factor for multiple sclerosis
__Recent immunization in general (i.e., flu vaccine, rabies, and strep): is a risk factor for Guillain-Barré syndrome

Trauma/Physical Injury
__Repeated hand-arm vibration injury (jackhammer and chainsaw operators): is a risk factor for scleroderma
__Neck trauma: is a risk factor for autoimmune thyroid disease
__Automobile accident: is a risk factor for autoimmune thyroid disease and multiple sclerosis

Stress
__Chronic physical stress: is a risk factor for all autoimmune diseases
__Chronic emotional stress: is a risk factor for all autoimmune diseases

■ Symptoms Checklist ■

Joint and Muscle Pain
__SUPER-SYMPTOM—JOINT/MUSCLE PAIN: Pain in the joints and muscles is one of the most common autoimmune disease symptoms and is a key symptom of rheumatoid

arthritis. Joint and muscle pain can be found in almost every autoimmune disease.

__**General pain, burning, aching, and soreness:** can be a symptom of fibromyalgia and multiple sclerosis

__**Moving pain:** that shifts from one joint to another without swelling or redness can be a symptom of chronic fatigue immune dysfunction syndrome

__**General bone pain:** can be a symptom of celiac disease

__**Joint pain, aches:** is a key symptom of rheumatoid arthritis, and is also a symptom of lupus, mixed connective tissue disease, sarcoidosis, Sjögren's syndrome, Reiter's syndrome, scleroderma, dysautonomia, Addison's disease, and autoimmune thyroid disease

__**Joint stiffness:** is a key symptom of rheumatoid arthritis, and is also a symptom of psoriasis, multiple sclerosis, and lupus

__**Muscle pains and aches:** can be found in most autoimmune diseases, particularly Addison's disease, autoimmune thyroid disease, lupus, sarcoidosis, and Sjögren's syndrome

__**Muscle cramping and twitching:** can be symptoms of fibromyalgia

__**Stiffness, particularly in the morning:** is a key symptom of rheumatoid arthritis, but can also be a symptom of fibromyalgia and Sjögren's syndrome

__**Swelling, warmth, and tenderness of joints:** is a key symptom of rheumatoid arthritis, and can be seen in most autoimmune diseases, but can also be a symptom of fibromyalgia, Sjögren's syndrome, ulcerative colitis, and lupus

__**Knee pain/stiffness:** is a key symptom in scleroderma, Reiter's syndrome, and fibromyalgia

__**Tendinitis in legs:** can be a symptom of autoimmune thyroid disease and rheumatoid arthritis

__**Joint stiffness in ankles and feet:** can be a symptom of Reiter's syndrome; pain in heels can be a symptom of ankylosing spondylitis

___**Achilles tendinitis/pain in Achilles tendon in foot:** can be a symptom of Reiter's syndrome

___**Plantar's fasciitis/pain in sole of foot:** can be a symptom of ankylosing spondylitis, Hashimoto's thyroiditis/hypothyroidism, and Reiter's syndrome

___**Throbbing in toes:** can be a symptom of Raynaud's phenomenon

___**Pain in hips:** can be a symptom of fibromyalgia and ankylosing spondylitis

___**Radiation of pain into the buttocks from the back:** can be a symptom of ankylosing spondylitis

___**Pain in the buttocks:** can be a symptom of fibromyalgia and Guillain-Barré syndrome

___**Back pain relieved by movement or exercise:** can be a symptom of ankylosing spondylitis

___**Pain in the lower back:** can be a symptom of fibromyalgia, Guillain-Barré syndrome, and Reiter's syndrome

___**Carpal tunnel syndrome:** including its symptoms of tingling in fingertips, weakness of hands/fingers, and pain in forearm, can be a symptom of Hashimoto's thyroiditis/hypothyroidism and scleroderma

___**Tendinitis in arms:** can be a symptom of Hashimoto's thyroiditis/hypothyroidism

___**Elbow pain:** can be a symptom of fibromyalgia and scleroderma

___**Wrist pain:** can be a symptom of scleroderma

___**Finger pain:** can be a symptom of scleroderma and Raynaud's phenomenon

___**Skull pain:** in back of skull, can be a symptom of fibromyalgia

___**Facial pain:** can be a symptom of scleroderma

___**Neck pain/stiffness:** can be a symptom of fibromyalgia and autoimmune thyroid disease

__Shoulder pain:__ can be a symptom of fibromyalgia, scleroderma, and mixed connective tissue disease

Muscle and General Weakness
__SUPER-SYMPTOM—GENERAL MUSCLE WEAKNESS:__ Feeling weak, particularly in muscles, is a common autoimmune disease symptom, and may be seen in most conditions.

__Muscle fatigue after exercise:__ can be a symptom of chronic fatigue immune dysfunction syndrome and myasthenia gravis

__General muscle pain:__ can be a symptom of chronic fatigue immune dysfunction syndrome

__Loss of arm or hand strength:__ can be a symptom of multiple sclerosis and Graves' disease/hyperthyroidism

__Loss of leg/thigh strength:__ can be a symptom of multiple sclerosis and Graves' disease/hyperthyroidism

__Facial weakness:__ can be a symptom of Guillain-Barré syndrome

__Sore hips:__ can be a symptom of mixed connective tissue disease

__Reduced or absent reflexes:__ can be a symptom of Guillain-Barré syndrome and Hashimoto's disease/hypothyroidism

__Increased reflexes:__ can be a symptom of multiple sclerosis and Graves' disease/hyperthyroidism

__Paralysis:__ can be a symptom of multiple sclerosis

Infections/Immune System/Resistance/Allergies
__SUPER-SYMPTOM—INFECTIONS:__ Greater susceptibility and more frequent infections—such as urinary tract, bladder, gum, skin, or vaginal infections, as well as viruses—and slower recovery from those infections are common symptoms of autoimmune disease.

__More frequent cold sores:__ can be a symptom of Sjögren's syndrome

__Development or worsening of allergies:__ can be a symptom of Hashimoto's thyroiditis/hypothyroidism and chronic fatigue immune dysfunction syndrome

__Chronic sinus infections:__ can be a symptom of Hashimoto's thyroiditis/hypothyroidism

__Chronic yeast infections:__ can be a symptom of Hashimoto's thyroiditis/hypothyroidism and Sjögren's syndrome

__Oral fungus or thrush:__ can be a symptom of Hashimoto's thyroiditis/hypothyroidism

Feelings/Senses/Cravings

__Heightened senses of smell, taste, and hearing:__ can be a symptom of Addison's disease

__Impaired smell:__ can be a symptom of pernicious anemia

__Cravings for salt:__ can be a symptom of Addison's disease

__Sensation in the legs that progresses up to the arms:__ can be a symptom of Guillain-Barré syndrome

__Sensation of warmth:__ can be a symptom of multiple sclerosis

__Sense of fullness:__ can be a symptom of pernicious anemia

__Feeling hot:__ can be a symptom of Graves' disease/hyperthyroidism

__Feeling cold:__ can be a symptom of chronic fatigue immune dysfunction syndrome and Hashimoto's disease/hypothyroidism

__Hot flashes:__ can be a symptom of autoimmune oophoritis/premature ovarian failure

__Intolerance to cold:__ can be a symptom of Addison's disease and Hashimoto's thyroiditis/hypothyroidism

__Sensitivity to heat:__ can be a symptom of Graves' disease/hyperthyroidism

__Hypersensitivity to temperatures, sounds, sensations, confu-sion:** can be a symptom of chronic fatigue immune dysfunc-tion syndrome

Walking/Balance/Posture/Flexibility

__Balance problems/clumsiness/unsteadiness:** can be a symp-tom of fibromyalgia, pernicious anemia, and multiple sclerosis

__Feeling of clumsiness in hands and fingers:** can be a symptom of Raynaud's phenomenon

__Difficulty walking:** can be a symptom of multiple sclerosis, ankylosing spondylitis, and Addison's disease

__Bent-over posture:** can be a symptom of ankylosing spondy-litis

__Difficulty bending the spine:** can be a symptom of ankylosing spondylitis and rheumatoid arthritis

__Fingers frozen in flexed position:** can be a symptom of sclero-derma

__Elbows frozen in flexed position:** can be a symptom of scle-roderma

__Wrists frozen in flexed position:** can be a symptom of sclero-derma

__Paralysis:** can be a symptom of multiple sclerosis

Skin Nodules and Lesions

__SUPER-SYMPTOM—RASHES:** Rashes and skin involve-ment are common symptoms of autoimmune diseases in gen-eral, particularly lupus, autoimmune thyroid disease, and sarcoidosis.

__Butterfly-shaped rash on the nose and cheeks:** can be a symp-tom of lupus and mixed connective tissue disease

__Discoid lesions:** disc-shaped lesions on the scalp, face, neck, and ears can be a symptom of lupus

__Red-purple areas on palms and fingers:__ can be a symptom of lupus and sarcoidosis

__Rashes, lesions on the face and extremities:__ can be a symptom of sarcoidosis

__Rash, blisters, and pustules on palms and soles:__ can be a symptom of Reiter's syndrome, psoriasis, and pemphigus

__Blisters/pustules:__ clear, soft, fluid-filled blisters that rupture and do not heal can be a symptom of pemphigus

__Skin lesions:__ can be a symptom of Crohn's disease and sarcoidosis

__Blisters:__ can be a symptom of pemphigus

__Sores on fingertips and knuckles:__ can be a symptom of scleroderma

__Scaly lesions:__ raised inflamed lesions covered with silvery white scale on knees, elbows, scalp, and trunk can be a symptom of psoriasis

__Smooth, inflamed lesions:__ in armpit, groin, under the breast, and in the folds of the skin can be a symptom of psoriasis

__Sores on fingertips and knuckles:__ can be a symptom of scleroderma

__Small red dots on the body trunk, arms, and legs, dots may have scales:__ can be a symptom of psoriasis

__Hives/urticaria:__ can be a symptom of Hashimoto's thyroiditis/hypothyroidism and Crohn's disease

__Spider veins or dilated blood vessels:__ on fingers, chest, and face can be a symptom of scleroderma

__Lesions and nodules under the skin:__ can be a symptom of sarcoidosis

__Calcium deposits:__ causing bumps on fingers, bony areas, and joints, can be a symptom of scleroderma

__Nodules near joints:__ skin bumps called rheumatoid nodules, located near joints, can be a symptom of rheumatoid arthritis

__**Sun sensitivity:** including sunburn or rash after exposure to sunlight, can be a symptom of lupus

__**Tendency to bruise:** can be a symptom of lupus

__**Itching:** can be a symptom of psoriasis, multiple sclerosis, alopecia, autoimmune thyroid disease, Type II diabetes, and scleroderma

__**Dry skin:** can be a symptom of Graves' disease/hyperthyroidism

__**Scaly patches:** can be a symptom of pemphigus

__**Hyperpigmentation:** areas of skin coloration, such as tan or freckles, in the skin and mucous membranes, can be a symptom of Addison's disease and scleroderma

__**Hypopigmentation:** areas of loss of pigmentation, frequently white spots, can be a symptom of vitiligo, Addison's disease, and scleroderma

__**Color changing:** skin on hands and feet that changes colors to white, blue, or red, can be a symptom of Raynaud's phenomenon

__**White patches:** of colorless skin, can be a symptom of vitiligo

__**Waxiness:** lemon-yellow waxy appearance to the skin, can be a symptom of pernicious anemia

__**Pallor/paleness:** can be a symptom of skin pernicious anemia

__**Taut, shiny, darker skin:** may appear to be tanned, can be a symptom of scleroderma

__**Thickened patches on shins and legs:** can be a symptom of Graves' disease/hyperthyroidism

__**Thickening and swelling of the ends of the fingers:** can be a symptom of scleroderma

__**Slow healing of cuts and bruises:** can be a symptom of diabetes

Fatigue

__SUPER-SYMPTOM—FATIGUE: Fatigue is one of the most common autoimmune disease symptoms and is found in most conditions, so it is considered a general symptom of all conditions.

__Extreme fatigue: can be a symptom of chronic fatigue immune dysfunction syndrome, autoimmune thyroid disease, multiple sclerosis, and Type II diabetes

__Unrefreshing sleep: fatigue right after you wake up, more common in chronic fatigue immune dysfunction syndrome and autoimmune thyroid disease

__Fatigue with or after normal activity: can be a symptom of chronic fatigue immune dysfunction syndrome and fibromyalgia

__Postexertional malaise: (fatigue after exercise, usually lasting more than twenty-four hours), can be a symptom of chronic fatigue immune dysfunction syndrome

Sleep Changes

__Insomnia: can be a symptom of autoimmune oophoritis/premature ovarian failure, Graves' disease/hyperthyroidism, and fibromyalgia

__Difficulty falling asleep: can be a symptom of autoimmune oophoritis/premature ovarian failure, Graves' disease/hyperthyroidism, and fibromyalgia

__Frequent waking: can be a symptom of autoimmune oophoritis/premature ovarian failure, Graves' disease/hyperthyroidism, and fibromyalgia

Fever/Temperature Changes

__SUPER-SYMPTOM—LOW-GRADE FEVER: seen in almost all autoimmune diseases

__Extremely high temperatures: can be a symptom of Addison's disease

___Fluctuations of body temperature:__ can be a symptom of Guillain-Barré syndrome

___Low basal body temperature:__ can be a symptom of Hashimoto's thyroiditis/hypothyroidism

Lymph Nodes/Glands

___Swollen lymph nodes/glands:__ can be a symptom of lupus, mixed connective tissue disease, sarcoidosis, rheumatoid arthritis, and chronic fatigue immune dysfunction syndrome

Sweating

___Night sweats:__ can be a symptom of sarcoidosis, autoimmune oophoritis/premature ovarian failure, and chronic fatigue immune dysfunction syndrome

___Sweating more than usual:__ can be a symptom of Graves' disease/hyperthyroidism and dysautonomia

Other Symptoms

___Breath that smells like nail polish remover:__ can be a symptom of Type I diabetes

___Ringing in the ears/tinnitus:__ can be a symptom of pernicious anemia

___Growth retardation in infants and children:__ can be a symptom of Crohn's disease, celiac disease, and Hashimoto's thyroiditis/hypothyroidism

___Cholesterol unresponsive to diet and medication:__ can be a symptom of Hashimoto's thyroiditis/hypothyroidism

___Reactivity to environmental exposures__ (i.e., increased sensitivity to chemicals, perfumes, odors, bug sprays, etc.): can be a symptom of chronic fatigue immune dysfunction syndrome

Hands and Feet

__SUPER-SYMPTOM—NUMBNESS/TINGLING IN HANDS/ FEET: can be seen in most autoimmune diseases

__Swelling in hands and fingers: can be a symptom of mixed connective tissue disease

__Cold hands and feet: can be a symptom of fibromyalgia, Hashimoto's thyroiditis/hypothyroidism, Raynaud's phenomenon, and scleroderma

__Color changes in hands and feet: can be a symptom of scleroderma

__Feeling of clumsiness in hands and fingers: can be a symptom of Raynaud's phenomenon

__Fingers frozen in flexed position: can be a symptom of scleroderma

__Sores on fingertips and knuckles: can be a symptom of scleroderma

__Thickening and swelling of the ends of the fingers: can be a symptom of scleroderma

Tremors and Seizures

__Restless leg syndrome: can be a symptom of fibromyalgia

__Seizures: can be a symptom of Type I diabetes

__Tremors: can be a symptom of multiple sclerosis

__Hand tremors: can be a symptom of Graves' disease/hyperthyroidism

Face

__Parotid gland inflammation and enlargement: can be a symptom of sarcoidosis

__Facial weakness: can be a symptom of Guillain-Barré syndrome

Eyes

__**SUPER-SYMPTOM—DRY EYES:** a symptom found in almost all autoimmune diseases, particularly Sjögren's syndrome

__**Swollen eyes:** can be a symptom of lupus, Reiter's syndrome, Hashimoto's thyroiditis/hypothyroidism, and ankylosing spondylitis

__**Pain/burning in eyes, or when eyes move:** can be a symptom of multiple sclerosis, ankylosing spondylitis, Sjögren's syndrome, Reiter's syndrome, and rheumatoid arthritis

__**Blurry vision:** can be a symptom of sarcoidosis, multiple sclerosis, diabetes, and dysautonomia

__**Tearing eyes:** can be a symptom of sarcoidosis and Reiter's syndrome

__**Red eyes:** can be a symptom of sarcoidosis and ankylosing spondylitis

__**Double vision:** can be a symptom of sarcoidosis, multiple sclerosis, myasthenia gravis, and Graves' disease/hyperthyroidism

__**Light sensitivity:** can be a symptom of Sjögren's syndrome, sarcoidosis, Reiter's syndrome, ankylosing spondylitis, and Graves' disease/hyperthyroidism

__**Gritty/itchy/sandy feeling:** can be a symptom of Sjögren's syndrome, Reiter's syndrome, rheumatoid arthritis, ulcerative colitis, and Graves' disease/hyperthyroidism

__**Ghosting:** a visual disturbance "ghost image" or flashes of light when the eyes move, can be a symptom of Sjögren's syndrome and multiple sclerosis

__**Bulging eyes:** can be a symptom of Graves' disease/hyperthyroidism

__**Drooping eyelids:** can be a symptom of myasthenia gravis

__**Jerky eye movements:** can be a symptom of multiple sclerosis

__**Weak eye muscles:** can be a symptom of myasthenia gravis

__**Weak eyelids:** can be a symptom of myasthenia gravis

__Dim vision:__ can be a symptom of multiple sclerosis

__Loss of central vision:__ can be a symptom of multiple sclerosis

__Color distortion:__ can be a symptom of multiple sclerosis

__Depth perception problems:__ can be a symptom of multiple sclerosis

__Partial blindness:__ can be a symptom of multiple sclerosis

Weight

__SUPER-SYMPTOM—WEIGHT LOSS:__ not extensive, but typically in the 10- to 15-pound range, can be a sign of numerous autoimmune diseases

__Weight loss, even with good appetite or overeating:__ can be a symptom of Type I diabetes and Graves' disease/hyperthyroidism

__Unusually large and/or rapid weight loss:__ can be a symptom of Type I diabetes and Graves' disease/hyperthyroidism

__Difficulty losing weight:__ can be a symptom of Hashimoto's thyroiditis/hypothyroidism

__Inappropriate weight gain:__ can be a symptom of Hashimoto's thyroiditis/hypothyroidism

Appetite/Thirst Changes

__Lack of appetite:__ can be a symptom of pernicious anemia, ankylosing spondylitis, Addison's disease, sarcoidosis, and Graves' disease/hyperthyroidism

__Extreme hunger:__ can be a symptom of Type II diabetes and Graves' disease/hyperthyroidism

__Increased thirst:__ can be a symptom of Sjögren's syndrome and diabetes

__Dehydration:__ can be a symptom of Addison's disease and ulcerative colitis

Hair/Nails/Scalp

__**SUPER-SYMPTOM—HAIR LOSS:** General hair loss is a common symptom of many autoimmune diseases.

__**Hair loss in round or oval patches:** can be a symptom of alopecia

__**Small patches of hair loss:** can be a symptom of mixed connective tissue disease

__**Loss of outer eyebrow hair:** can be a symptom of Hashimoto's thyroiditis/hypothyroidism

__**Decreased body hair in women:** can be a symptom of Addison's disease

__**Fine, brittle hair:** can be a symptom of Graves' disease/hyperthyroidism

__**Dry, tangled, or coarse hair:** can be a symptom of Hashimoto's thyroiditis/hypothyroidism

__**Tenderness of the scalp:** can be a symptom of fibromyalgia

__**Premature whitening of the hair:** can be a symptom of pernicious anemia

__**Brittle fingernails:** can be a symptom of Hashimoto's thyroiditis/hypothyroidism

__**Pitting, yellowing, and thickening of nails:** can be a symptom of alopecia and psoriasis

__**Hyperpigmentation in nails:** can be a symptom of Addison's disease

Mouth/Oral

__**SUPER-SYMPTOM—DRY MOUTH:** Having a dry mouth is a common symptom in many autoimmune diseases.

__**Mouth pain:** can be a symptom of pemphigus, Reiter's syndrome, lupus, pernicious anemia, and Sjögren's syndrome

__**Burning sensation in mouth:** can be a symptom of Sjögren's syndrome

__Spider veins or dilated blood vessels on lips and tongue:__ can be a symptom of scleroderma

__Bleeding gums and gum infection:__ can be a symptom of pernicious anemia and diabetes

__Loosening of teeth:__ can be a symptom of scleroderma

__Recurrent cavities:__ can be a symptom of Sjögren's syndrome

__Difficulty chewing and swallowing:__ can be a symptom of Sjögren's syndrome and myasthenia gravis

__Breath that smells like nail polish remover:__ can be a symptom of diabetes

Respiratory/Throat/Neck

__SUPER-SYMPTOM—SHORTNESS OF BREATH:__ Generally and upon exertion, is a common symptom of many autoimmune conditions, and may also be manifested as feeling the need to yawn to get a full breath, or heaviness in the chest that makes breathing more difficult.

__Cough:__ can be a symptom of sarcoidosis, Sjögren's syndrome, scleroderma, and mixed connective tissue disease

__Deep, rapid breathing:__ can be a symptom of Type I diabetes

__Difficulty chewing and swallowing:__ can be a symptom of Sjögren's syndrome, myasthenia gravis, mixed connective tissue disease, and scleroderma

__Hoarseness/raspy voice:__ can be a symptom of mixed connective tissue disease, sarcoidosis, scleroderma, and Hashimoto's thyroiditis/hypothyroidism

__Tonsillitis:__ can be a symptom of sarcoidosis

__Parotid gland inflammation and enlargement:__ can be a symptom of sarcoidosis

__Sore throat:__ can be a symptom of chronic fatigue immune dysfunction syndrome and autoimmune thyroid disease

__**Full or sensitive feeling in the neck:** can be a symptom of Hashimoto's thyroiditis/hypothyroidism

__**Enlarged salivary or parotid glands:** can be a symptom of Sjögren's syndrome

__**Enlarged thyroid gland:** can be a symptom of autoimmune thyroid disease

Chest/Heart/Blood Pressure/Pulse Rate

__**SUPER-SYMPTOM—PALPITATIONS:** Feeling missed heartbeats, changes in rhythm, skipped beats, irregular heart rhythms, and other types of palpitations are common autoimmune disease symptoms.

__**Rapid heart rate/tachycardia:** can be a symptom of ulcerative colitis, pernicious anemia, dysautonomia, sarcoidosis, and Graves' disease/hyperthyroidism

__**Chest pain:** can be a symptom of lupus, sarcoidosis, scleroderma, and fibromyalgia

__**Atrial fibrillation:** a special type of abnormal heart rhythm, can be a symptom of Graves' disease/hyperthyroidism

__**Fluctuations in heart rate and blood pressure:** can be a symptom of Guillain-Barré syndrome

__**Low blood pressure:** with its associated symptoms of dizziness and fainting, can be a symptom of dysautonomia, Addison's disease, and Hashimoto's thyroiditis/hypothyroidism

__**Neurally mediated hypotension** (when you stand up, your blood pressure drops, which can make you feel dizzy, nauseous, your heart rate drops, and you can even faint): can be a symptom of chronic fatigue immune dysfunction syndrome and Addison's disease

__**Increased blood pressure:** can be a symptom of Graves' disease/hyperthyroidism and scleroderma

__**High heart rate:** can be a symptom of Graves' disease/hyperthyroidism

Abdominal/Digestive

__Abdominal pain/cramps/tenderness:__ can be a symptom of mixed connective tissue disease, celiac disease, ulcerative colitis, Addison's disease, Type I diabetes, pernicious anemia, ulcerative colitis, Crohn's disease, and Sjögren's syndrome

__Bloating:__ can be a symptom of chronic fatigue immune dysfunction syndrome, fibromyalgia, and celiac disease

__Heartburn:__ can be a symptom of mixed connective tissue disease, scleroderma, and pernicious anemia

__Nausea:__ can be a symptom of Sjögren's syndrome, Addison's disease, and pernicious anemia

__Vomiting:__ can be a symptom of Type I diabetes, Addison's disease, and pernicious anemia

Urinary Tract/Bowel Habits

__Diarrhea:__ can be a symptom of scleroderma, Addison's disease, fibromyalgia, Graves' disease/hyperthyroidism, pernicious anemia, chronic fatigue immune dysfunction syndrome, Crohn's disease, celiac disease, and Reiter's syndrome

__Bloody diarrhea:__ can be a symptom of ulcerative colitis

__Constipation:__ can be a symptom of scleroderma, pernicious anemia, chronic fatigue immune dysfunction syndrome, fibromyalgia, multiple sclerosis, and Hashimoto's thyroiditis/hypothyroidism

__Bowel-control problems:__ can be a symptom of multiple sclerosis

__Bowel urgency:__ can be a symptom of ulcerative colitis

__Stools with a foul odor:__ can be a symptom of celiac disease

__Tan or gray stools:__ can be a symptom of celiac disease

__Oily or frothy stools:__ can be a symptom of celiac disease

__Watery or semiformed stools:__ can be a symptom of celiac disease

__Excessive or explosive gas:__ can be a symptom of celiac disease and pernicious anemia

__Bladder infections:__ can be a symptom of Sjögren's syndrome

__Frequent urination:__ can be a symptom of fibromyalgia, multiple sclerosis, and Type I diabetes

__High volume of urine:__ can be a symptom of Type I diabetes

__Bladder-control problems:__ can be a symptom of multiple sclerosis and pernicious anemia

__Difficulty urinating:__ can be a symptom of multiple sclerosis and Guillain-Barré syndrome

__Painful urination:__ can be a symptom of Reiter's syndrome

__Bedwetting in children:__ can be a symptom of Type I diabetes

__Inflamed and painful prostate:__ can be a symptom of Reiter's syndrome

Gynecological/Reproductive/Fertility/Sex Drive

__SUPER-SYMPTOM—RECURRENT MISCARRIAGE:__ Recurrent miscarriage is a very common symptom in various autoimmune diseases

__Infertility:__ can be a symptom of Graves' disease/hyperthyroidism, Hashimoto's thyroiditis/hypothyroidism, celiac disease, and autoimmune oophoritis/premature ovarian failure

__Absence of menstrual periods:__ can be a symptom of celiac disease, Addison's disease, Graves' disease/hyperthyroidism, and autoimmune oophoritis/premature ovarian failure

__Delayed start of menstrual periods in adolescents:__ can be a symptom of celiac disease and Hashimoto's thyroiditis/hypothyroidism

__Periods are lighter, less frequent:__ can be a symptom of Graves' disease/hyperthyroidism

__Heavier, longer, more painful menstrual periods:__ can be a symptom of autoimmune oophoritis/premature ovarian failure, Hashimoto's thyroiditis/hypothyroidism, and fibromyalgia

__Irregular periods:__ can be a symptom of autoimmune oophoritis/premature ovarian failure and autoimmune thyroid disease

__Reduced or low sex drive:__ can be a symptom of Hashimoto's thyroiditis/hypothyroidism, Addison's disease, and autoimmune oophoritis/premature ovarian failure

__Difficulty reaching orgasm:__ can be a symptom of multiple sclerosis

__Difficulty getting an erection:__ can be a symptom of scleroderma

__Impotence in men:__ can be a symptom of Addison's disease, pernicious anemia, multiple sclerosis, and celiac disease

__Lack of sensation in the vagina:__ can be a symptom of multiple sclerosis

__Vaginal discharge:__ can be a symptom of Reiter's syndrome

__Vaginal dryness:__ can be a symptom of autoimmune oophoritis/premature ovarian failure

__Pelvic pain:__ can be a symptom of fibromyalgia

__Painful sex:__ can be a symptom of autoimmune oophoritis/premature ovarian failure

__Pain and discharge from the penis:__ can be a symptom of Reiter's syndrome

Neurological

__Dizziness/vertigo:__ can be a symptom of sarcoidosis, Addison's disease, multiple sclerosis, and celiac disease

__Headaches:__ can be a symptom of lupus, sarcoidosis, scleroderma, Type I diabetes, pernicious anemia, and fibromyalgia

__Headaches of a new type, pattern, or severity:__ can be a symptom of chronic fatigue immune dysfunction syndrome

__Fainting:__ can be a symptom of celiac disease, dysautonomia, and Addison's disease

__Seizures:__ can be a symptom of lupus

Mental Health

__**SUPER-SYMPTOM—DEPRESSION:** is a common symptom in most autoimmune conditions

__**Anxiety:** can be a symptom of Graves' disease/hyperthyroidism, fibromyalgia, and dysautonomia

__**Panic attacks:** can be a symptom of Graves' disease/hyperthyroidism

__**Excessive irritability:** can be a symptom of chronic fatigue immune dysfunction syndrome, Type I diabetes, pernicious anemia, and Graves' disease/hyperthyroidism

__**Ill-tempered behavior in children:** can be a symptom of Type I diabetes and Addison's disease

__**Erratic behavior/ personality changes:** can be a symptom of pernicious anemia and Graves' disease/hyperthyroidism

__**Mood/emotional changes:** can be a symptom of multiple sclerosis, Addison's disease, and autoimmune oophoritis/premature ovarian failure

__**Mental confusion:** can be a symptom of fibromyalgia, Addison's disease, chronic fatigue immune dysfunction syndrome, diabetes, and autoimmune thyroid disease

__**Psychosis/delusions/hallucinations:** can be a symptom of lupus and pernicious anemia

Swelling

__**Swollen legs/ankles:** can be a symptom of lupus and Hashimoto's thyroiditis/hypothyroidism

__**Swollen eyes:** can be a symptom of lupus and Hashimoto's thyroiditis/hypothyroidism

__**Swollen face:** can be a symptom of Hashimoto's thyroiditis/hypothyroidism

__**Swollen arms:** can be a symptom of Hashimoto's thyroiditis/hypothyroidism

__Sense of tissues feeling swollen:** can be a symptom of Hashimoto's thyroiditis/hypothyroidism and fibromyalgia

Cognitive/Thinking

__SUPER-SYMPTOM—CONCENTRATION/MEMORY PROB-LEMS:** sometimes referred to as "brain fog," is a common autoimmune disease symptom that appears in most conditions

__Difficulty speaking or putting words in order (dysphasia):** can be symptoms of Guillain-Barré syndrome, multiple sclerosis, myasthenia gravis, and chronic fatigue immune dysfunction syndrome

__Forgetfulness/memory problems:** can be a symptom of fibromyalgia, chronic fatigue immune dysfunction syndrome, pernicious anemia, and multiple sclerosis

__Short attention span:** can be a symptom of Graves' disease/hyperthyroidism

Finding and Working with the Right Practitioner

Unfortunately, there is currently no specialist known as an autoimmunologist—although there should be—who can look at the broad spectrum of autoimmune symptoms, run the appropriate tests, and make a diagnosis of one or more autoimmune diseases. Usually, you will start your search for diagnosis and treatment with a primary care doctor—frequently a general practitioner, internist, or, for some women, a primary care gynecologist.

But proper diagnosis and treatment of autoimmune diseases will likely require a team approach, involving a primary care practitioner, specialists (i.e., endocrinologist, rheumatologist, neurologist, dermatologist, etc.) and other practitioners such as nutritionists, alternative and holistic experts, herbalists, physical therapists, and so on, to round out your health care team. If you have a more holistically oriented general practitioner, that's even better, because he or she can help you integrate the conventional and any alternative therapies.

■ Holistic/Alternative Practitioners

I tend to believe autoimmune disease patients should have at least one holistic practitioner on the team because most of these conditions are particularly tricky—and sometimes barely treatable—by conventional medicine. My family doctor is a holistic MD in general practice. She is also a licensed acupuncturist and is trained in osteopathy. She has been a tremendous asset in helping to integrate alternatives into my own treatment for Hashimoto's thyroiditis.

Of course, if you feel well and back to normal on the standard treatment for your condition, then conventional doctoring can work well for you. But for everyone else, a more integrative, holistic approach may be necessary to devise a program that will optimize health. When looking for a holistic general practitioner, you can look for either an osteopathic physician or a holistic doctor.

Women's health and hormonal expert and author Sherrill Sellman urges autoimmune disease patients to get off the "treadmill of allopathic medicine":

> *Going from traditional doctor to traditional doctor to specialist is like rearranging the deck chairs on the* Titanic. *You have to get responsible, get educated, learn the keys to good health. Then you have to be willing to do whatever is required, changing diet, lifestyle, and seeking out holistic health practitioners who have an understanding of how to heal the body at the root cause level.*

Osteopathic Physicians

Currently, it's estimated that there are more than 30,000 American-educated and -licensed osteopathic physicians practicing in the United States. The majority of osteopathic physicians are in primary care—family medicine, pediatrics, internal medicine, and obstetrics-gynecology. Osteopaths have DO after their names instead of MD. Doctors of osteopathic medicine (DOs) are "complete" physicians, fully trained and licensed to prescribe medication and to perform surgery. Licensed in the same way as doctors, osteopaths attend an osteopathic medical school and do internships and residencies. The main difference is in the philosophy of osteopathy versus conventional medicine. Osteopaths typically address people holistically, and instead of treating each symptom separately, they look for the overall cause and attempt to treat the whole person.

Holistic Doctors

Holistic doctors focus on the whole person and how he or she interacts with the environment, rather than illness, disease, or specific body parts. A small number of MDs and a larger percentage of DOs practice holistic medicine following some general principles. They believe in prevention of disease when possible and in dealing with the underlying cause of a problem versus just treating symptoms. They want to understand the patient as much as the disease or illness, and they diagnose patients as individuals rather than as members of a disease category. They encourage patient autonomy, a doctor–patient relationship that considers the patient's needs as much as the doctor's, and use of the healing power of love, hope, humor, and other positive forces.

Herbal Medicine Experts

When it comes to finding the right herbal practitioner, master herbalist and author Alan Tillotson believes it's important to find a practitioner who has substantial experience, good clientele, a good reputation in the community, who has demonstrated clear knowledge, and is not someone just trying to sell supplements. According to Dr. Tillotson, you can't particularly go looking for someone who is an "expert in autoimmune disease," because there really aren't many herbal "specialists." It goes against the general idea of herbalism, which is holistic:

> *The ability to deal with holistic, complex conditions means that a trained herbalist may in fact be far more suited to deal with autoimmune disease than a conventional practitioner. Autoimmune diseases are later stage, complex, they didn't start yesterday, they may have begun in childhood, they reflect alterations in the immune system, and because of all those factors, they are complex to repair.*

According to Dr. Tillotson, members of the American Herbalists Guild are typically the type of herbalists who are up to the task of tackling autoimmune disease. In addition, he counsels:

> *Naturopathic physicians are often competent. Many Chinese doctors and Ayurvedic doctors have a strong history and good philosophical basis with which to treat autoimmune disease. And some European phytotherapists can be of help with these diseases. But Western-trained alternative medicine physicians, herbalists, and naturopaths may be the real leaders, in that these diseases are more common in the West.*

■ Specialists

In addition, based on your condition, you will probably want or need to have a specialist on your team. Some of the key specialists involved in autoimmune diseases include the following:

- **Endocrinologists:** specialize in diseases of the endocrine system, including autoimmune diseases such as diabetes, thyroid conditions, adrenal problems, oophoritis, and ovarian decline. Endocrinologists typically have the initials FACE after their names, standing for Fellow, American College of Endocrinology. Some endocrinologists identify themselves with particular conditions, so you can also have self-identified diabetologists, thyroidologists, and reproductive endocrinologists.

• **Rheumatologists:** specialize in diagnosing and treating arthritis and other diseases of the joints, muscles, and bones. Rheumatologists treat rheumatoid arthritis, osteoarthritis, lupus, other autoimmune diseases, and some specialize in chronic fatigue syndrome and fibromyalgia. Rheumatologists have to be detectives, as some of these diseases are difficult to diagnose, and early diagnosis and treatment are important. There is a small subspecialty of rheumatologists who are integrating alternative therapies into Western medical practice. Integrative rheumatologists are likelier to be more receptive of holistic and alternative therapies, and more knowledgeable about how they can best apply to your own health.

• **Dermatologists:** specialize in skin, hair, and nail disorders. Autoimmune conditions treated by dermatologists include psoriasis, scleroderma, alopecia, pemphigus, vitiligo, and others.

• **Gastroenterologists:** focus on diseases of the esophagus, stomach, liver, pancreas, small intestine, and colon. Autoimmune specialties frequently include celiac disease, Crohn's disease, pernicious anemia, and ulcerative colitis.

• **Nephrologists:** specialists in the treatment of kidney diseases, and may be called upon when a condition such as lupus affects the kidneys.

• **Pulmonologists:** specialize in the diagnosis and treatment of the respiratory tract. This includes diseases such as emphysema, chronic bronchitis, pneumonia, respiratory failure and asthma, and in the autoimmune arena, lung involvement from conditions such as sarcoidosis.

• **Neurologists:** specialize in disorders of the nervous system, including the brain, spinal cord, nerves, and muscles. In the autoimmune arena, neurologists frequently treat Guillain-Barré syndrome, multiple sclerosis, and myasthenia gravis. Some neurologists specialize in fibromyalgia.

• **Gynecologists:** focus on the diagnosis and treatment of diseases of the female reproductive organs, and some are specialists in hormonal medicine and conditions such as premature ovarian decline.

• **Ophthalmologists:** physicians trained in all aspects of eye care, who may be called upon to treat Sjögren's syndrome, diabetic eye disease, or uveitis related to autoimmune disease, among other conditions.

• **Urologists:** specialists in the male and female urinary tract and the male reproductive organs. They frequently work with kidney disease.

• **Cardiologists:** experts in the heart and its actions and diseases, including cardiomyopathy, myocarditis, and pericarditis that can result from autoimmune disorders, as well as complications of lupus, sarcoidosis, and other conditions.

• **Immunologists:** study the causes of immunity and immune responses. Most immunologists focus on research, however, and not on patient practice, but some are clinical practitioners.

• **Orthopedists:** work on the correction or prevention of skeletal deformities, and some treat conditions such as rheumatoid arthritis and other autoimmune conditions that affect the joints.

• **Vascular surgeons:** deal with the treatment of circulatory diseases. Raynaud's phenomenon, among other autoimmune conditions, may be treated by some of these specialists.

■ Problem Solving with Challenging Doctors

Since autoimmune diseases are difficult to diagnose, you may find yourself with a primary care doctor who won't take your symptoms seriously. If you face this situation, there are some steps you can take, according to Virginia Ladd, founder of the American Autoimmune Related Diseases Association:

Many times, especially with women, we tend to be enablers. When we fail to find out what's the matter, we try to help the diagnostician, we list everything, we make our list longer, adding every single twitch and cramp, in order to enable the diagnosis. This ends up confusing people even more. So, take a step back from the frenzy of trying to find out what's the matter and list your major symptoms. If you have suspicions that you have a particular autoimmune condition, based on your own knowledge or information from a friend or family member, then contact the organizations that represent that disease, gather your information, and go into the physician knowledgeable. Then be an advocate for yourself . . . present the list to the physician. If you have a family history of autoimmune disease, don't forget to present that first, because it's not asked on the medical record, and there is a genetic component.

Dr. Marie Savard, patient advocate and author of the bestselling book *The Savard Health Record,* also believes that family history is vital, especially when a doctor is considering autoimmune illness:

The best way to get your family history is to fill out a tree called a genogram—I have one in my Savard Health Record *patient binder—which is critical for patients with autoim-*

mune diseases to fill out and show everyone . . . taking a family history takes time, which doctors rarely have, so the family history is a quick jot-down of a few key things like cancer and heart disease . . . other illnesses are often forgotten and often the patient doesn't know what parts of the history are important, so it is crucial to get the family history taken by everyone in the family once, then share with every family member and show to every practitioner, giving copies of the tree or genogram to all. . . . It saves time in the long run and contains a lifetime of critical information. Make it a family project, teaching everyone the importance of their history to all the others, keep it up to date, etc. It's not like the old days where no one talked about anything. Today, family history often holds the key to future problems.

If you go in to the doctor with some tests already in mind that you'd like to have run, or you'd like to be referred to a specialist, you may find some doctors resistant. Sometimes, they are protecting their ego and want the tests or referral to be their idea. In other cases, they may be reacting to management or cost-containment measures that discourage some tests. When faced with a doctor who refuses to run appropriate tests or refuses to refer you to a specialist, the best option is to find another doctor, even if you have to pay for it yourself. But if you have no options, here are a few tips:

• If a doctor suggests your problem is psychosomatic or nonexistent, says Alexandria, Virginia, women's health expert Dr. Donna Hurlock, you can request the "SED" rate test (the formal name is the erythrocyte sedimentation rate, or ESR). Dr. Hurlock explains, "If a SED rate is sky high, it's a good way to pick up inflammation. A physician cannot dismiss it as psychosomatic. You can get at least some idea that something is going on."

• Be persistent. Ask for various tests. Show the doctor articles about autoimmune disease that reflect your symptoms.

• Bring your Autoimmune Disease Risk Factors and Symptoms Checklist (see Chapter 15) to an appointment and ask that it be included in your medical chart after the doctor signs it, dates it, and indicates that he or she has read the checklist and discussed it with you. Make sure you get a signed and dated copy for yourself. Send a copy to the HMO's or insurance company's ombudsman or consumer liaison, along with your request that testing be approved.

• Write a simple letter stating that for the various reasons listed (and list them) you have specifically requested medical testing, and that this doctor has refused. Ask the doctor to sign it, place a copy in your charts, and give you a copy. (You can then use this copy with the HMO in your request for a referral to another doctor, if needed.) Most doctors will order tests rather than officially document their decision to refuse a patient's request.

• While it's a last resort, you can complain when necessary. According to a Norwegian survey, dissatisfied patients who threatened their doctor with negative publicity or said they might file a complaint could demonstrably affect their course of treatment:

According to the research, 44 percent of physicians will act in a defensive way to protect themselves legally when dealing with a case where relatives threaten to go to the press if the doctor doesn't order further tests for a family member's chest pain. Without the threat, only 30 percent would order the tests. In the same study, 57 percent of doctors would make a referral for a patient with severe headaches who threatened to file a formal medical complaint if not referred to a neurologist, versus only 25 percent of doctors who were not threatened.

What if you cannot change your health maintenance organization (HMO) and aren't satisfied with your current doctor? Tracee

Cornforth, a writer and educator on women's health issues who runs a popular women's health website, recommends that patients start by checking with their HMO or preferred provider organization (PPO) about its rules for changing primary physicians: "In most cases, HMOs do allow you to switch your primary care provider during any month, with the changes effective on the first of the next month (depending on how late it is in the current month when you make your request)." Cornforth also suggests looking into changing plans:

> Most HMOs/PPOs are employee-related benefits that have an open enrollment period only once a year. It's only during this open enrollment period that you can change HMOs/PPOs. However, patients who receive Medicare benefits often have an option of choosing a local HMO for coverage instead of basic Medicare at no additional cost. For these patients, there is no open enrollment period and they can switch HMOs, or back to regular Medicare, during any month of the year.

Cornforth was personally able to choose her doctor simply by calling him and asking, "Which HMOs do you accept?" She switched to the HMO he accepted and had the doctor she wanted.

■ Finding a Great New Doctor

Finding the right specialist, or even primary care doctor, is truly the best step toward getting better treatment—or even in getting diagnosed in the first place. To find a great doctor, there are a few key steps to follow.

Qualities and Features

Decide what qualities and features you are looking for in a doctor. You spend time finding a good auto mechanic, tax preparer, or babysitter. You need to at least make as much of an effort to find the right doctor for you. Before you set out to choose a doctor, consider your main priorities and selection criteria.

- **Male/female:** It's important to consider whether a male or female doctor is best for you. Men and women doctors tend to have different ways of interacting with patients. Women doctors, for example, tend to spend more time with patients than their male colleagues. One study found that women spent, on average, eight minutes (or 29 percent) longer with patients than male doctors. In Dutch research, almost 33 percent of visits with female physicians were longer than ten minutes, versus almost 26 percent with male doctors. Generally, studies suggest that women doctors tend to be more successful at involving patients in decisions and explaining things.

- **Cost/coverage:** For some people, going outside the HMO or insurance plan is simply not a financial option. It's helpful to make this decision up front so that you can narrow your search accordingly. If you are limited to selecting doctors from a preapproved list provided by your HMO or health plan, you may want to start by asking your HMO plan or insurance company if it offers any help in choosing from the lists, or if it has further information on available doctors. Otherwise, many of the other resources we'll discuss here can be used to help "qualify" the doctors you do have available via your HMO or insurance plan.

- **Experience:** Younger doctors may be more open to alternative medicine, whereas older doctors may be more set in their ways but more seasoned, experienced, and with a better bedside manner.

- **Credentials:** In some cases, you may want a doctor who graduated from a top conventional or osteopathic medical school. This isn't always an indicator of a good doctor, but the top-echelon medical schools usually manage to weed out some of the worst students.

• **Certification:** Being board-certified means a doctor has had several additional years of training in a particular specialty and passed a competency exam. Again, this doesn't guarantee that the doctor will be a success for you, but you're getting assurance of extra education in the particular specialty.

• **Other factors:** Some other important factors include

Record: Some people want to make sure there are no disciplinary actions filed against a doctor.

Cutting edge: Some people want a doctor who is innovative and on the cutting edge, who reads all the journals and health reports.

Conventional or alternative focus: Some people balk at having a doctor who suggests acupuncture or herbal remedies, whereas others wouldn't want a doctor who wasn't open to alternative therapies.

Flexibility: Some people want a doctor who has evening or weekend hours, or who can see patients on short notice, or who will consult by phone.

Success: Most people want a doctor who has successfully treated other patients with the same condition. This is usually information you can get only from other patients, or perhaps from another doctor.

Recommendations: You might want to talk to other patients who are satisfied customers of this doctor. If a doctor is not willing to provide patient references, look somewhere else.

Referrals or peer recommendations: You might want a doctor who has been recommended by other doctors. There are a variety of sources of this information that you can access.

Choose a Style That Works Best for You

Your doctor's style can have a profound effect on the success of your relationship, and ultimately your health. No style or relationship is necessarily good or bad. The success depends on your personality and needs, the nature of your illness, and the skills you bring to the relationship with your doctor. It's worth thinking about some of the styles you might encounter and which ones would fit best for you.

Father figures tend to be older male doctors (although there are definitely women physicians who fit this category). These doctors tend to feel that patients should be respectful of their prestigious position, and patients should follow instructions without question. You'll find this type of doctor both in private practice and in HMOs, where many older physicians have found themselves due to rising costs of private practice and insurance. Some people, in particular older patients, find that the formality and authoritativeness of this style of doctor can inspire confidence in a patient, which can be a positive factor in recovery and wellness. On the downside, father-figure doctors may not respond well to being asked too many questions or asked to explore alternatives to their recommended treatments. If you like to be involved in the decision-making process, this may not be the ideal type of doctor for you.

The *dictator* style of doctor may have gone out of fashion, but you can still find some of these more authoritarian, old-school doctors. Think of Dr. Romano, the imperious surgeon from the TV series *ER*. (Surgeons are frequently known to fall into this category.) On the positive side, some of the greatest minds in medicine can fall into this personality style. It may be well worth putting up with a more difficult personality if this doctor is considered particularly expert or talented in treating your condition. On the downside, if interacting with this type of doctor is too difficult, it may not be conducive to recovery. Unless the doctor is considered a renowned expert in treating your particular condition and offers such great technical ability or medical skill that the negative personality traits are worth putting up with, it may be better to consider another physician.

The *partner/colleague/consultant* tends to appeal to the new breed of informed/empowered patients. This style of doctor believes that treating you is a partnership. Likely to be younger, these physicians act as consultants who offer their expertise to help you in your health care decisions. Many alternative physicians tend to fall into this category, and women physicians also seem more likely than men to adopt this style. On the downside, these doctors may leave too many decisions up to you. If you want this type of physician, you must be willing to delve in, research, read, and educate yourself *and* the doctor.

The *revolving door doctors* are common in HMOs, the military medical system, and in the national health systems of Canada and the United Kingdom. In these situations, the doctor you see this week may not be the same doctor you see next week. Of course, having medical coverage and access to a physician is almost always better than not having any care at all. But to make the best of a situation where you may see a different doctor every visit, your strategy should be to plan ahead. Write up a one-page extremely concise and bulleted summary of your entire health history so that each doctor can quickly review your situation. Have all your questions prepared in advance and prioritized, and bring an extra copy to share with the physician the minute you walk into the examining room. However, if you are not making progress working within the system, if at all possible, it's worth going "out of plan" for some answers. For the cost of an office visit and a lab test, you may be able to forego years of ill health. I am reminded of a military dentist who had a long list of thyroid symptoms, but the military doctor she saw assured her that because he couldn't feel an enlarged thyroid, she didn't have a problem. After numerous fruitless visits to the doctor assigned to her case and months of ill health, she finally went to see a civilian endocrinologist, who in one visit ran TSH (thyroid-stimulating hormone) and antibody tests, and easily diagnosed a case of Hashimoto's thyroiditis—total bill, $150.

The *innovators* are frequently pursuing holistic or alternative medicine and breaking new ground. These doctors are often writing the books, talking on television, hosting radio shows, and may be the ones willing to try innovative therapies for your condition. On the downside, they are frequently so busy with their various engagements and become so popular that they have limited time to see patients. You may have to wait four to six months for a new-patient visit. Even then, they may also be expensive and not covered by insurance.

Appendix A has a number of helpful organizations, referral services, and websites that can help you find potential doctors.

Identify Candidates

Identify several candidates. Once you know what type of doctor or specialist you are looking for, ask friends and relatives, medical specialists, and other health professionals for the names of practitioners they highly recommend. Ask about the person's experiences and what they like or don't like about a practitioner.

Once you've narrowed down your selections and have a short list of possible doctors, it's time to have a brief screening interview with the doctor or office manager by phone, during which you might want to ask the following sorts of questions:

- Are you accepting new patients, and, if so, is a referral required?
- Are you an individual or group practice? If I have an appointment with you, is there a possibility I may be seen by another doctor without advance notice?

- Who covers for you when you're unavailable?
- On average, how long does a patient have to wait for an appointment? (How long in advance must I make an appointment?)
- Do you charge for missed appointments?
- Do you accept patient phone calls? Do you restrict them to any particular time of day? How soon do you typically return calls? Do you have your nurses return calls on your behalf?
- Is advice given over the phone?
- Do you accept patient emails?
- Do you accept patient faxes?
- What are your customary fees?
- Do you accept my health insurance coverage or Medicare?
- Is full payment (or deductibles, copayments) required at the time of the appointment?
- Do you take the time to explain treatment options, answer questions, and generally involve patients in their own treatment?
- Are lab work and x-rays performed in the office? Do you send your blood out for TSH tests, or do you perform them in house?
- What hours are you available?
- Do you refer patients to alternative treatments?
- Can you provide several patient references?

If a doctor's office isn't interested in at least providing you with some of this information in advance, I'd suggest moving on. Doctors who don't recognize that patients are clients to whom they provide a service often aren't productive in the long run.

Verify Credentials

Look at reference sources for verification. *The Official American Board of Medical Specialties Directory of Board Certified Medical Specialists* is available at many libraries, and they have a free online search service as well. See Appendix A for more information.

Don't assume, however, that the doctor is right for you just because he or she is on a hospital or magazine's "Best Doctors" list or is well known in your area. Dina found that sometimes even the most lauded of physicians are not a good match:

> *I went to see an endocrinologist at Stanford Medical Center with the belief that some of the best doctors in the world taught there, so I would have the best care. I couldn't have been farther from wrong if I tried. I did get an excellent doctor, but I was only permitted to be in his glorified presence a total of forty-five minutes over the two-and-a-half-year span of our "relationship." His idea of treatment was to tell me that in some cultures an enlarged thyroid is a sign of beauty and wealth. While this tidbit of information was indeed interesting, it was neither comforting nor pertinent. I don't live in "some cultures." I live in northern California and I'm not wealthy.*

Learn About the Doctors

Learn more about the doctors you are considering. Call their offices. The office staff can be a good source of information about the doctor's education and qualifications, office policies, and payment procedures. Pay attention to the office staff—you will have to deal with them often! You may want to set up an appointment to talk with a doctor. He or she is likely to charge you for this visit.

There are other questions about your possible doctor that unfortunately can't usually be answered until you are a patient. You may be able to get some ideas from other patients, but it's more likely you'll need to assess the doctor firsthand. However, keep your ears and eyes open when talking to other patients, or when talking on the phone to the doctor's office, or during the initial visit, as some of the answers to these questions can be answered fairly early on.

- Does your doctor patiently explain reasons for all tests and treatments?
- Does your doctor offer you any options?
- Does your doctor seem interested in educating you or just in giving orders to be followed?
- Does your doctor encourage you to participate in decisions about your health care?
- Does your doctor believe in alternative or complementary therapies?
- Does your doctor take time to learn about you, your background, your lifestyle, and how you truly feel?
- Does your doctor really listen?
- Does your doctor answer your questions satisfactorily?
- Does your doctor's receptionists, nurses, and other staff treat you and other patients politely and respectfully?
- Does your doctor and his or her staff let you dress and undress in private?
- Does your doctor or his or her staff gossip or share private information about other patients?
- Does your doctor admit or indicate that he or she just "isn't comfortable" with assertive or informed patients?
- Does your doctor take an authoritarian or dictatorial approach to the doctor-patient relationship?
- Does your doctor become irritated, act impatient, or ignore you when you ask for further explanation of your diagnosis, procedures to be performed, or drugs prescribed?

- Does your doctor return phone calls within a reasonable amount of time, or tell you that he or she has left messages or tried to call when it's evident that this isn't true?
- Does your doctor keep you waiting and usually run late for your appointments?
- When you mention some major health finding you heard about on the evening news, does your doctor seem to be aware of it?
- Will your doctor read anything you provide to him or her as far as background information?
- Does your doctor categorically dismiss the Internet as a source of quack information?

Make Your Selection and Evaluate

The final step is to make your selection. After your first appointment, evaluate whether you feel comfortable and can work well with this doctor. If you weren't satisfied, consider visiting one of the other doctors on your short list.

■ Your First Appointment

At an initial visit to evaluate autoimmune disease, a variety of factors should be reviewed and discussed.

■ Autoimmune Disease: Initial Evaluation Checklist ■

- ☑ Your history of allergies
- ☐ Personal or family history of autoimmune and rheumatic diseases
- ☐ Unusual occupational exposures to allergic or toxic substances
- ☐ Any out-of-the-ordinary childhood diseases

❑ Your current or past alcohol and tobacco use
❑ Any previous hospitalizations and surgeries
❑ Current prescription medications
❑ Past prescription medications
❑ Your current or past use of herbs and supplements

General Symptoms Evaluation
❑ Fever
❑ Malaise
❑ Fatigue
❑ Weight gain or loss
❑ Sleep difficulties

Head/Neck Evaluation
❑ Eyes, including eye pain, dry eyes, vision disturbances
☑ Dry mouth, dental problems such as frequent cavities
☑ Frequent sinus infections
❑ Feeling of fullness in neck, pain in neck or throat area

Heart/Lung Evaluation
❑ Asthma
❑ Breathing problems
❑ Pleurisy (pain taking a deep breath)
❑ History of or current heart murmur, palpitations, irregular heart-
beat, rapid heartbeat, or very slow heart rate

Gastrointestinal Evaluation
❑ Nausea and vomiting
❑ Diarrhea
❑ Constipation
❑ Ulcers
❑ Gallstones

Genitourinary Evaluation
❑ Venereal disease
❑ Pregnancies
❑ Miscarriages
❑ Breast disorders
❑ Menstrual problems
❑ Low sex drive
❑ Urinary incontinence, frequency, or discomfort

Blood/Immune System Evaluation
❑ Bruises easily
❑ Anemia
❑ Frequent infections
❑ Swollen glands

Mental Health Evaluation
❑ Depression
❑ Mood
❑ Cognitive dysfunction

Neurological Evaluation
❑ Headaches
❑ Seizures
❑ Numbness
❑ Tingling
❑ Dizziness
❑ Fainting

Joints/Muscle Evaluation
❑ Joint pain
❑ Joint stiffness
❑ Joint swelling

❑ Gout
❑ Muscle or joint weakness

Endocrine Evaluation

❑ Thyroid function evaluation
❑ Diabetes/blood sugar evaluation
❑ Cholesterol check

Vascular Evaluation

❑ Phlebitis—inflammation of veins
❑ Blood clots
❑ Stroke
❑ Raynaud's phenomenon

Hair/Skin Evaluation

❑ Sun sensitivity
❑ Hair loss
❑ Mouth sores
❑ Butterfly rash, etc.
❑ Hyper- or hypopigmentation
❑ Unusual rashes

■ Effective Communications with Your Practitioners

Keeping a Health Record and Symptoms Diary

Dr. Marie Savard feels that medical information is the most valuable information a doctor has to rely on to make an accurate diagnosis and recommend the best treatment: "Unfortunately that information is *never* all in one place and available when you need it most—whether in the ER, visiting a specialist or new doctor. The patient is the only person who can reasonably be the central repository of all the information." Dr. Savard's health information organizer/book and binder, known as the *Savard System,* provides a health information tracking tool for patients. Generally, she advocates keeping track of key information:

> *Ask for all laboratory tests—give the doctor a self-addressed stamped envelope to send test results . . . they appreciate it and it makes the point you are serious—ask for the copies of the original, not the doctor's handwritten summaries of the information. Include bloodwork, x-ray reports, pathology and special study results, typed consultation reports from specialists, all heart testing and procedures, discharge summary and operative summary if hospitalized. Remember to keep this information organized by date; store all lab work, consultations, etc., in their own section for a doctor to easily review.*

Keeping this sort of health and symptoms record and diary between appointments can help you get the most out of appointments and keep your health information organized. You can do this in a notebook, on the computer, or in folders. The main concern is keeping track of appointments, copies of test results, and other pertinent information.

- *Doctor information:* Include the name, address, phone, fax, and email address for every doctor you see, even periodically. Keep track of receptionists' names. And also store directions to offices you don't visit frequently.
- *Pharmacy information:* Include the prescription numbers and number of refills available for all current prescriptions, plus phone numbers for your pharmacy or pharmacies.
- *Lab/treatment facility information:* Include the name,

address, and phone number of any labs or treatment facilities (radiology labs, testing locations, physical therapists, etc.)

The diary should also keep track of your key health events, including illnesses, surgeries, and other pertinent information. A detailed health diary includes

- Dates of visits to the doctor
- Dates when you've received any injections, vaccinations, or special treatments
- Dates and locations of diagnostic procedures (TSH tests, x rays, MRI, bone scan)
- Dates starting and stopping a medication, and dosage levels
- Blood test results—ask for a photocopy for your folder
- Major emotional and physical stresses

According to Dr. Savard, in addition to copies of medical records, you need to keep your own progress notes. Here are some of the key questions to answer in a symptom diary:

- When do symptoms occur? Do you wake up having certain symptoms? Do they strike at certain times of the day? Are there particular activities, foods, or locations that precede your symptoms?
- What makes your symptoms slow down or stop? Are there particular remedies that work better than others?
- Do your symptoms have any connection to your moods?
- How do symptoms affect your life? Are they affecting your ability to work, exercise, your sex life, and so forth?
- If you have pain, how would you describe it—burning, stabbing, throbbing? Sharp or dull? On a scale of 1 to 10, with 10 being the worst, how would you rate the pain? Does the

pain's location, type, or intensity vary at different times of the day?

- When does pain occur? Are there particular activities, foods, or locations that precede pain?
- What makes your pain decrease or stop? Are there particular remedies that work better than others?
- Does your pain have any connection to your moods?

Preparing for Your Appointment

A productive doctor's appointment is one during which you have a chance to cover your key concerns with the doctor. In many doctors' offices, time is at a premium, so a successful appointment requires advance preparation.

- Write down the names and dosages of all medications that you are taking, including supplements and herbs.
- Prioritize your concerns. According to the American Autoimmune Related Diseases Association, studies show that many patients will go to the doctor with several complaints, but they will wait to mention the one that is of most concern until the end of the visit, when the doctor is about to leave the exam room. If your doctor knows all the specific concerns you have when he or she enters, then you can have an appropriate discussion.
- Ideally, once you've considered your main concerns, write them down and bring this list to the doctor, with the most important problem listed first. Put your concerns into the form of an agenda for your doctor's visit and bring two copies. Be sure you include on your agenda all key questions, concerns, or unusual health symptoms.
- Share your research ahead of time. If you have articles or information—more than your one-page list of concerns—that you would like to share with your doctor, mail or fax it ahead of time, with a note regarding the date and time of your appointment, and

the fact that you'd like to discuss this at that time. If you bring these materials to the appointment without sending them in advance, your doctor may not have time to review them, or may spend the entire appointment reading rather than communicating with you.

- Get in business mode. Act as if your appointment is a business meeting. You're the client and the doctor is the contractor, so to speak. Doctors treat patients more respectfully when the patients dress professionally for the appointment and when patients stay calm, relaxed, and unemotional, and do not act apologetic or passive.

- Be sure to arrive on time. If you arrive in advance, don't spend time reading old magazines. Spend the time reviewing your agenda and mentally preparing for your appointment.

- Take notes. It's hard to remember what the doctor says after an appointment, so jot down notes, names of things, instructions, and other information so that you have a reference. Tape record your conversation if you aren't confident that you will remember everything the doctor says.

- Bring a friend. This can help you feel more relaxed with the doctor. If your doctor gives you a hard time about having a friend with you, this is a red flag. You're the patient, you're paying the bill, and you should be able to decide who you'd like in the examining room with you. Choose a friend who is able to speak up but is diplomatic. Friends who are health professionals—or even doctors themselves—can be of particular help. Be sure your friend knows the agenda for the appointment so that he or she can remind you of points to cover and can help remember details of what your doctor said or agreed to do.

- Ask questions. It's important to ask questions at your appointment when you don't understand something or want to further explore solutions. This advice is particularly important for men. Studies have shown that men tend to internalize health fears and concerns, and even when worried, are reluctant to admit to concerns or problems. One study found that the average man asked his doctor no questions during an office visit, versus the average woman, who asked six.

More than anything, remember that your doctor needs to be your partner in wellness decisions, so ideally you need to find a compassionate, informed practitioner who is willing to work with you—not dictate to you—to find the right diagnosis, treatment, and solutions that will allow you to achieve optimal health.

17

Putting Together Your Autoimmune Repair Plan

For more than six years, I've been on a journey—a mission to be cured of my own autoimmune thyroid problem. I have Hashimoto's thyroiditis and am hypothyroid. Down deep in my heart, I've always had the belief that somewhere out there is the right practitioner, endocrinologist, herbalist, alternative therapy, or mind-body technique—the one that offers the "cure."

What do I mean by the cure? Because there is, after all, thyroid hormone replacement therapy, which may not be a cure but is, according to most doctors, all the "treatment" I need for my condition. By cure, what I really mean is returning to the way I used to feel. Feeling well. Losing the extra weight. Not being so easily fatigued. Having thicker hair and healthier skin again. Arms and legs that don't tingle and ache. More regular periods.

For many thyroid patients, thyroid hormone replacement is not a cure. It's a treatment. It keeps you alive and functioning, but it doesn't solve all the problems. It's the same with other conditions. Insulin doesn't "cure" diabetes; it treats the disease. Interferon drugs don't "cure" multiple sclerosis; they try to minimize the frequency and intensity of flares. In the best of circumstances, a patient will get relief of some symptoms, and perhaps ward off worsening damage, or minimize flares. But conventional medicine really doesn't offer much in the way of durable or realistic "cures" for autoimmune diseases.

So I've been looking for a cure. On my journey, I've read hundreds of books, interviewed hundreds of practitioners, surfed thousands of websites, answered many thousands of emails, seen three endocrinologists, one internist, an infectious disease specialist, a naturopath, a master herbalist, half a dozen holistic MDs, multiple hormonal experts, and a reiki practitioner. I've tried herbs, supplements, acupuncture, homeopathic medicine, yoga, meditation, and tai chi, among other alternative therapies. I've talked to everyone. I've tried nearly everything.

The certainty that the cure was out there somewhere is what spurred me to start my thyroid website, to write my last book, *Living Well with Hypothyroidism,* to become a patient advocate, and to expand my mission to understanding and writing about autoimmune disease. Well, I've discovered that cures *are* out there for some autoimmune disease patients. And, even when there's no clear cure, there are treatments that can significantly improve symptoms, prevent recurrences and flares, and minimize or prevent further damage to organs, joints, and tissues—treatments that can offer more hope and a better quality of life than standard conventional treatments. But the cure or help for each condition is not standardized—it is unique to each person.

There are many factors that go into why you get an autoimmune disease. Your immune function, your genetic background and heritage, your diet and nutritional status, your level of stress, and your environment and toxic exposures all play a role in how and where you get an autoimmune condition. And, since there are so many factors at play—factors unique to your own situation—in developing an autoimmune disease, crafting the optimal solution is an equally complex process that is also unique to you. Your own autoimmune repair plan will, by nature, have to be holistic—it must incorporate a variety of elements, including traditional medicine, alternative approaches, diet/nutrition, mind-body techniques, stress reduction, and more.

Because some of the autoimmune conditions can be life-threatening if not treated, it's important to note that I'm not advocating that you abandon traditional treatments and drugs in favor of only alternatives. As a thyroid patient, even though I'm taking herbs and supplements to help support my immune system and heal imbalances, I did not stop taking thyroid hormone replacement. Over time, though, the alternative treatments I've pursued have enabled me to, with supervision from my doctor, cut back on thyroid hormone medicine dosages, and effectively deal with troublesome symptoms, such as weight gain and fatigue, without taking more prescription drugs. Similarly, I don't think it would be responsible to suggest that someone with rheumatoid arthritis should bypass recommended disease-modifying antirheumatic drugs (DMARDs) in favor of a totally herbal or natural approach, as DMARDs may be able to prevent joint damage. The real key is creating a program that adds to, supports, and mitigates the negative effects of—but does not subtract from—conventional treatment.

In his highly recommended book *Cancer as a Turning Point*, renowned psychotherapist Lawrence LeShan describes holistic medicine as resting on four basic, interrelated ideas:

1. The person exists on many levels, all of which are equally real and important. Physical, psychological, and spiritual levels are one valid way of describing the person, and none of these can be "reduced" to any other. To move successfully toward health, all must be treated.
2. Each person is unique. A valid program of treatment, whether it focuses primarily on nutrition, meditation, chemotherapy, or exercise, must be individualized for

each person. A standardized approach to a condition is not valid under this concept.

3. The patient should be a part of the decision-making team. Each person in a program of holistic health is given as much knowledge and authority as he or she will accept.

4. The person has self-healing abilities.

Some experts have referred to a healing program as a pie, and it's a useful comparison to use when thinking about your plan. Each component of your plan is a piece of the pie. How large each piece of the pie ends up is unique to you, your condition, your own style, and your needs. You may find that your condition is in total remission after you implement a program that involves 50 percent of your pie dedicated to prescription drug treatments, 25 percent to prayer, and 25 percent to tennis and other exercise. Another person may find that she can reduce antibody levels and return to generally normal health with a pie that includes 25 percent conventional drugs, 25 percent diet, 15 percent herbs and supplements, 15 percent yoga, 10 percent acupuncture, and 10 percent reiki. And a third patient may find that his condition is managed and flares are rare on a program consisting of 50 percent diet and nutrition, 25 percent yoga, 15 percent conventional drugs, and 10 percent exercise. Yet others may find that the actual mix is not as easily defined, and rather involves a regularly changing mix of components, based on how they feel and what's going on in their lives and health at the time. The key is to find the right approach for you, then to identify what pieces should be in your pie—to develop your *own* autoimmune repair plan.

■ Start with the Right Attitude

The most important part of your plan is approaching it with the right attitude. And that may mean first recognizing and dealing with the anger and sadness that comes with a chronic disease diagnosis. Dr. Christina Puchalski, director of the George Washington Institute for Spirituality and Health in Washington, DC, encourages us to grieve for lost health, if necessary:

People will say, "Keep a stiff upper lip, have hope." But it's appropriate to feel sadness; it's appropriate to grieve. I'm thinking of someone with rheumatoid arthritis, for example—someone who can't cook or write the way they did before. To say "hang in there" is fine, but there's a certain amount of grieving to do. People shouldn't feel guilty about the anger and sense of loss. But to try to move through that, seek counseling, go to support groups—some people find spiritual or medical support groups helpful—plus look within yourself and don't let your illness define you.

Make sure you keep a sense of hope. Dr. Puchalski believes that attitude and spirit can have a profound impact on health:

Initially, when people are diagnosed with anything, there's a hope for a cure. It's not abnormal, and it's very logical. As people begin to see that their diagnosis is clear, it's important to not lose hope. But hope may not be for a cure, but for as few exacerbations as possible, or to alleviate pain. Look for hope in other ways. Hope for a good quality of life. Being able to cope with exacerbations as part of life, but not as the critical part of the disease. And not defining yourself as the disease.

Dr. Puchalski raises an important point—that we may need to make healing our objective rather than a "cure." We shouldn't give up hope that the body can do amazing things but should focus our energy on the act of healing, in a broader sense. Says holistic healer Phylameana lila Desy:

Being cured would, to most people, suggest that all symptoms disappear. A cure would indicate that a person is now in "ease" rather than in "dis-ease." But the first step in being healed is understanding that something is amiss. Delving deeper into what brought about a particular ailment would naturally follow. Then, finally, seeking how to change that pattern so it will bring peace and balance back into your life is the last step. Being healed does not mean that all symptoms disappear but only that you recognize that there are reasons for the suffering and you seek relief. Pain is our body's language. It is its way of communicating with us about how we are honoring ourselves. Every experience we have from birth to the present becomes a part of who we are. How we deal or choose not to deal with each drama and trauma in our lives can surface several years later as an illness. We are given the choice of confronting our issues or burying our heads in the sand and ignoring dis-eases. Healing occurs when the "looking for a cure" journey becomes one where the person learns to embrace the hurdles and mishaps they stumble across along with the wonderful teachings they represent.

■ Find the Best Practitioners for Your Wellness Team

Chapter 16 is dedicated to finding and working with your practitioners. There are also many resources available in Appendix A that can help you find the best doctors, specialists, herbalists, nutritionists, and other practitioners. But the most important aspect of your team is that it is made up of practitioners who bring the right expertise, who are supportive of your objectives, and who have the right personality and style for you.

Keep in mind that in almost all cases you are the coach of your wellness team. You will need to make sure that the various practitioners communicate with each other and are aware of the elements of your treatment. To that end, here are a few helpful tips:

- Have all your practitioners periodically summarize your status in a brief report and give you a copy. (If you can't get them to write a report, then summarize your notes from visits yourself.) You can then make photocopies and share these reports with your other practitioners.
- Always make sure each practitioner has a current list of your prescription drugs, nutritional supplements, and alternative treatments.
- If there is a disagreement among practitioners regarding recommendations, encourage them to speak with each other, ideally with you as part of the discussion whenever possible. Three-way calling is useful for these sorts of discussions.

Above all, remember that practitioners are part of your team. If you leave a visit with a doctor or practitioner feeling demoralized, ill-informed, or hopeless, this is a clear sign that it's time to seek out another practitioner. On the other hand, if visits to your practitioner leave you feeling calmer, more confident, and better able to face the challenges of your health condition, this is a positive sign that you've found a caring, talented practitioner worth keeping on your team.

■ Investigate and Choose Your Conventional and Alternative Options

With the assistance and direction of your practitioners, plus books and website information, as well as support group input, you need to develop a plan that includes the various approaches you will use to treat your condition. Keep in mind that over time, this mix of treatments and approaches will change in response to your health condition and improvements. Your plan can include the following general categories:

- Conventional treatments and drugs
- Diet/nutritional approaches
- Supplements/herbal remedies
- Alternative treatments (e.g., acupuncture)
- Exercise (e.g., yoga, tai chi, tennis, biking, aerobics, treadmill, etc.)
- Relaxation response/spirituality/mind-body (e.g., prayer, meditation, breathing, guided imagery)
- Healing therapies (e.g., reiki)

Here's a sample form you can use to develop your plan. A downloadable version of this form is also available online, at http://www.autoimmunebook.com/plan.

■ Autoimmune Repair Plan Outline ■

My Practitioners
Name, Specialty: _____
Name, Specialty: _____
Name, Specialty: _____
Name, Specialty: _____
Name, Specialty: _____

Conventional Treatments and Drugs

Drug, Dosage, Since When: _____

Drug, Dosage, Since When: _____

Drug, Dosage, Since When: _____

Drug, Dosage, Since When: _____

Drug, Dosage, Since When: _____

Drug, Dosage, Since When: _____

Diet/Nutritional Approaches

Dietary Approach: _____

Dietary Approach: _____

Dietary Approach: _____

Dietary Approach: _____

Dietary Approach: _____

Supplements/Herbal Remedies

Item, Dosage: _____

Item, Dosage: _____

Item, Dosage: _____

Item, Dosage: _____

Item, Dosage: _____

Item, Dosage: _____

Item, Dosage: _____

Item, Dosage: _____

Alternative Treatments

Treatment:_____

Treatment:_____

Treatment:_____

Treatment:_____

Treatment:_____

Treatment:_____

Exercise
Approach: _____
Approach: _____
Approach: _____

Relaxation Response/Spirituality/Mind-Body
Approach: _____
Approach: _____
Approach: _____
Approach: _____

Healing Therapies
Approach: _____
Approach: _____
Approach: _____
Approach: _____

Other Notes:

_____

_____

_____

_____

_____

_____

■ Mary Shomon's Own
Autoimmune Repair Plan Outline ■

Practitioners
- Dr. Kate Lemmerman, general practitioner, acupuncture, osteopathy
- Dr. Mark Sklar, endocrinologist
- Melanie, nutritionist/diet consultant
- Alan Tillotson, herbalist
- Dr. Donna Hurlock, hormonal balance
- Angela, reiki healer and massage therapist
- Dr. Stephen Langer, Dr. Richard Shames, Dr. Larrian Gillespie, Gillian Ford, Sherrill Sellman—for other advice, ideas, and health suggestions

Conventional Treatments and Drugs
- Armour Thyroid, natural thyroid medication, daily
- Antibiotics, periodically, for rheumatoid symptoms
- Mild tranquilizer, periodically, for dysautonomia symptoms

Diet/Nutritional Approaches
- Following low-glycemic diet
- Increased water consumption, 64+ ounces daily, mostly bottled
- Eating fish, two times a week
- Eliminated most starches and processed foods
- Switched from saccharine and aspartame to natural sweetener stevia

Supplements/Herbal Remedies
- Chinese herbal powder, customized formula created for me by Alan Tillotson
- Essential fatty acid supplements
- DHA supplements

- Vitamin E supplements
- Grapefruit seed extract
- Probiotics
- Ginseng
- Calcium/magnesium
- Chromium picolinate/garcinia

Alternative Treatments
- I've personally had several Body Restoration Technique (BRT) treatments, and so far, the results have seemed positive. After being cleared for sensitivity to mycoplasma and the presence of lupus and rheumatoid factor, I've had a fairly noticeable reduction in joint pain and aches, especially morning stiffness. I was also cleared for an allergy to apples, and have found myself able to eat some fresh apples, where before, I had a severe allergic reaction.
- Periodic osteopathic manipulation and acupuncture for joint/muscle aches

Exercise
- Yoga, home, with tape one or two times a week
- Treadmill, for thirty minutes two or three times a week
- Resistance exercise (exercise bands), for fifteen minutes two times a week

Relaxation Response/Spirituality/Mind-Body
- Practicing guided imagery, using audiotapes, weekly
- Following breathing techniques, learned in yoga pranayama class, periodically
- Crocheting/needlework, for acute stress, as needed

Healing Therapies

- Reiki, once or twice a month, one-hour session. I've become a fan of reiki and can attest to the unexpected power of this healing art in the hands of a good practitioner. I've gone in to reiki sessions with major pain, stiffness, and fatigue, and left an hour later feeling as if I'd slept eight hours, with every kink and pain worked out, not to mention an overwhelming sense of mental and spiritual peace and comfort.

Since being diagnosed in July 1995 with Hashimoto's disease, and evolving into following this repair plan, I've managed to lose 30 pounds, stop my hair from falling out, get my periods almost back to normal, have a successful pregnancy, and have enough energy to raise my daughter and write a book, hold down a full-time job, and launch a new business—all at the same time. And this is after a period from 1993 to 1995 when there were times I could sleep twelve hours a night and wake up exhausted, couldn't even move off the couch, and actually had to take a two-month leave of absence from work due to a period of terrible chronic fatigue.

Am I cured? Not by traditional definitions, as I still have a thyroid condition and take some thyroid hormone replacement. But I am healed. I'm generally in better health than ever before. I usually have good energy; I eat well, and usually feel well. My hair is thick, my mood is usually good, and my periods are fairly normal. And while I still worry sometimes that I may develop another autoimmune disease, or have periodic spurts of negative symptoms, I also know enough to realize that an occasional bout of dry eyes, or some tingling in the arms and legs, are probably more likely to be related to my existing autoimmune condition than ominous signs of new diseases.

I've stopped beating myself up during those times when I may need some extra rest, and I just get the extra rest I need. I've stopped feeling sorry for myself or cursing the fates when I realize I have to work harder to lose weight than my friends.

I prefer doctors who have a warm, participatory style, and are open to alternative and complementary therapies, so my primary care physician, Kate, is a "partner/colleague/consultant." I occasionally bring in experts for specialized consultations, but they are always practitioners who treat me as a partner in my own health care. I've been known to fire a doctor here and there, but I usually do enough research up front to avoid the bad doctors in the first place!

It's taken me a few years to get to this plan, and even then, it changes and evolves over time. But please remember, I share my plan with you not to suggest that you adopt my particular program or take the same supplements that I take. Your plan must be unique to you. I am hoping that by seeing my plan, however, you can get some idea of the different practitioners and approaches that have worked for me, and see how such a plan might look.

I hope that the information, resources, and ideas in this book will inspire you to find your optimal wellness team and create your own autoimmune repair plan! I encourage you to write to me anytime with questions, thoughts, ideas, comments about the book, or if you want to share your own personal story or experiences with autoimmune disease. You can reach me by email at mshomon@thyroid-info.com, or regular mail, at P.O. Box 0385, Palm Harbor, FL 34682.

Our education about autoimmune disease shouldn't stop with this book. We're all on an ongoing search for answers, information, and new developments to help diagnose, treat—and even potentially cure—our autoimmune diseases. Every day, I review medical journals, news sources, websites, and conventional and alternative health resources, looking for information that can be of help to people with autoimmune conditions. I feature links to the best information on the web, summarize important information at my website, and publish key information and news in my newsletter, *The Autoimmune Report*. If you're interested in continuing the journey with me, find out how to subscribe to my newsletter in Appendix A of this book.

I'd like to close with a favorite quote from a pioneer in mind-body medicine, Norman Cousins: "Drugs are not always necessary, but belief in recovery always is." May you always believe!

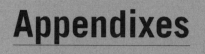

Appendixes

APPENDIX A: RESOURCES

When it comes to autoimmune disease, information is critical. I've put together the following list of resources to help you find the information and support you need regarding your condition.

Resources sections, are, by their very nature, subject to change. You may, therefore, run into a phone number or web address that has changed since publication. If you come across out-of-date information and would like the updated information, please visit my website: http://www.autoimmunebook.com. You'll find updates for organizations and their contact information, current website addresses, links to online sources where you can get more information about books that are mentioned, and other helpful resources.

If you just have email access, you can get an updated resources listing by emailing me at mshomon@thyroid-info.com, or if you don't have web or email access at home, work, or the library, please feel free to write to me at: Mary Shomon, P.O. Box 0385, Palm Harbor, FL 34682.

■ General Autoimmune Disease Information

American Autoimmune Related Diseases Association
National Office
22100 Gratiot Ave. E.
Detroit, MI 48021
(810) 776-3900

http://www.aarda.org/

Email: aarda@aol.com

> Information about more than fifty different autoimmune disorders.
> This website and organization provide general information about
> autoimmune disorders and profiles of specific diseases.

National Institutes of Health

Bethesda, MD 20892-2350

http://www.niaid.nih.gov/publications/autoimmune/autoimmune.htm

> Excellent site explaining the nuts and bolts of the immune system.

The Autoimmune Diseases

Edited by Noel R. Rose and Ian R. MacKay

Academic Press, 1998

> The definitive medical textbook on all facets of autoimmune dis-
> ease, from the "father of autoimmune disease research" (Dr. Rose).

Human Trials: Scientists, Investors, and Patients in the Quest for a Cure

By Susan Quinn

Perseus Books, 2001

> An intense, exciting account of the world of experimental drug tri-
> als—in this case, drugs that offer hope for relief from autoimmune
> diseases such as multiple sclerosis and rheumatoid arthritis—along
> with the scientists, researchers, venture capitalists, and patients
> whose careers and lives are on the line.

AutoimmuneBook.com

http://www.autoimmunebook.com

> The home page of this book, *Living Well with Autoimmune Dis-
> ease,* and a starting point and central portal for all your web
> research related to autoimmune disease, both conventional and
> alternative. Features a free email newsletter with updates about the
> latest news on autoimmune disease.

The Autoimmune Report

http://www.autoimmunebook.com/report

A print newsletter for autoimmune disease patients, dedicated to the latest conventional and alternative news and information about living well with autoimmune disease. For more information, send a self-addressed stamped envelope to *Autoimmune Report*, P.O. Box 0385, Palm Harbor, FL 34682.

Autoimmune Conditions Support Forum

http://www.delphiforums.com/autoimmunehelp

An online support group featuring information exchange, support, and online community.

Rare Diseases

http://rarediseases.about.com

Information about some of the rare autoimmune diseases is featured at Mary Kugler's site.

■ Lupus/Systemic Lupus Erythematosus

Patient Support Organization

Lupus Foundation of America, Inc.
1300 Piccard Dr., Suite 200
Rockville, MD 20850-4303
(301) 670-9292 or (800) 558-0121
http://www.lupus.org/

Medical Organization

American College of Rheumatologists
1800 Century Place, Suite 250
Atlanta, GA 30345
(404) 633-3777
http://www.rheumatology.org/index.asp

Websites

Lupus Around the World
http://www.mtio.com/lupus/

According to this website, "30,000 people a month from 80 countries use this site." It's easy to see why. In addition to the usual medical information, the site features personal stories by people dealing with lupus, a forum for patients under 21, fast facts on lupus, a place for parents of children with lupus, and a buddy program for adults and kids alike.

Lupus Foundation of America, Inc.
http://www.lupus.org/

Listing of local chapters, link to check on bills before Congress affecting lupus patients, FAQ, information on coping with the disease, and so on.

Hamline University, St. Paul, MN
http://www.hamline.edu/lupus/index.html

Good basic site with links to articles, addresses, and phone numbers of national, state, and international lupus organizations, information about lupus conferences, and a Spanish-language lupus page.

Lupus Listserv
http://listserv.acor.org/archives/lupus.html

Patient support—in the form of a moderated listserv—for those with lupus and their families.

Lupus Canada
http://www.lupuscanada.org/en/index.html

Features numerous medical articles, basic primer for those trying to understand the immune system, facts on lupus and how it affects various parts of the body, and so on.

Kids with Lupus
http://members.home.net/mplaw/LGirl
> Hip, cool site for kids and young adults with the disease, created by
> university student Jaclyn Law and her partner, Jacob Mouka. There
> are personal stories about what it's like to live with the disease at a
> young age, plus non-lupus-related writings.

Books

The Lupus Book: A Guide for Patients and Their Families
By Daniel J. Wallace
Oxford University Press, 2000
> The author, a world expert on lupus, has revised this key resource
> using the latest research and information on state-of-the-art treat-
> ment, yet maintaining an informal, patient-oriented format. It is the
> only book for nonspecialists that is recommended by the Lupus
> Foundation of America.

**Coping with Lupus: A Practical Guide to Alleviating the Challenges of
Systemic Lupus Erythematosus**
By Robert H. Phillips, Ronald I. Carr, and Harry Spiera
Avery Penguin Putnam, 2001
> This revised edition offers informed and compassionate advice
> about living and coping with the disease. Topics include the impor-
> tance of choosing the right medication, pain control, diet, exercise,
> and ways to manage the emotional problems of living with this
> chronic illness.

ABC of Asthma, Allergies, and Lupus: Eradicate Asthma Now!
By Fereydoon Batmanghelid
Global Heath Solutions, 2000
> This book introduces a unique theory that lupus and other degener-
> ative diseases are caused by long-term, unintentional dehydration.
> Readers will learn how to prevent and treat lupus by ensuring they
> consume adequate water and salt.

Lupus: Alternative Therapies That Work
By Sharon Moore
Inner Traditions Intl. Ltd., 2000
   After suffering from lupus for fourteen years, the author used conventional and complementary (alternative) treatment and recovered. She devotes an entire chapter to caring for your spirit as part of a mind, body, and spirit approach.

■ Reiter's Syndrome

Patient Support Organizations

Reiter's Information and Support Group
1105 D 15th Ave., #172
Longview, WA 98632-3068
Message phone (360) 423-9374
Toll-free in U.S. and Canada (877) 800-RISG or (877) 800-7474
Email: rick@risg.org
http://www.risg.org/infosupp/

Reiters Information and Support Group
http://www.risg.org
   A good site for anyone suffering from not only Reiter's syndrome but from related diseases such as ankylosing spondylitis and psoriatic arthritis. Features discussion forums, articles on new advances, medications, and the like.

Spondylitis Association of America
P.O. Box 5872
Sherman Oaks, CA 91413
(818) 981-1616 or (800) 777-8189
http://www.spondylitis.org/

Arthritis Foundation
1330 W. Peachtree St.
Atlanta, GA 30309
(404) 872-7100 or (800) 283-7800
http://www.arthritis.org/

Medical Organization

American College of Rheumatology
60 Executive Park South, Suite 150
Atlanta, GA 30329
(404) 633-3777
http://www.rheumatology.org/

Websites

Reiter's Info and Support Group
http://www.risg.org/infosupp/
> Extensive site on Reiter's and other related diseases. Features medical information, support, discussions, chats and message boards, tips on pain management, and so forth. Use the mammoth table of contents to find what you're looking for.

Arthritis at About.com
http://arthritis.about.com/msub18.htm
> Under the main arthritis site, About.com offers several articles on Reiter's syndrome.

National Institute of Arthritis, Musculoskeletal and Skin Diseases
http://www.niams.nih.gov/hi/topics/reiter/reiters.htm
> Features an informative page about Reiter's syndrome, including methods of treatment.

National Arthritis Foundation
http://www.arthritis.org/Answers/DiseaseCenter/reiters.asp
    Fact sheet about the disease and its treatment.

■ Sarcoidosis

Patient Support Organizations

National Sarcoidosis Research Center
P.O. Box 1593
Piscataway, NJ 08855-1593
(732) 699-0733
http://www.nsrc-global.net/

Sarcoidosis Research Institute
3475 Central Ave.
Memphis, TN 38111
(901) 766-6951
http://www.sarcoidosisresearch.org/
Email: paula@sarcoidosisresearch.org

Sarcoid Networking Association
6424 151st Ave. East
Sumner, WA 98390-2401
(253) 891-6886
http://www.sarcoidnetworkingassociation.org/
Email: sarcoidosis_network@prodigy.net

National Sarcoidosis Foundation at St. Michael's Medical Center
268 Martin Luther King Blvd.
Newark, NJ 07102
(800) 223-6429 (voice)
http://www.healthy.net/pan/cso/cioi/TNSFSMMC.HTM

Foundation for Sarcoidosis Research
P.O. Box 577849
Chicago, IL 60657
(773) 665-2400
http://www.fightsarcoidosis.org
Email: fsr@fightsarcoidosis.org

Medical Organizations

American College of Rheumatology
60 Executive Park South, Suite 150
Atlanta, GA 30329
(404) 633-3777
http://www.rheumatology.org/

NIH/National Institute of Arthritis and Musculoskeletal and Skin Diseases
1 AMS Circle
Bethesda, MD 20892-3675
(301) 496-8188 or (877) 226-4267
TDD: (301) 565-2966
http://www.nih.gov/niams/
Email: NAMSIC@mail.nih.gov

American Lung Association
1740 Broadway
New York, NY 10019
1-800-LUNG-USA
http://www.lungusa.com

National Heart, Lung and Blood Institute
National Institutes of Health
Bethesda, MD 20892-2350
http://www.nhlbi.nih.gov

Websites

Jay Lloyd
http://www.blueflamingo.net/sarcoid/
> Clearinghouse of Internet information on the disease. Should be your first stop on the way to search the Internet for sarcoidosis facts.

National Sarcoidosis Research Center
http://www.nsrc-global.net/
> Support in the form of chats, online newsletter, physician referrals, and so forth.

World Sarcoidosis Society
http://www.worldsarcSOCIETY.com/
> Information on the disease by doctors, support, "cyberpal" program, mailing lists, good page on sarcoidosis in children.

Dr. Norman Soskel, MD
http://www.sarcoidcenter.com/
> This pulmonologist with a longstanding interest in sarcoidosis has created an informative site with lots of medical information, links to other sites, and lists of drugs frequently used to treat the disease. If you've just been diagnosed with the disease, be sure to read the excellent information page at: http://www.sarcoidcenter.com/sarjames.htm.

Sarcoidosis Worldwide Support Group
http://www.geocities.com/HotSprings/Spa/9139/
> Patient support galore, plus huge listing of sarcoidosis websites, chat rooms, and archived newsletter.

Becky Mitchell
http://noairtogo.tripod.com/sarcoid.htm
> Good, solid, informative page gives an overview of the disease, its treatment, and the emotional side of coping with sarcoidosis.

Books

Sarcoidosis Resource Guide and Directory
By Sandra Conroy
PC Publications, 1992

> This pre-Internet savvy book was the first patient-oriented book on the disease, using the author's own pioneering research after she was diagnosed in 1984. She founded the National Sarcoidosis Research Center in 1992.

Model Patient: My Life as an Incurable Wise-Ass
By Karen Duffy
Cliff Street Books, 2000

> The author describes how her life as a successful MTV presenter, model, and actress was drastically affected by sarcoidosis. Her refreshingly determined and sassy response brings hope to other patients.

■ Sjögren's Syndrome

Patient Support Organization

Sjögren's Syndrome Foundation
366 North Broadway
Jericho, NY 11753
(516) 933-6365
Information requests: (800) 475-6473
http://www.sjogrens.org/

Medical Organizations

American College of Rheumatologists
1800 Century Place, Suite 250
Atlanta, GA 30345
(404) 633-3777
http://www.rheumatology.org/index.asp

American Optometric Association
243 North Lindbergh Blvd.
St. Louis, MO 63141
(314) 991-4100
http://www.aoanet.org/

National Institute of Dental and Craniofacial Research
National Institutes of Health
Bethesda, MD 20892-2190
http://www.nidcr.nih.gov

National Institute of Arthritis and Musculoskeletal and Skin Diseases
National Institutes of Health
Bethesda, MD 20892-2190
http://www.niams.nih.gov/

Websites

SJSWorld
http://www.sjsworld.org/index.htm
Patients with Sjögren's looking to discuss symptoms, share stories,
and provide and receive support should definitely visit this site,
which is chock-full of articles, message boards, a chat room, and
links. The site is particularly focused on the neurological effects of
the disorder.

National Institute of Arthritis, Musculoskeletal and Skin Diseases
http://www.nih.gov/niams/healthinfo/sjogrens/index.htm
> Easy-to-navigate site featuring symptoms, diagnosis, treatment, and tips for coping with the disease. Excellent sections on how different parts of the body can be affected by Sjögren's.

Sjögren's/Arthritis at About.com
http://arthritis.about.com/cs/sjogrens/
> Features links to other articles and contains information about new advances in coping with the disease.

University of Washington
http://www.orthop.washington.edu/arthritis/types/sjogrens/01
> The Department of Orthopedics and Sports Medicine hosts an informative page on the disorder.

Sjögren's Research Centre at Malmo University Hospital
http://www.medforsk.mas.lu.se/ssrc/index.html
> Excellent, wide-ranging site on Sjögren's syndrome, offering an overview, symptoms, diagnosis, treatment, and advice.

Lynne Messina
http://users.tp.net/tonym/
> Good personal site featuring overview of the disease, tips for coping, personal stories, links, and products (nonendorsed).

Dry.org
http://dry.org/
> Site is a good starting point for those searching for Internet resources about Sjögren's, including support sites and mailing lists. Be sure to read *Dr. Robert Fox's Guide for Patients* at: http://www.dry.org/ss95gui.html.

Books

The New Sjögren's Syndrome Handbook
By Steven Carson and Elaine K. Harris
Oxford University Press, 1998
> This book is extensively revised, giving a comprehensive and informed guide produced by the Sjögren's Syndrome Foundation. Some patients have given copies to their medical personnel, because it provides hard-to-find information.

Understanding Sjögren's Syndrome
By Sue Dauphin
Pixel Print, 1993
> This is a good practical guide for people with the disease, offering everything from personal experiences, to a definition of the disease, to a comprehensive survey of the symptoms, immunology, and diagnosis. Treatment options and support groups are also covered.

■ Thyroid Disease

Patient Support Organizations

Thyroid Foundation of America
410 Stuart St.
Boston, MA 02116
(617) 534-1500 or (800) 832-8321
http://www.tsh.org *(A Patient's Guide to Thyroid Disease)*
http://www.allthyroid.org (Thyroid Foundation of America)
> The main U.S. organization involved in thyroid education and outreach. Primarily run by doctors and medical interests, and funded in part by pharmaceutical companies, this organization stays fairly close to the official party line, but does offer decent conventional introductory information on thyroid disease.

American Foundation for Thyroid Patients
P.O. Box 820195
Houston, TX 77282
http://www.thyroidfoundation.org/
Email: thyroid@flash.net
> A patient founded this thyroid organization. Primary activities
> include a newsletter.

Medical Organizations

The Endocrine Society
4350 East West Highway, Suite 500
Bethesda, MD 20814-4426
(301) 941-0200
http://www.endo-society.org
Email: endostaff@endo-society.org
> The Endocrine Society is the world's largest professional organiza-
> tion of endocrinologists, and their primary focus is on disseminat-
> ing state-of-the-art research in endocrinology-related topics. The
> Endocrine Society also publishes some of the world's key journals
> covering endocrinology topics, including: the *Journal of Clinical
> Endocrinology & Metabolism; Endocrinology; Molecular
> Endocrinology;* and *Endocrine Reviews.* Their website highlights
> recent research and new findings.

American Association of Clinical Endocrinologists
1000 Riverside Ave., Suite 205
Jacksonville, FL 32204
(904) 353-7878
http://www.aace.com
> The American Association of Clinical Endocrinologists (AACE) is a
> professional medical organization devoted to clinical endocrinology.
> At their website they sponsor an online "Specialist Search Page," at
> http://www.aace.com/directory, which allows you to identify AACE
> members by geographic location, including international options. A
> unique feature of this page is the ability to select by subspecialty.

American Thyroid Association
6066 Leesburg Pike
P.O. Box 1836
Falls Church, VA 22041
(703) 998-8890
http://www.thyroid.org
   Features patient information sheets and a doctor referral service.

Websites

Thyroid-Info.com
http://www.thyroid-info.com
   Comprehensive links, information about thyroid books and
   newsletters.

Thyroid Support Online Forum
http://forums.delphi.com/thyroidinfo
   An online forum for patient support and exchange of information.

IThyroid
http://www.ithyroid.com
   The Internet's only website totally dedicated to nutritional treatments for thyroid disease.

Endocrineweb
http://www.endocrineweb.com
   Comprehensive, doctor-developed website covering thyroid disease
   and other endocrine topics.

Thyroid Manager
http://www.thyroidmanager.org
   Comprehensive, technical, online medical thyroid textbook.

Books

Living Well with Hypothyroidism: What Your Doctor Doesn't Tell You . . . That You Need to Know
By Mary J. Shomon
HarperCollins, 2000

> Most thyroid patients end up hypothyroid, and this best-selling book offers both conventional and alternative advice on how to find the best prescription treatments, the right doctors, and alternative approaches that help with weight loss, depression, fertility, and more. Features a detailed resources chapter for more help and information.

Graves' Disease: A Practical Guide
By Elaine Moore and Lisa Moore
MacFarland & Company, 2001

> Excellent, comprehensive, and well-researched overview of Graves' disease that offers conventional and alternative information on diagnosis and treatment.

Solved: The Riddle of Illness
By Stephen E. Langer and James F. Scheer
McGraw Hill–NTC, 3rd edition, 2000

> Highlights the authors' tremendous knowledge of nutritional medicine, and the relationship between thyroid disease and many conditions, such as arthritis, obesity, depression, diabetes, heart disease, cancer, sexual problems, and much more.

Thyroid Power: Ten Steps to Total Health
By Richard Shames and Karilee Halo Shames
Harper Resource, 2001

> Puts some basics of hypothyroidism's causes, tests, diagnosis, and treatment into a ten-step program of information that can help patients get properly diagnosed and treated. Interesting chapter on the psychology behind the "common characteristics" of people with autoimmune hypothyroidism.

The Thyroid Solution: A Mind-Body Program for Beating Depression and Regaining Your Emotional and Physical Health
By Ridha Arem
Ballantine Books, 1999
> A solid overview of thyroid disease from a doctor who focuses on the connection between thyroid disease and depression.

Healing Options: A Report on Graves' Disease Treatments
By Kate Flax
Sally Breer, 1998
> One of the only sources of information on alternative approaches for Graves' disease, providing options and alternatives beyond the usual radioactive iodine or surgical approaches.

Thyroid Sourcebook
By M. Sara Rosenthal
McGraw Hill–NTC, 4th edition, 2000
> A good introductory book covering the general basics on thyroid cancer, hyperthyrodism, surgery, and hypothyroidism.

■ Diabetes

Patient Support Organizations

American Diabetes Association
1701 N. Beauregard St.
Alexandria, VA 22311
(800) DIABETES/(800) 342-2383
http://www.diabetes.org/

Juvenile Diabetes Association
120 Wall St.
New York, NY 10005-4001
(212) 785-9595 or (800) 533-2783 (in U.S.)
http://www.jdf.org/

National Diabetes Information Clearinghouse
1 Information Way
Bethesda, MD 20892-3560
(301) 654-3327 or (800) 860-8747
http://www.niddk.nih.gov/health/diabetes/ndic.htm
Email: ndic@info.niddk.nih.gov

Medical Organizations

The Endocrine Society
4350 East West Highway, Suite 500
Bethesda, MD 20814-4426
(301) 941-0200
http://www.endo-society.org
Email: endostaff@endo-society.org

The Endocrine Society is the world's largest professional organization of endocrinologists, and their primary focus is on disseminating state-of-the-art research in endocrinology-related topics. The Endocrine Society also publishes some of the world's key journals covering endocrinology topics, including: the *Journal of Clinical Endocrinology & Metabolism; Endocrinology; Molecular Endocrinology;* and *Endocrine Reviews.* Their website highlights recent research and new findings.

National Institute of Diabetes & Digestive & Kidney Disorders
National Institutes of Health
31 Center Dr. MSC 2560
Bethesda, MD 20892-2560
http://www.niddk.nih.gov/index.htm

American Association of Clinical Endocrinologists
1000 Riverside Ave., Suite 205
Jacksonville, FL 32204
(904) 353-7878
http://www.aace.com/indexjava.htm

Websites

National Diabetes Information Clearinghouse
http://www.niddk.nih.gov/health/diabetes/ndic.htm

Offers phone, fax, mail, and email responses to questions about diabetes, as well as pamphlets, books, and brochures on dealing with the disease.

About.com Diabetes Site
http://diabetes.about.com

Contains extensive information about diabetes, including primer of basic facts about diabetes, information about diet, insulin therapy, risks of uncontrolled diabetes, advocacy pages, information about support groups, conditions associated with diabetes, exercise tips and articles, and so on.

American Diabetes Association
http://www.diabetes.org/

One-stop shopping for information about the disease. Excellent site for both the newly diagnosed and long-timers.

Diabetes Station
http://www.diabetesstation.org/

An online "radio station," where the listener can hear live and archived talks by physicians and others in the diabetic community, as well as drop in to talk to others coping with the disease. Features latest information about new drugs, immunology, insulin pumps, health care policies about diabetes, and so on.

Children with Diabetes
http://www.childrenwithdiabetes.com/index_cwd.htm

Good meeting place for children and parents to talk with others in the same situation, via virtual chat rooms and message boards. Also features information for schools and day care providers on dealing with diabetic children, nutrition info, questions and answers, information about diabetic supplies, and so forth.

Aventis

http://www.diabeteswatch.com

Provides support, basic information about the disease, personal stories, a build-your-own self-care journal, diabetes in the news, physician questions and answers, chat rooms, and so forth. Sponsored by a pharmaceutical company.

Diabetes Monitor

http://www.diabetesmonitor.com/main.htm

Excellent stepping stone to online sites devoted to diabetes. According to the home page, the site is dedicated to "monitoring diabetes happenings everywhere in cyberspace."

Insulin-Free World Foundation

http://www.insulinfree.org

Good site to explore medical articles, insurance advice, new research, and an online directory of pancreatic and islet transplant specialists. The Insulin-Free World Foundation promotes the need to cure, rather than just manage, the disease.

Diabetes Living

http://www.diabetesliving.com/

Excellent site that touts itself as "a comprehensive reference manual for day-to-day living with diabetes."

Books

Diabetes for Dummies

By Alan L. Rubin

Hungry Minds Inc., 1999

The author has managed to provide a great deal of detailed and useful information while maintaining the accessible, amusing style of the *Dummies* series. The book contains links to diabetes websites, recipes from famous restaurants, and plenty of encouragement for the bewildered diabetic or family member.

Growing Up with Diabetes: What Children Want Their Parents to Know
By Alicia McAuliffe
John Wiley & Sons, 1998

The author is a diabetic 21-year-old chiropractic student who has
been working with young diabetics for many years. Aimed at parents, this book expresses the young diabetics' need for a normal
and optimistic life.

**Living with Juvenile Diabetes: A Practical Guide for Parents and
Caregivers of Children with Type I Diabetes Mellitus**
By Victoria Peurrung
Hatherleigh Press, 2001

This detailed and organized book offers practical information and
support for frightened parents who have just discovered their child
has a serious disease. It offers coping strategies. Victoria Peurrung
has firsthand experience with her 12-year-old daughter and 10-
year-old son, who both have Type I diabetes.

My Own Type I Diabetes Book
By Sandra J. Hollenberg
Grandma Sandy, 2000

The author wrote this book after her 6-year-old grandson was diagnosed with diabetes. It is a beautifully illustrated book for children
of all reading levels and their caregivers.

■ Addison's Disease

Patient Support Organization

National Adrenal Disease Foundation
505 Northern Blvd., Suite 200
Great Neck, NY 11021
(516) 487-4992
http://www.medhelp.org/nadf/

Medical Organizations

National Institute of Diabetes and Digestive and Kidney Diseases
National Institute of Health
31 Center Dr. MSC 2560
Bethesda, MD 20892-2560
http://www.niddk.nih.gov/index.htm

American Association of Clinical Endocrinologists
1000 Riverside Ave., Suite 205
Jacksonville, FL 32204
(904) 353-7878
http://www.aace.com

Websites

National Adrenal Diseases Foundation
http://www.medhelp.org/nadf/
Good site featuring facts, treatment information, new research, support groups, and the like.

National Institute of Diabetes and Digestive and Kidney Diseases
http://www.niddk.nih.gov/health/endo/pubs/addison/addison.htm
Basic information on how Addison's disease develops and what parts of the body are affected. Covers diagnosis and treatment, special situations such as pregnancy, patient education, and a recommended reading list.

Aspen Johnson
http://www.HEALINGLIGHT.COM/autoimmune/
Features information about the disease, personal stories, a message board, recommended doctors, and so on.

■ Oophoritis/Premature Ovarian Decline and Failure

Patient Support Organization

POF Support Group
P.O. Box 23643
Alexandria, VA 22304
(703) 913-4787
http://www.pofsupport.org/
Email: Info@POFSupport.org

Medical Organizations

American College of Obstetricians and Gynecologists
409 12th St., S.W.
P.O. Box 96920
Washington, DC 20090-6920
http://www.acog.com

American Society for Reproductive Medicine
Formerly the American Fertility Society
1209 Montgomery Highway
Birmingham, AL 35216-2809
(205) 978-5000 or (205) 978-5005
http://www.asrm.com/index.html
Email: asrm@asrm.org

Websites

Premature Ovarian Failure Support Group
http://www.pofsupport.org/
> An excellent place to turn to for support, whether you've just been
> diagnosed or have been struggling with the condition for years. Fea-
> tures articles, one-to-one support, chat rooms, research, and more.

Daisy Network

http://www.daisynetwork.org.uk

U.K. site that features a support group, news about premature ovarian failure and infertility, in vitro fertilization treatments, and so on.

Early Menopause.com

http://www.earlymenopause.com

Comprehensive site about all the different causes of early menopause, including premature ovarian failure. Includes message board, chats, and section on vitamins and natural remedies.

About.com's Infertility Site

http://infertility.about.com/

Large site dealing with all the aspects and causes of infertility.

Books

Taking Charge of Your Fertility: The Definitive Guide to Natural Birth Control and Pregnancy Achievement

By Toni Weschler

Harper Perennial Library, 1995

This book clearly describes the fertility awareness method using natural signs of fertility to increase the possibility of conception. There is also a simple explanation of the role of hormones, the menstrual cycle, fertility tests and treatment.

Six Steps to Increased Fertility: An Integrated Medical and Mind/Body Approach to Promote Conception

By Robert L. Barbieri, Alice D. Donmar, and Kevin R. Loughlin

Simon & Schuster, 2000

Although it is written by a Harvard Medical School team, this book draws on both natural and conventional medicine in a refreshing style. The details of conception, possible problems, and the full gamut of fertility treatment are covered, interspersed with experiences of other couples.

Screaming to Be Heard: Hormonal Connections Women Suspect, and Doctors Still Ignore, 2nd Edition
By Elizabeth Lee Vliet
M. Evans and Company, Inc., 2001
   A comprehensive look at hormonal imbalances, including ovarian problems, and their autoimmune connections to fibromyalgia, thyroid disease, and more.

■ Chronic Fatigue Immune Dysfunction Syndrome (CFIDS)

Patient Support Organizations

Chronic Fatigue and Immune Dysfunction Syndrome Association of America
P.O. Box 220398
Charlotte, NC 28222-0398
Toll-free information line: (800) 442-3437
Resource line: (704) 365-2343
http://www.cfids.org/
Email: info@cfids.org

Chronic Syndrome Support Association, Inc.
801 Riverside Dr.
Lumberton, NC 28358-4625
http://www.cssa-inc.org/

National CFIDS Foundation
103 Aletha Rd.
Needham, MA 02492
(781) 449-3535
http://www.ncf-net.org/

American Fibromyalgia Association
6380 E. Tanque Verde, Suite D
Tucson, AZ 85715
http://www.afsafund.org/
> Despite its name, addresses issues affecting both fibromyalgia and chronic fatigue syndrome. Especially dedicated to promoting more research and raising public awareness about the two conditions.

Medical Organization

American Association for CFS
325 Ninth Ave., Box 359780
Seattle, WA 98104
(206) 521-1932
http://www.aacfs.org/
> The association is composed of physicians, research scientists, and others.

Websites

EndFatigue.com
http://www.endfatigue.com
> Jacob Teitelbaum, MD's website, featuring information on his book, *From Fatigued to Fantastic!*, and his various innovative programs for fibromyalgia, chronic fatigue, and hypometabolism treatment.

Roger Burns
http://www.cfs-news.org/
> News, links, research articles, answers to frequently asked questions about chronic fatigue syndrome and related diseases. Site is run by Roger Burns, who publishes the *CFS Newsletter.*

Edelson Center for Environmental and Preventive Medicine
http://www.ephca.com/cfs.htm
> Interesting page discussing the history of CFS diagnosis, symptoms, treatment, and possible causes.

CFS Files
http://www.geocities.com/cfsdays/cfsfiles.htm
   Good compedium of links and articles about CFS.

Chronic Fatigue and Immune Dysfunction Syndrome Association
http://www.cfids.org/
   Site features wealth of information on the disorder, plus tips on
   choosing the right doctor, information on research, patient support
   and online resources, disability and health information, and advocacy.

National CFIDS Foundation
http://www.ncf-net.org/
   Site features everything you need to know on CFIDS and other
   related conditions.

National Fibromyalgia Awareness Foundation
2415 N. River Trail Rd., #200
Orange, CA 92865
(714) 921-0150
http://www.fmaware.org/

Chronic Syndrome Support Association, Inc.
http://www.cssa-inc.org/
   Information for the patient and medical professional alike. The
   association also publishes a highly regarded quarterly newsletter.

Books

**Running on Empty: The Complete Guide to Chronic Fatigue Syndrome
(CFIDS)**
By Katrina H. Berne
Hunter House, 1995
   This book provides a detailed history of chronic fatigue syndrome, the
   possible causes, a survey of medical research and effective treatments

including alternative health sources. There are interviews with patients, which help readers with the disease feel that they are not alone. The insights described also help the families and friends understand the plight of the patients.

Chronic Fatigue Syndrome, Fibromyalgia, and Other Invisible Illnesses
By Katrina Berne
Hunter House, 2001

This revised and expanded book provides the latest research on chronic fatigue syndrome, fibromyalgia, and allied diseases such as Gulf War syndrome. There is also information about the interaction of the immune system with brain function and the emotional state of the patient.

The CFIDS/Fibromyalgia Toolkit: A Practical Self-Help Guide
By Bruce F. Campbell
iUniverse.com, 2000

This is a practical book that encourages patients to take control of their lives and to improve quality of life despite the fact that there is not yet a cure for these medical conditions. Information about the illnesses and suggestions on alleviating symptoms allow the patient to create an individualized self-help program.

Voices from the Hidden Epidemic of Chronic Fatigue Syndrome
Edited by Peggy Munson
Haworth, 2000

The author concentrates on the social and political aspects of this debilitating condition by recounting the personal odyssey of twenty-nine chronic fatigue patients. The struggles with the symptoms and the search for professional help are often moving.

■ Fibromyalgia and Fibromyositis

Patient Support Organizations

National Fibromyalgia Awareness Foundation
2415 N. River Trail Rd., #200
Orange, CA 92865
(714) 921-0150
http://www.fmaware.org/

American Fibromyalgia Syndrome Association, Inc.
6380 E. Tanque Verde, Suite D
Tucson, AZ 85715
(520) 733-1570
http://www.afsafund.org/

National Chronic Fatigue Syndrome and Fibromyalgia Association
P.O. Box 18426
Kansas City, MO 64133
(816) 313-2000 (Voice)
http://www.ncfsfa.org
Email: KEAL55A@prodigy.com

Websites

EndFatigue.com
http://www.endfatigue.com
   Jacob Teitelbaum, MD's website, featuring information on his book, *From Fatigued to Fantastic!,* and his various innovative programs for fibromyalgia, chronic fatigue, and hypometabolism treatment.

American Fibromyalgia Association
http://www.afsafund.org/
   Addresses issues affecting both fibromyalgia and chronic fatigue syndrome. Especially dedicated to promoting more research and raising public awareness about the two conditions.

Fibromyalgia Network

http://www.fmnetnews.com/

Offers good coping tips, interviews with experts, links to medical journals, political advocacy, drug and nondrug therapies, and so on.

FMS

http://www.tidalweb.com/fms/

Personal site that includes bulletin boards, support groups, self-graphing pain charts and pain scales to use in doctor examinations, bookstore, overview of fibromyalgia, medications, and fibromyalgia diet information.

FMS Discussion/Support Board

http://fmpsc.org/wall/wallinks.htm

Discussion board and support for people with fibromyalgia and related illnesses.

Dr. Lowe/Fibromyalgia Research Foundation

http://www.drlowe.com

Dr. John C. Lowe is a fibromyalgia, thyroid, and metabolism researcher. He is also a board-certified pain management specialist. As director of research for the Fibromyalgia Research Foundation, he has spearheaded the scientific study of two related subjects: the metabolic bases of fibromyalgia and the metabolic rehabilitation of fibromyalgia patients.

Books

From Fatigued to Fantastic!: A Proven Program to Regain Vibrant Health, Based on a New Scientific Study Showing Effective Treatment for Chronic Fatigue and Fibromyalgia
By Jacob Teitelbaum, MD
Avery Penguin Putnam, 2001

One of the most authoritative books on chronic fatigue syndrome and fibromyalgia, this book covers nutrition, stress, medications, and both conventional and alternative approaches.

Fibromyalgia: A Handbook for Self-Care and Treatment
By Janet A. Hulme
Phoenix Publishing, 2001

This comprehensive guide to fibromyalgia covers research and new subcategories of symptoms for which patients can be tested and then treated. There is information on diet, exercise, physiological quieting, and daily routines to help sufferers feel more relaxed yet energetic and free of pain.

The Fibromyalgia Relief Handbook
By Chet Cunningham
United Research Pub., 2001

This book covers the problems associated with the symptoms of fibromyalgia and offers fresh information about alternative and traditional treatments. It is written in an easy-to-read style and format.

Alternative Medicine Guide to Chronic Fatigue, Fibromyalgia and Environmental Illness
Edited by Burton Goldberg
Future Medicine Publishing, 1998

This book describes the treatment programs used by twenty-six leading physicians to bring complete recovery to patients with these illnesses. They all employ a combination of nontoxic alternative medicine.

What Your Doctor May Not Tell You About Fibromyalgia: The Revolutionary Treatment That Can Reverse the Disease
By R. Paul St. Amand and Claudia Craig Marek
Warner Books, December 1999

Describes an innovative, reportedly highly effective treatment using guaifenesin, a common ingredient in cough medicine. This is part of the author's program to prevent and treat fibromyalgia. He claims that symptoms were reversed in 80 percent of his patients.

Speeding Up to Normal: Metabolic Solutions to Fibromyalgia
Edited by John C. Lowe and Jackie G. Yellin
McDowell Pub. Co., 2001

> A presentation of Dr. Lowe's innovative theories about the role of
> metabolism and thyroid function in fibromyalgia.

■ General Skin Information

Books

Skin Disorders Sourcebook: Basic Information About Common Skin and
Scalp Conditions, Caused by Aging, Allergies, Immune Reactions, Sun
Exposure, Infections
Edited by Allan R. Cook
Omnigraphics, Inc., 1997

> This book is an easy-to-read reference for most skin disorders. It is
> useful for the layperson who wants authoritative information on
> various skin conditions from children's rashes, through dermatitis,
> psoriasis, and early melanoma.

■ Scleroderma/Crest Syndrome

Patient Support Organizations

Scleroderma Foundation
12 Kent Way, Suite 101
Byfield, MA 01922
(978) 463-5843
Info line: (800) 722-HOPE (4673)
http://www.scleroderma.org/
Email: sfinfo@scleroderma.org

Scleroderma Research Foundation
2320 Bath St., Suite 315
Santa Barbara, CA 93105
(805) 563-9133 or (800) 441-CURE
http://www.srfcure.org/
Email: rfcure@srfcure.org

Medical Organizations

American Academy of Dermatology
930 N. Meacham Rd.
P.O. Box 4014
Schaumburg, IL 60168-4014
(847) 330-0230
http://www.aad.org/

**National Institute of Arthritis and Musculoskeletal and Skin Diseases,
National Institutes of Health**
Bethesda, MD 20892-2190
http://www.niams.nih.gov

American College of Rheumatologists
1800 Century Place, Suite 250
Atlanta, GA 30345
(404) 633-3777
http://www.rheumatology.org/index.asp

Websites

Scleroderma Foundation
http://www.scleroderma.org/
  Overview of the disease, links and advocacy, patient education,
  weekly coping tips, and so on.

Shelley Ensz, Scleroderma Webmasters Association
http://www.sclero.org/
> Everything you've ever hoped to know about scleroderma is here. Offers over 500 pages of information (in eleven different languages) on scleroderma and its issues.

About.com Arthritis Site
http://arthritis.about.com/cs/sclero/index.htm
> Extensive medical information and links to articles about scleroderma.

Sherry Messick's Scleroderma Support
http://www.sclerodermasupport.com/
> Great site on all the different aspects—medical, practical, emotional—of coping with the chronic disease.

Amie Yaussy
http://www.ihavescleroderma.com
> Touching, tragic, and inspiring stories of people with scleroderma.

Ed Harris
http://www.synnovation.com/sclerodermafaq.html
> Detailed page about the disease, its treatment, and how it affects various parts of the body.

Books

The Scleroderma Book: A Guide for Patients and Families
By Maureen D. Mayes
Oxford University Press, 1999
> This informative and easy-to-read book is based on twenty years of clinical experience with scleroderma patients.

Scleroderma: The Proven Therapy That Can Save Your Life
By Henry Scammell
M. Evans & Co., 1998
This book describes this painful disease and its treatment. It provides the results of a landmark clinical trial of the only therapy to report reversal and remission of this condition.

Scleroderma: Caring for Your Hands and Face
By Jeanne L. Melvin
American Occupational Therapy Association, Inc., 1994
Although this slim paperback was published in 1994, it is still an excellent resource for learning how to maintain and improve flexibility of the hands and face when systemic scleroderma causes swelling or hardening. The exercises in the book can be done alone or with an occupational therapist.

■ Alopecia Areata

Patient Support Organization

National Alopecia Areata Foundation (NAAF)
P.O. Box 150760
San Rafael, CA 94915-0760, or
710 C St., Suite 11
San Rafael, CA 94901
(415) 456-4644
http://www.naaf.org/
Email: info@naaf.org

Professional Organization

American Academy of Dermatology
930 N. Meacham Rd.
P.O. Box 4014
Schaumburg, IL 60168-4014

(847) 330-0230
http://www.aad.org/
Find a Doctor: http://www.aad.org/findaderm_intro.html

Websites

National Alopecia Areata Foundation
http://www.naaf.org/
Good, all-encompassing site on alopecia and what it involves. Special section on ongoing research studies.

AlopeciaKids
http://www.alopeciaKIDS.org/
Excellent site just for children and their families.

Keratin.com
http://www.keratin.com/ad/adindex.shtml
Site offers products for sale on its main home page but is notable for its wealth of information on alopecia: common questions, new research, explanation of the role of autoimmunity, genetics, stress.

Alopecia Page
http://alopecia.mcg.edu/alopecia/main.html
Well-organized site featuring medical information, tips on coping, personal stories, and advice on coping with problems. Especially good for parents of children with alopecia areata.

Books

Alopecia Areata: Understanding and Coping with Hair Loss
By Wendy Thompson, Jerry Shapiro, and Vera H. Price
Johns Hopkins University Press, 2000
Jerry Shapiro is a hair-loss expert in the United States. This book is an easy-to-read handbook that explains the condition, new drug treatments, and current research.

The Hair Loss Cure: How to Treat Alopecia and Thinning Hair
By Elizabeth Steel
Thorsons Publishing, 1999

Hair loss is increasing, especially among women. This practical guide to the condition offers information about treatment and remedies in a sympathetic tone.

The Truth About Women's Hair Loss: What Really Works for Treating and Preventing Thinning Hair
By Spencer David Kobren and Angela Christiano
McGraw Hill, 2000

This book gives a comprehensive and objective survey of information on hair loss in women and its treatment against a background of a mostly unregulated hair restoration industry.

■ Psoriasis

Patient Support Organization

National Psoriasis Foundation
http://www.psoriasis.org/a000.htm
6600 SW 92nd Ave., Suite 300
Portland, OR 97223-7195
(503) 244-7404 or (800) 723-9166
Email: getinfo@npfusa.org

Medical Organization

American Academy of Dermatology
930 N. Meacham Rd.
P.O. Box 4014
Schaumburg, IL 60168-4014
(847) 330-0230
http://www.aad.org/

Websites

National Psoriasis Foundation

http://www.psoriasis.org

The National Psoriasis Foundation provides information to doctors and patients regarding the latest research, developments in treatments, and support groups for people with psoriasis.

American Academy of Dermatology—Find a Doctor

http://www.aad.org/findaderm_intro.html

Psorheads

http://www.psorheads.com/

Excellent site. Offers support, forums, surveys, and chat rooms for those dealing with the disease.

Ed Anderson

http://pinch.com/skin/p.html

Provides shortcuts to information about psoriasis, including how to join an online newsgroup. Don't miss the useful page cautioning readers to be wary of "sure-cure" remedies to psoriasis, located at http://www.pinch.com/skin/pshame.html.

Ed Dewke

http://www.flakehq.com/

Entertaining and educational website that features personal stories sent in by readers, articles about treatment and research, archives, and what not to say to a psoriasis sufferer.

American Academy of Dermatology and Fujisawa Healthcare, Inc.

http://www.skincarephysicians.com/psoriasisnet

A patient education guide detailing treatments, new research, patient stories, glossary of psoriasis terms, and so on.

Books

Healing Psoriasis: The Natural Alternative
By John O. A. Pagano
Pagano Organization, 1991

> This book offers a novel approach to a painful, disfiguring condition. Those who have stayed on the regime and tried to lower the stress in their lives have shown signs of improvement.

Coping with Psoriasis: A Patient's Guide to Treatment
By David L. Cram and Gail Zimmerman
Addicus Books, 2000

> Dr. Cram has years of experience with psoriasis patients and understands the physical and psychological problems caused by this condition. He discusses the possible causes and progress of the disease, choosing a doctor, treatment, and diet. The importance of the patient's self-acceptance is emphasized.

The Psoriasis Cure: A Drug-Free Guide to Stopping and Reversing the Symptoms of Psoriasis
By Lisa Levan
Avery Penguin Putnam, 1999

> Ms. Levan provides a nutritional approach to treatment for psoriasis. She teaches the patient to eliminate allergic reactions and adds nutritional supplements to a drug-free diet.

■ Vitiligo

Patient Support Organizations

American Vitiligo Research Foundation, Inc.
P.O. Box 7540
Clearwater, FL 33758

(727) 461-3899
http://vitiligosearch.org/
Email: info@vitiligosearch.com

National Vitiligo Foundation, Inc.
611 South Fleishel Ave.
Tyler, TX 75701
(903) 531-0074
http://www.nvfi.org/
Email: vitiligo@trimofran.org

Medical Organizations

American Academy of Dermatology
930 N. Meacham Rd.
P.O. Box 4014
Schaumburg, IL 60168-4014
(847) 330-0230
http://www.aad.org/

National Institute of Arthritis and Musculoskeletal and Skin Diseases, National Institutes of Health
Bethesda, MD 20892-2190
http://www.niams.nih.gov/

Websites

Vitiligo Support.com
http://www.vitiligosupport.com/
The first place to visit when seeking support for vitiligo. Offers live chats, message boards, patient and public information, physician referrals, and so forth. You must sign up to access the information on the site.

Vitiligo Society, UK

http://www.vitiligosociety.org.uk/index.html

> British foundation that aims to increase public awareness and "promote a positive approach to living with vitiligo." Good basic information for the newly diagnosed, and excellent resources for parents and children.

American Vitiligo Research Foundation, Inc.

http://vitiligosearch.org/

> Excellent, wide-ranging site for adults and children alike. Features medical information and overview of the disease, discussion of treatment options, and so on.

National Vitiligo Foundation, Inc.

http://www.nvfi.org/

> Check out the good "treatment library" section for a large collection of articles.

Vitiligo Switchboard

http://web.onramp.ca/cadd/vitiligo.htm

> A useful little site offering numerous links to articles, as well as corporations and doctors who offer vitiligo treatments.

Vitiligo Friends Network

http://www.vitnet.org/index.html

> Much of the site is currently under construction, but what's there looks promising.

Inigo Garcia

http://www.astro.rug.nl~iruiz/vitiligo/

> Good overview of medical, adjunctive, and alternative therapies for vitiligo.

■ Pemphigus

Patient Support Organization

National Pemphigus Foundation
Atrium Plaza, Suite 203
828 San Pablo Ave.
Albany, CA 94706
(510) 527-4970
http://www.pemphigus.org

■ Irritable Bowel Syndrome, Crohn's Disease, and Ulcerative Colitis

Patient Support Organization

Crohn's and Colitis Foundation of America
386 Park Ave. South
New York, NY 10016-8804
(800) 932-2423
http://www.ccfa.org/
Email: info@ccfa.org

Medical Organizations

National Institute of Diabetes and Digestive and Kidney Diseases,
National Institute of Health
31 Center Dr., MSC 2560
Bethesda, MD 20892-2560
http://www.niddk.nih.gov/index.htm

American College of Gastroenterology
4900 B S. 31st St.
Arlington, VA 22206-1656
(703) 820-7400
http://www.acg.gi.org/

American Gastroenterological Association
7910 Woodmont Ave.
7th Floor
Bethesda, MD 20814
(301) 654-2055
http://www.gastro.org/

Websites

IBS/Crohn's Site at About.com
http://ibscrohns.about.com

> An important library to turn to, whether you've just been diagnosed or have been living with Crohn's for years. Features articles on new research and treatment, information on drugs and side effects, alternative and homeopathic treatments, links to recipes and nutritional information, traveling with Crohn's disease, and so forth.

Crohn's and Colitis Foundation of America
http://www.ccfa.org/

> Site offers education and support, weekly feature articles, doctor-locating service, "ask-the-specialist" questions and answers, resource pages for physicians, news about legislative affairs, and a bookstore.

Healingwell.com
http://www.healingwell.com/ibd/

> Good site to turn to for chats, information on books about Crohn's disease, new research and treatments, and tips on practical and emotional challenges of living with Crohn's.

Prometheus Labs

http://www.patientcommunity.com/

Comprehensive site that includes articles about new research, a chat room, a library, features (some written in highly clinical language, some not), discussion boards, a doctor locator, and more. Sponsored by a pharmaceutical company.

My Crohn's

http://mycrohns.freeservers.com/

Decent personal website devoted to support and education for people with Crohn's disease. Includes personal stories, books, chat room, and a good section on emotional issues in coping with the disorder.

Books

The New Eating Right for a Bad Gut: The Complete Nutritional Guide to Ileitis, Colitis, Crohn's Disease and Inflammatory Bowel Disease
By James Scala
Plume, 2000

This revised and updated book provides Crohn's disease patients with a new drug-free dietary plan that can help the condition go into remission. There is an easy testing program, identification of safe foods, fitness and stress-relief techniques.

Crohn's Disease and Ulcerative Colitis Fact Book
By National Foundation for Ileitis and Colitis, and Daniel H. Present;
Edited by Peter A. Banks
Hungry Minds, Inc., 1984

This book was the first thorough and comprehensive guide to Crohn's disease and remains a very useful reference for newly diagnosed patients and those who are still trying to understand the nature of their illness.

Positive Options for Crohn's Disease: Self-Help and Treatment
By Joan Gomez
Hunter House, 2000

> This guide provides detailed information on the symptoms, possible causes/risk factors, latest research, treatment, and dietary needs, all in a style accessible to nonspecialists.

Irritable Bowel Syndrome & the Mind-Body/Brain-Gut Connection: 8 Steps for Living a Healthy Life with a Functional Bowel Disorder or Colitis
By William B. Salt II
Parkview Publishing, 1999

> An eight-step program that combines mind and body approaches to help deal with chronic digestive disorders. Focuses on prevention, medications, and mind-body approaches.

Irritable Bowel Syndrome: A Natural Approach
By Rosemary Nicol
Ulysses Press, 1999

> Diet and stress are examined as contributing factors to irritable bowel syndrome. Provides natural solutions and dietary alternatives and methods to help deal with the condition.

Breaking the Vicious Cycle: Intestinal Health Through Diet (Millennium Edition)
By Elaine G. Gottschall, Patricia Wilson, and Marilyn Jones
Kirkton Print, 1994

> This book is essential reading for anyone with ulcerative colitis. The simple, natural diet guide of "do eat" and "don't eat" foods has shown marked improvement in the condition of many patients.

Crohn's Disease and Ulcerative Colitis
By Fredric G. Sabil
Firefly Books, 1997

This book is recommended by the National Association for Colitis and Crohn's Disease, United Kingdom, because it is comprehensive, well laid out, and readable by the layperson. The latest drug and surgical techniques and the role of diet are discussed. There are clear diagrams and a glossary of medical terms.

■ Celiac Sprue Dermatitis

Patient Support Organizations

Celiac Disease Foundation
13251 Ventura Blvd., Suite 1
Studio City, CA, 91604-1838
(818) 990-2354
http://www.celiac.org/
Email: cdf@celiac.org

Celiac Sprue Association—USA, Inc.
P.O. Box 31700
Omaha, NE 68131-0700
http://www.csaceliacs.org/

Gluten Intolerance Group
15110 10th Ave. SW, Suite A
Seattle, WA 98166
(206) 246-6652
http://www.gluten.net/

American Celiac Society
59 Crystal Ave.
West Orange, NJ 07052
(973) 325-8837
Email: amerceliacsoc@netscape.net

Medical Organizations

National Institute of Diabetes and Digestive and Kidney Diseases,
National Institutes of Health
31 Center Dr., MSC 2560
Bethesda, MD 20892-2560
http://www.niddk.nih.gov/index.htm

National Center for Nutrition and Dietetics
American Dietetic Association
216 W. Jackson Blvd., Suite 800
Chicago, IL 60606-6995
(800) 366-1655
http://www.eatright.org/

Websites

Celiac Disease Foundation
http://www.celiac.org/
> Virtually everything you would ever want to know about celiac disease, including causes and treatment, support, bulletin board, newsletter, and more.

About.com's Allergies Site
http://allergies.about.com/library/weekly/aa020899.htm
> General look at the disease, its symptoms and causes, plus links to gluten-free recipes and vendors.

National Institute of Diabetes and Digestive Diseases and Kidney Disease
http://www.niddk.nih.gov/health/digest/pubs/celiac/index.htm
> Good site for getting health information; interesting graphics on how many products contain gluten.

Celiac Sprue Association
http://www.csaceliacs.org/

Starting place for the newly diagnosed; features loads of well-organized information on understanding and coping with the disorder, nutrition, and recipes.

Celiac Database
http://www.celiacdatabase.org/

Getting nutritional information from food packaging is important for the rest of us, but for those with celiac disease, it's crucial. This website allows patients with celiac disease to find out what products contain gluten and the name of the manufacturer. Type in, for example, "pasta" under the product search category and you'll get a listing of which pastas are gluten-free.

Gluten Intolerance Group
http://www.gluten.net/

In addition to the usual information about the disease, diet, and treatment, this site aims to increase public awareness of the disorder. Also supports a Kids Camp for children with celiac disease.

Books

The Gluten-Free Diet Book: A Guide to Celiac Sprue, Dermatitis Herpetiforms and Gluten-F
By Peter Rawcliffe and Ruth Rolph
Hungry Minds, 1985

This book is based on the premise that certain people are allergic to gluten and thus should avoid it. It advocates a change of diet relying on alternate gluten-free foods.

The Gluten-Free Kitchen: 135 Delicious Recipes for People with Gluten Intolerance or Wheat Allergy
By Roben Ryberg
Prima Communications, Inc., 2000

The recipes are easy to follow and use affordable ingredients. The results are said to be delicious.

■ Pernicious Anemia

Medical Organization

National Heart, Lung and Blood Institute (NHLBI)
6701 Rockledge Dr.
P.O. Box 30105
Bethesda, MD 20824-0105
(301) 592-8573
http://www.nhlbi.nih.gov/

Websites

Encyclopedia Brittanica
http://www.britannica.com/eb/article?eu=60787
    Good overview of the condition.

Cynthia Donlan
http://www.geocities.com/Athens/Acropolis/6338/pernicious.html
    A good page written by a sufferer of pernicious anemia. Includes a
    basic explanation of what the disease is, common symptoms, and
    treatment.

■ Rheumatoid Arthritis

Patient Support Organizations

Arthritis Trust
7111 Sweetgum Rd., Suite A
Fairview, TN 37602-9384
http://www.arthritistrust.org/

Arthritis Foundation of America
1330 W. Peachtree St.
Atlanta, GA 30309
(404) 872-7100, ext. 6271 (Voice), or (800) 283-7800 (Voice)
http://www.arthritis.org
  Toll-free national hotline for Joint Effort Against Rheumatoid
  Arthritis at (800) 538-7799.

Medical Organization

American College of Rheumatology
1800 Century Place, Suite 250
Atlanta, GA 30345
(404) 633-3777
http://www.rheumatology.org

Websites

Arthritis Site at About.com
http://arthritis.about.com/cs/ra/index.htm
  A gold mine of information about living with rheumatoid arthritis,
  new advances in treating the disease, tips on coping, the effects of
  diet on the disease, patient support, and more.

Arthritis Insight
http://www.arthritisinsight.com/
  Wonderful site featuring medical information, patient support and
  discussions, pain management, physician locator, alternative therapies, and so on.

Arthritis Foundation
http://www.arthritis.org
  Visit the foundation's well-done website for a look at all issues—
  medical, emotional, and practical—in dealing with the disease.

Nancy Etchemendy
http://www.sff.net/people/etchemendy/arthritis/
Nice personal website; includes a look at conventional and alternative therapies, stress reduction, guided imagery, acupuncture, and so forth.

Books

Conquering Rheumatoid Arthritis: The Latest Breakthroughs and Treatments
By Thomas F. Lee
Prometheus Books, 2001
The author writes from his own experience as a rheumatoid arthritis patient. He provides an excellent resource using the latest research and websites for further information and updates.

The Arthritis Foundation's Guide to Good Living with Rheumatoid Arthritis
By Gretchen Henkel, Arthritis Foundation, and John H. Klippel; Edited by T. Pincus
Longstreet Press, 2001
This book is edited by eminent physicians in rheumatology and rheumatoid arthritis under the auspices of the Arthritis Foundation. It is a comprehensive book that offers plenty of information and easy exercises, diet, and other tips to improve the quality of life.

Finding Ways: Recovering from Rheumatoid Arthritis Through Alternative Medicine
By Barbara Jay Nies
Synchrony Publishing, 1997
The author has been living and struggling with this chronic, debilitating disease for thirty years. This book is about her unsatisfactory journey through the tortuous maze of conventional medicine before she discovered success with alternative treatments. It is well written and moving.

The Arthritis Foundation's Guide to Alternative Therapies
By Judith Horstman, William J. Arnold, Matthew H. Liang, and J. Roger Hollister
Longstreet Press, 1999
> This book aims to be a "common-sense guide through the maze of the most-used complementary therapies for arthritis, to help you choose wisely among the many options available." It covers twenty-two different complementary therapies from acupuncture and yoga to magnets and bee stings. In addition, forty herbs and supplements are discussed.

Overcoming Arthritis
By David Brownstein
Medical Alternatives Press, 2001
http://www.drbrownstein.com
> An excellent resource on alternative therapies for arthritis, including antibiotic therapy.

■ Juvenile Arthritis

Patient Support Organization

American Juvenile Arthritis Organization
Arthritis Foundation of America
1330 W. Peachtree St.
Atlanta, GA 30309
(404) 872-7100, ext. 6271 (Voice), or (800) 283-7800 (Voice)
http://www.arthritis.org/communities/children_young_adults.asp

Medical Organization

American College of Rheumatology
1800 Century Place, Suite 250
Atlanta, GA 30345

(404) 633-3777
http://www.rheumatology.org

Websites

JRA World
http://jraworld.arthritisinsight.com/
> Excellent site; loads of medical information as well as support and
> message boards, tons of suggestions on coping and living well with
> the disease, pain management, physician locator, and more.
> Includes a section on alternative therapies.

Rheumatic Arthritis
http://rheumatic.org/
> Site promotes the use of antibiotic therapies to treat juvenile and
> rheumatoid arthritis, as well as several other related diseases. Also
> includes information for patient and doctor, support group, and
> links to scientific journal articles.

Pediatric Rheumatology Home Page
http://www.goldscout.com/
> Well-organized site for kids with JA, their families, and the doctors
> who treat them. Offers pages for the layperson and for their physi-
> cians.

Books

Juvenile Arthritis (Perspective on Disease and Illness)
Judith Peacock
Lifematters, 2000
> This clearly written book is designed to inform those 13 years of
> age and older without frightening the readers. The main thrust is to
> learn to live with this chronic disease. The resulting emotional
> responses are handled with compassion and hope.

Nicole's Story: A Book About a Girl with Juvenile Rheumatoid Arthritis
By Virginia Tortorica Aldape and Lillian S. Kossacoff
Lerner Publications Company, 1996
> Aimed at the reading level of 4 to 8 years of age, this book describes juvenile rheumatoid arthritis in some detail. The reader begins to understand how this disability affects normal life through the eyes of 8-year-old Nicole.

Your Child with Arthritis: A Family Guide for Caregiving
By Lori B. Tucker, Bethany A. Denardo, and Judith A. Stebulis
Johns Hopkins University Press, 2000
> This book is designed to give parents information about the medical, social, and emotional issues that confront the suffering child and those around him or her. There are forms to compile medical records, a resource section for further research, and an important message that these children should be encouraged to join in all activities and have some fun.

■ Ankylosing Spondylitis

Patient Support Organization

Spondylitis Association of America
14827 Ventura Blvd., #222
Sherman Oaks, CA 91403
(818) 981-1616 or (800) 777-8189 (U.S. only)
http://www.spondylitis.org/

Medical Organization

American College of Rheumatology
1800 Century Place, Suite 250
Atlanta, GA 30345

(404) 633-3777
http://www.rheumatology.org/

Websites

KickAs.org
http://kickas.org/
http://www.kickas.org/direct_assistance.shtml

This is an excellent site filled with medical information, treatment options, forums, diet and nutrition information, special forums for women and teens with AS, and personal stories.

About.com's Spondylitis Page
http://arthritis.about.com/cs/spondy

Index to articles about the disease, as well as links to other spondylitis pages.

Spondylitis Association of America
http://www.spondylitis.org

Good, basic site featuring news about medical advances in the disease, message boards, and so on.

National Ankylosing Spondylitis Society (Great Britain)
http://www.nass.co.uk/

Excellent compendium of information on the disease, including basic questions and explanations, tips on coping, exercises, and practical advice.

Book

Straight Talk on Spondylitis
By Spondylitis Association of America
SAA http://www.spondylitis.org

This is a comprehensive site developed by the Spondylitis Association of America for patients and their families to help them understand and manage the disease. A full-size pull-out exercise chart is included. Both the *Journal of Rheumatology* and the *Journal of the American Physical Therapy Association* gave it good reviews.

■ Multiple Sclerosis

Patient Support Organizations

Multiple Sclerosis Foundation, Inc.
Kitty Burofsky, Program Services Administrator
6350 N. Andrews Ave.
Fort Lauderdale, FL 33309
(954) 776-6805 (Voice) or (800) 441-7055 (Voice)
http://www.msfacts.org

Multiple Sclerosis Association of America
706 Haddonfield Rd.
Cherry Hill, NJ 08002-2652
(609) 488-4500 (Voice) or (800) LEARNMS (Voice)
http://www.msaa.com/

National Multiple Sclerosis Society
733 3rd Ave.
New York, NY 10017-3288
(212) 986-3240 (Voice) or (800) FIGHTMS (Voice)
http://www.nmss.org

International Multiple Sclerosis Foundation
PMB #291
9420 E. Golf Links Rd.
Tucson, AZ 85730-1340
http://www.msnews.org/
Email: jean@imssf.org

Medical Organizations

NIH Neurological Institute
P.O. Box 5801
Bethesda, MD 20824
(800) 352-9424

American Academy of Neurology
1080 Montreal Ave.
St. Paul, MN 55116
(651) 695-1940
http://www.aan.com/

Websites

Understanding MS.com/MS Active Source
http://www.understandingms.com/
  Good site to turn to after receiving a diagnosis of MS. Features
  overview of the disease and treatment, coping strategies, new
  research, and webcasts on MS topics.

Multiple Sclerosis International Federation
http://www.ifmss.org.uk/
  Interesting international site, featuring medical information, personal stories of encouragement, pages for physicians, section for
  the newly diagnosed, pages on MS and intimacy/sexuality, and
  more.

MS World
Teva Neuroscience
http://www.msworld.org/index.htm
  Provides forums, chat rooms, information on new research and
  medications, overview of the disease, kids' pages, links, MS magazine, financial aid sites, and book reviews, among other things.

Multiple Sclerosis Education Network
http://www.htinet.com/msen/index.html
> Good information featuring patient education, personal stories of living with the disease, new treatments on the horizon, treatment of side effects, and coping with the emotional side of the disease.

National Multiple Sclerosis Society
http://www.nmss.org/
> Nicely designed website featuring a compendium of MS information and avenues of support.

Multiple Sclerosis University
http://www.mswatch.com
> Online MS resources and courses. Freshman courses teach students all they need to know about the human body. Sophomore and upper-class courses focus more specifically on MS and its treatments.

Books

Multiple Sclerosis Fact Book, 2nd Edition
By Richard Lechtenberg
F. A. Davis Company, 1995
> This extensively revised edition is a guide for people with MS and their families. It differs from other MS handbooks because it includes a wide discussion of current drug therapies. Another unique section is a bibliography from the medical literature. This book is recommended by the National Multiple Sclerosis Society.

Alternative Medicine and Multiple Sclerosis
By Allen C. Bowling
Demos Medical Publishing, 2001
> This book contains accurate and unbiased information on an extensive range of complementary and alternative medical therapies and

medicines that can help manage MS and improve general well-being. Patients will find unusual treatments and information on subjects such as the risk of interactions between medical and alternative therapies.

The Multiple Sclerosis Diet Book: A Low-Fat Diet for the Treatment of M.S.
By Roy L. Swank and Barbara Brewer Dugan
Doubleday, 1987 (revised and expanded)
This completely revised edition of an old favorite complies with the latest medical research. There are hundreds of recipes that keep to the dietary rules.

■ Guillain-Barré Syndrome

Patient Support Organization

Gullain-Barré Syndrome Foundation International
P.O. Box 262
Wynnewood, PA 19096
(610) 667-0131
http://www.webmast.com/gbs

Medical Organization

American Academy of Neurology
1080 Montreal Ave.
St. Paul, MN 55116
(651) 695-1940
http://www.aan.com/

Websites

Gullain-Barré Syndrome Support Group
http://www.gbs.org.uk/index.html
> Features a little bit of everything for the patient with a Gullain-Barré diagnosis: treatment, support, personal stories, kids' pages, discussion boards, and pages for health professionals.

Gullain-Barré Syndrome Association of New South Wales
http://www.ozemail.com.au/~guillain/
> General overview of GBS for the layperson and for the physician, personal stories, and more.

GBS Syndrome
http://www.gbsyndrome.com/eng/default.asp
> Personal page featuring overview of GBS, including treatment and possible causes, support, discussion board, and personal stories.

National Institute of Neurological Disorders and Stroke
http://www.ninds.nih.gov/health_and_medical/disorders/gbs.htm
> Fact sheet on Gullain-Barré disease.

Books

Bed Number Ten
By Sue Baier and Mary Zimmeth Schomaker
CRC Press, 1989
> This true story is seen through the eyes of someone who became completely paralyzed with Guillain-Barré. She remained in the hospital for eleven months, where she experienced both sensitive and insensitive treatment.

No Time for Tears: Transforming Tragedy into Triumph
By Dorris R. Wilcox
Corinthian Books, 2000
> The author made a 95 percent recovery from Guillain-Barré syn-

drome against all expectations, which she attributes to self-education, nutritional supplements, positive thinking, and an unswerving belief in God's healing power. She advocates her approach in this book and includes a useful appendix of sources for further information.

Masks
Gloria Hatrick
Orchard Books, 1996
> This book is aimed at the young adult level. It is a fictional story about what happens when the narrator's older brother becomes paralyzed by Guillain-Barré very suddenly.

■ Myasthenia Gravis

Patient Support Organizations

Myasthenia Gravis Foundation of America, Inc.
5841 Cedar Lake Rd., Suite 204
Minneapolis, MN 55416
(952) 545-9438 or (800) 541-5454
http://www.myasthenia.org/
Email: myastheniagravis@msn.com

Muscular Dystrophy Association
MDA Headquarters
3300 E. Sunrise Dr.
Tucson, AZ 85718-3208
(520) 529-2000 (Voice) or (800) 572-1717 (Voice)
http://www.mdausa.org
> The MDA offers health services to people with muscular disorders, including myasthenia gravis.

Medical Organizations

NIH Neurological Institute
P.O. Box 5801
Bethesda, MD 20824
(800) 352-9424
http://www.ninds.nih.gov/index.htm

American Academy of Neurology
1080 Montreal Ave.
St. Paul, MN 55116
(651) 695-1940
http://www.aan.com/

Websites

Myasthenia Gravis Foundation of America, Inc.
http://www.myasthenia.org/
    Good starting point for information and support about MG.
    Offers medical information, videocasts of MG talks, new research,
    and more.

Myasthenia Gravis Association
http://www.mgauk.org/
    This British MG site offers extensive information, including a good
    section on various aspects of coping with the disease under the
    heading "MGA General Information Leaflets."

Donna Whittaker and MG Friends
http://pages.prodigy.com/lifewithmg/
    Patient support site bringing people with MG together to share
    experiences, plus daily coping strategies.

Prodigy Myasthenia Page
http://pages.prodigy.net/stanley.way/myasthenia/mgmail.htm
    Information on joining an automated email list of MG patients.

■ Raynaud's Phenomenon

Patient Support Organization

Raynaud's Foundation
P.O. Box 346176
Chicago, IL 60634-6176
(773) 622-9220
http://members.aol.com/Raynauds/

Medical Organizations

American College of Rheumatologists
1800 Century Place, Suite 250
Atlanta, GA 30345
(404) 633-3777
http://www.rheumatology.org/index.asp

National Institute of Arthritis and Musculoskeletal and Skin Diseases
National Institutes of Health
Bethesda, MD 20892-2350
http://www.niams.nih.gov/

National Heart, Lung and Blood Institute
National Institutes of Health
Bethesda, MD 20892-2350
http://www.nhlbi.nih.gov

Websites

Raynaud's Foundation
http://members.aol.com/Raynauds/
　　Terrific site to find everything you've ever wanted to know about
　　Raynaud's phenomenon, and then some. Good section on autoim-
　　mune diseases and why they are related.

National Institute of Arthritis and Musculoskeletal and Skin Diseases
http://www.niams.nih.gov/hi/topics/raynaud/ar125fs.htm
> Detailed and informative site on Raynaud's, its causes, diagnosis, treatment, and self-care tips.

Raynaud's and Scleroderma Association (Great Britain)
http://www.raynauds.demon.co.uk/
> British site features discussion of the two diseases, photos, and information about ongoing research.

■ Cardiomyopathy

Patient Support Organization

Hypertrophic Cardiomyopathy Association
P.O. Box 306
Hibernia, NJ 07842
Call 8am to 8pm Eastern time (973) 983-7429
http://www.kanter.com/hcm/index.html
> Website has a pretty good overview of the disease and damage it can do to the heart, plus information on diagnosis and treatment.

Medical Organization

American Heart Association
National Center
7272 Greenville Ave.
Dallas, TX 75231
http://www.americanheart.org

Websites

Cardiomyopathy Association (Great Britain)
http://www.cardiomyopathy.org/homepage.htm
   Excellent discussion about the disorder, plus information for medical professionals on identifying and treating the disease.

Johns Hopkins University
http://www.med.jhu.edu/heart/
   Offers information on the possible causes, treatment, and procedures of cardiomyopathy and other heart disorders, new research and techniques, and more.

About.com
http://heartdisease.about.com/cs/cardiomyopathy
   Features information on different types of cardiomyopathy, plus links to other sites.

■ Eosinophilia-Myalgia

Patient Support Organization

National Eosinophilia-Myalgia Syndrome Network
P.O. Box 1095
Bryson City, NC 28713-9998
http://www.nemsn.org/

Website

Yahoo!Groups: EosinophiliaMyalgiaInformation
http://groups.yahoo.com/group/EosinophiliaMyalgiaInformation

■ Dietary, Nutritional, and Herbal Medicine Approaches

Books

The One Earth Herbal Sourcebook: Everything You Need to Know About Chinese, Western, and Ayurvedic Herbal Treatments
By Alan Keith Tillotson, with Nai-shing Hu Tillotson and Robert Abel Jr.
Kensington Publishing, 2001

> The definitive, comprehensive guide about herbal medicine. A must-have manual for anyone interested in nutritional approaches and supplements, from one of the nation's premier herbalists.

Herbal Defense: Positioning Yourself to Triumph Over Illness and Aging
By Robyn Landis, with Karta Purkh Singh Khalsa
Warner Books, 1997

> An excellent guide to the use of herbal medicine to prevent or treat specific illnesses, from another of the nation's most respected herbalists.

Prescription for Natural Healing
By James F. Balch and Phyllis A. Balch
Avery Penguin Putnam, 2000

> A comprehensive reference featuring nutritional supplements, vitamins, and recommendations.

Dr. Atkins' Vita-Nutrient Solution: Nature's Answers to Drugs
By Robert D. Atkins
Simon & Schuster, 1998

> Excellent overview, with specific recommendations regarding supplements, including dosages, for different autoimmune conditions and other health issues.

Organizations

American Herbalists Guild
Herbalist Referral page:
http://www.americanherbalist.com/referral_search.htm
> Enter your state in the search box and hit submit, and you'll see AHG herbalists in your area. You can call (770) 751-6021.

Herb Research Foundation
1007 Pearl St., Suite 200
Boulder, CO 80302
Herbal Hotline: (303) 449-2265
(800) 748-2617
http://www.herbs.org
> Information on herbal support specifically for particular autoimmune diseases is available in a detailed packet. The packet is $7 for nonmembers. Individual memberships are also available for $35 a year and include a free information packet and a subscription to the foundation's magazine. To order a packet or find out more about membership, contact: Herb Research Foundation at (303) 449-2265. They also have a specialized Herbal Hotline to answer specific questions for a small fee. You need a Visa/Mastercard to use this service.

American Dietetic Association's Nationwide Nutrition Network
(800) 366-1655
Database: http://www.eatright.org/finddiet.html
> This organization offers referrals to registered dietitians and a searchable online database of registered dietitians.

American Association of Naturopathic Physicians
2366 Eastlake Ave. E, Suite 322
Seattle, WA 98102
Referral Line: (206) 298-0125
(206) 323-7610

Website database: http://www.naturopathic.org/find_d.htm
   This group offers a referral line, directory, and brochures explaining naturopathic medicine.

Websites

Nutrition Website
http://nutrition.about.com
   Rick Hall's excellent site provides a comprehensive web-based starting point for nutritional information.

Whole World Botanicals
P.O. Box 322074
Fort Washington Station
New York, NY 10032
(888) 757-6026
http://www.wholeworldbotanicals.com
   An excellent source of organic, wildcrafted South American herbs.

Great Smokies Diagnostic Laboratory
63 Zillicoa St.
Asheville, NC 28801
(800) 522-4762
http://www.gsdl.com
Email: cs@gsdl.com
   The nation's top lab for functional medicine testing.

■ Chinese Medicine/Acupuncture

American Association of Oriental Medicine
433 Front St.
Catasauqua, PA 18032
(610) 266-1433 or (888) 555-7999

http://www.aaom.org

Email: AAOM1@aol.com

AAOM provides referrals to practitioners who are state licensed or certified by various respected certifying organizations. They also have an online state-by-state referral search for TCM and acupuncture practitioners at http://www.aaom.org/referral.html.

Acupuncture and Oriental Medicine Alliance

14637 Starr Road SE

Olalla, WA 98359

(253) 851-6883

http://www.acuall.org

Practitioner Search: AOMA also offers a practitioner search at the HealthyNet website, http://www.healthy.net.

National Certification Commission for Acupuncture and Oriental Medicine

Department 0595

Washington, DC 20073-0595

(202) 232-1404

The NCCAOM awards the title Dipl.Ac. to acupuncture practitioners who pass its certification requirements. You can get a list of diplomates of acupuncture in your state from them for $3.

American Academy of Medical Acupuncture

(800) 521-2262

The AAMA, which provides referrals, requires that its members, who are all physicians, undergo at least 220 hours of continuing medical education in acupuncture.

Accreditation Commission for Acupuncture and Oriental Medicine

(301) 608-9680

This organization can verify which American schools of acupuncture and Oriental medicine have a decent reputation.

Dr. Patrick Purdue's Website
http://www.PatrickPurdue.com
　　Excellent website featuring information from this renowned traditional Chinese medicine practitioner.

Acupuncture.com
http://www.acupuncture.com/Referrals/ref2.htm
　　Acupuncture.com offers a list of licensed acupuncturists by state.

■ Antibiotic Therapies

Road Back Foundation
P.O. Box 447
Orleans, MA 02653
(614) 227-1556
http://roadback.org/Index1.html
　　Information on antibiotic therapy for patients with rheumatoid arthritis, scleroderma, lupus, polymyositis, Reiter's syndrome, psoriatic arthritis, ankylosing spondylitis, fibromyalgia, and juvenile rheumatoid arthritis, based on the work of Dr. Thomas McPherson Brown. Includes advocacy page, online support, recommended reading, self-care information, and more.

■ NAET/JMT/BRT

Jaffe-Mellor Technique (JMT) Website
http://www.jmt-jafmeltechnique.com
　　Features information about the technique, plus a partial list of JMT practitioners.

Official NAET Website
http://www.naet.com/subscribers/index3.html
　　Features NAET information and a practitioners' list.

Dr. Eric Berg's Healthy Self Wellness Center
http://www.nutrition-n-wellness.com/

■ Hormones

Listening to Your Hormones
By Gillian Ford
Prima Publishing, 1997
http://www.gillianford.com
http://www.menopausesolutionsonline.com
> One of the best, most comprehensive, and practical books on hormones, the interplay, and how they impact a woman's life and health. An absolute requirement on every woman's bookshelf.

Hormone Heresy: What Women Must Know About Their Hormones
By Sherrill Sellman
GetWell International, 2000
http://www.ssellman.com
> The dramatic physical, psychological, and emotional effects of hormone replacement therapy on women are explored in this book, which dares to challenge the prevailing dogma of hormonal therapy.

Screaming to Be Heard
By Elizabeth Lee Vliet
M. Evans & Company, 2001
> An excellent, comprehensive manual that discusses the relationship of hormones to PMS, fibromyalgia, weight gain, palpitations, and much more, by one of America's foremost hormonal physicians.

The Menopause Diet, The Goddess Diet, and The Gladiator Diet
Larrian Gillespie
> A series of excellent books that focus on how to work with hormones to ensure better health and weight loss.
> http://www.goddessdiet.com

■ Alternative Medicine—General

**Pocket Guide to Natural Health: Proven Remedies for
More Than 125 Ailments**
By Stephen Langer, MD and James F. Scheer
Kensington Publishing, 2001

> An excellent resource that offers alternative remedies for a variety
> of conditions that affect autoimmune disease patients, including
> allergies, candida/yeast, dry eye syndrome, fatigue, as well as many
> specific autoimmune conditions themselves. Under each condition,
> signs, causes, alternative supplements, diet, lifestyle, and mind-body
> approaches are covered.

**Intelligent Medicine: A Guide to Optimizing Health and Preventing
Illness for the Baby-Boomer Generation**
By Ronald Hoffman
Fireside, 1997

> A bridge between traditional and alternative medicine approaches,
> this excellent book looks at preventive and treatment options for
> many common ailments, including some autoimmune conditions.

Tired All the Time: How to Regain Your Lost Energy
By Ronald Hoffman
Pocket Books, 1996

> The twelve leading causes of fatigue, including autoimmune disease,
> are discussed in this helpful book that also guides patients through
> how to develop a personalized energy plan.

■ Traditional Mental Health Support

For traditional mental health support, such as a psychologist, a
counselor, or general support groups, contact:

National Mental Health Association
1021 Prince St.
Alexandria, VA 22314-2971
(800) 969-NMHA
> Provides referrals to state and regional mental health associations and resources.

National Mental Health Consumers Self-Help Clearinghouse
1211 Chestnut St., Suite 1000
Philadelphia, PA 19107
(800) 553-4539
Email: info@mhselfhelp.org
> Offers articles and books on consumer-oriented and mental health issues; and a reference file on relevant groups, organizations, and agencies.

Mental Health Site
http://mentalhealth.about.com
> Dr. Leonard Holmes's comprehensive site on mental health.

■ Spirituality

George Washington Institute for Spirituality and Health
George Washington University Medical Center
Warwick Building, Room 336
2300 K St., NW
Washington, DC 20037
(202) 994-0971
http://www.gwish.org
> Excellent organization pioneering integration of spirituality into medical education and practice.

■ Mind-Body Support

Stress Reduction
http://stress.about.com
> Dr. Melissa Stöppler's excellent site on stress reduction.

Mind Body Medical Institute
110 Francis St.
Boston, MA 02215
(617) 632-9530
http://www.mbmi.org
> Dr. Herbert Benson's Harvard-based organization that has pioneered the study and practice of mind-body medicine.

Center for Mind/Body Medicine
P.O. Box 1048
La Jolla, CA 92038
(619) 794-2425
> Developed under the guidance of Dr. Deepak Chopra. Offers both residential and outpatient programs, as well as education and training programs in Ayurveda.

American Chronic Pain Association
P.O. Box 850
Rocklin, CA 95677
(916) 632-0922
> This group manages a list of over 500 support groups internationally, and publishes workbooks and a newsletter.

Center for Attitudinal Healing
33 Buchanan
Sausalito, CA 94965
(415) 331-6161
> Support groups throughout the nation for people with chronic or serious illness.

Wellness Community
2716 Ocean Park Blvd., Suite 1040
Santa Monica, CA 90405
(310) 314-2555
> Chapters throughout the nation offer support groups for people with chronic or serious illness.

■ Reiki Information

Holistic Healing Site and Spiral Visions
http://healing.about.com
http://www.spiralvisions.com
> Websites of Usui Reiki Master Phylameana lila Désy, offering comprehensive reiki information, articles, community, and links.

Essential Reiki: A Complete Guide to an Ancient Healing Art
By Diane Stein
Crossing Press, 1995
> A definitive overview of reiki.

■ Patient Empowerment

DrSavard.com
> Marie Savard's site, featuring helpful downloadable charts and forms, plus information on Dr. Savard's health tracking systems.
> http://www.drsavard.com

Your Doctor in the Family.com
http://YourDoctorintheFamily.com
> Dr. Richard Fogoros's excellent site that empowers patients and provides helpful information.

■ Holistic/Complementary/Alternative Practitioners

American Osteopathic Association
142 East Ontario St.
Chicago, IL 60611
(800) 621-1773
http://www.aoa-net.org
Email: www@aoa.nat.org

> The American Osteopathic Association has referral lists for
> osteopaths in all fifty states.

American Board of Medical Specialties "Certified Doctor" Service
(800) 776-2378
http://www.abms.org

> This online service allows you to browse for doctors by specialty
> and locale and get certification information on doctors. These are
> conventional doctors.

American Medical Association (AMA) "Physician Select"
http://www.ama-assn.org/aps/amahg.htm

> The AMA's Physician Select program allows you to browse its data-
> base for AMA member doctors, almost always conventional doctors.
> It offers medical school and year graduated, residency training, pri-
> mary practice, secondary practice, major professional activity, and
> board certification for all doctors who are licensed physicians.

American Holistic Health Association
P.O. Box 17400
Anaheim, CA 92817-7400
(714) 779-6152
http://www.ahha.org/
Email: ahha@healthy.net

> The American Holistic Health Association offers an online referral
> to its members, who are holistic doctors.

American Holistic Medical Association
6728 Old McLean Village Dr.
McLean, VA 22101
(703) 556-9728
Patient Information number: (703) 556-9728
http://www.holisticmedicine.org
Email: info@holisticmedicine.org

The American Holistic Medical Association publishes a referral
directory of member MDs and DOs.

■ General Doctor Referral Services

American Board of Medical Specialties
Online search: http://www.abms.org/newsearch.asp
1007 Church St., Suite 404
Evanston, IL 60201-5913
Phone verification: (866) ASK-ABMS
(847) 491-9091

Hospital Referrals

If a good hospital in your area has a referral service, this can be a
decent source of information and referrals to doctors. If the hospital's reputation is good, the doctors typically are going to be of
higher caliber. Some of the more sophisticated hospital referral services offer educational and practice style information about doctors
in their databases.

**U.S. News and World Report "Best Graduate Schools"/Medical School
Evaluation**
(800) 836-6397
http://www.usnews.com/usnews/edu/beyond/gradrank/med/gdmedt1.htm

You can evaluate whether your doctor went to a good medical
school by checking the med school rankings provided by *U.S. News
and World Report*. The information is available on the web. You

can also order their *Best Graduate Schools Directory,* for $5.95, at the website, or by calling their 800 number.

Doctor Ratings

Find out if any of your local magazines rate doctors. *Washingtonian* magazine, for example, periodically asks doctors to pick those other Washington, DC/Maryland/Virginia–area doctors they'd most recommend in particular specialties, and publishes the results. It's always a comfort to me to see a doctor I've been referred to appear on this list, although it doesn't always guarantee I'll *like* that doctor!

Best Doctors
(888) DOCTORS
http://www.bestdoctors.com

Best Doctors has a Family Doc-Finder at their website, where for a small fee you can find recommended primary care physicians in your area. You'll find only conventional doctors via this service. Best Doctors also conducts specialized physician searches for rare, catastrophic, or serious illnesses. The highly specialized search, which costs approximately $1500, is only merited in the direst situations, but it's worth knowing about if you find yourself seriously in need of a specialist or expert.

■ Checking Out Bad Doctors

Questionable Doctors Listing
http://www.questionabledoctors.org

Check on whether your doctor has been listed in the "16,638 Questionable Doctors" report, which was produced by the consumer advocacy group Public Citizen. The book, also available in CD form, lists more than 20,000 doctors who were disciplined by state medical boards or federal agencies. Among these doctors were those accused of sexual abuse, substandard care, incompetence or negligence, criminal conviction, misprescribing drugs, and substance abuse. Interestingly, up to 69 percent of these doctors are still practicing medicine.

Medical Board Charges or Actions

You can find out if disciplinary action has ever been taken with your doctor, or if charges are pending against him or her, by calling your state medical board. A good list of all medical boards is found at http://www.fsmb.org/members.htm. You can also search at the Association of State Medical Board Executive Directors "DocFinder" service: http://www.docboard.org/.

■ Disability Issues

Talking About Disability Issues Site
http://www.aboutdisabilityissues.net
Gary Presley's excellent site covering disability issues and rights.

Please note: If you have new resources you'd like to recommend for future updates, or if you know of updates to the information in this section, please drop me a line by email, mshomon@thyroid-info.com, or regular mail, at P.O. Box 0385, Palm Harbor, FL 34682.

APPENDIX B: FEATURED EXPERTS

The following experts were interviewed for or generously provided information and input for this book:

Eric Berg, DC, is a certified doctor of chiropractic and certified in NAET and JMT, creator of the BRT technique, and founder of the Healthy Self Wellness Center.
Healthy Self Wellness Center
4609-D Pinecrest Office Park Dr.
Alexandria, VA 22312
(703) 354-7336
http://www.nutrition-n-wellness.com/
Email: welnes1@aol.com
Dr. Berg holds free workshops in the Washington, DC, area on energy, menopause, hormones and PMS, thyroid disease, and other topics. For more information, contact his office at (703) 354-7336. If you're a practitioner interested in training in BRT, please contact Dr. Berg's office for more information about upcoming training sessions. Dr. Berg also publishes a free email newsletter, *HealthySelf*. To subscribe, send an email to welnes1@aol.com with the subject "Subscribe Dr. Berg's Newsletter."

David Brownstein, MD, a family physician who integrates conventional and alternative therapies in his practice, is the author of *Overcoming Arthritis* and *The Miracle of Natural Hormones*. In this interview, he talks about the relationship between arthritis, arthritis symptoms, and thyroid conditions, and treatments that can help. He serves as the medical director for the Center for Holistic Medicine in West Bloomfield, Michigan, and is a

clinical assistant professor of medicine at Wayne State University School of Medicine.
Office: (248) 851-1600
Publications: Medical Alternatives Press
(888) 647-5616
http://www.drbrownstein.com

Kim Carmichael-Cox is a reporter and writer who has autoimmune thyroid disease. Kim is also a volunteer for the American Autoimmune Related Diseases Association in Virginia Beach, Virginia. Anyone who wishes to contact her for autoimmune disease support may reach her by email at PrufrockMedia@aol.com

Tracee Cornforth is a writer and educator on women's health issues. She also runs a popular women's health website at http://womenshealth.about.com.

Phylameana lila Désy is a Usui reiki master, who offers healing services—including reiki classes, reiki healings, and chakra cleansings—in the Burlington, Iowa, area. She also runs the popular holistic healing website at About.com, located at http://healing.about.com, which features articles, information, and an international support community interested in healing and holistic health.
(319) 752-9548
http://healing.about.com
http://www.spiralvisions.com
Email: phylameana@spiralvisions.com

Laura Dolson, MA, has a background in physical therapy and psychology. She also runs a popular website at http://gyncancers.about.com, and has been on a gluten-free diet for more than three years to successfully treat gluten intolerance.

John V. Dommisse, MD, FRCPC, is a nutritional, metabolic, and psychiatric physician in Tucson, where he runs a patient practice that offers a pioneering approach to hypothyroidism.

1840 E. River Rd., Suite 210
Tucson, AZ 85718-5892
(520) 577-1940
http://johndommissemd.com
Email: John@JohnDommisseMD.com

Carol Eustice was diagnosed with rheumatoid arthritis at age 19 and has more than twenty-six years of personal experience with a variety of treatments, medications, and joint surgeries. Carol is a rheumatoid arthritis patient advocate and educator, and runs the popular arthritis website http://arthritis.about.com.

Richard Eustice, a rheumatoid arthritis sufferer for over thirteen years, has worked as a restaurant manager, tax accountant, real estate investor, and is now on disability. Along with his wife, Carol, he helps create the arthritis site at About.com, located at http://arthritis.about.com.

Richard "Dr. Rich" Fogoros, MD, is a former professor of medicine, and a longtime practitioner, researcher, and author in cardiology and cardiac electrophysiology. Dr. Rich runs the popular heart disease site at http://heartdisease.about.com, and YourDoctorintheFamily.com, an online guide to understanding and surviving the American health care system.
http://heartdisease.about.com
http://YourDoctorintheFamily.com

Gillian Ford has worked for more than two decades as a women's health and hormonal educator, advocate researcher, clinician, and speaker. She is the author of the best-selling book *Listening to Your Hormones*.
P.O. Box 70
Caloundra, Q. 4551
Australia
http://www.gillianford.com
http://www.menopausesolutionsonline.com
Email: gford1@bigpond.net.au

Paula Ford-Martin is a health writer and diabetes educator who runs the popular diabetes site at About.com, located at http://diabetes.about.com.

Larrian Gillespie, MD, is an expert on hormones and weight loss, and author of a number of health best-sellers, including *You Don't Have to Live with Cystitis, The Menopause Diet, The Goddess Diet,* and *The Gladiator Diet.* For more information on her work, see her website at http://www.goddessdiet.com or call 1-800-554-3335.

Rick Hall, MS, RD, is a registered dietitian and nutrition educator, living in Phoenix, Arizona. He is a member of the American Dietetic Association, the American College of Sports Medicine, and two dietetic practice groups: Sports, Cardiovascular and Wellness Nutritionists (SCAN), and Nutrition in Complementary Care. He also runs the popular website http://nutrition.about.com.

Ronald Hoffman, MD, is founder of the Hoffman Center, which focuses on internal medicine with an integrative approach to chronic health concerns, combining conventional and natural therapies. Dr. Hoffman hosts a popular radio show on WOR radio in the New York City area, and is author of a number of books, including *Tired All the Time: How to Regain Your Lost Energy* and *Intelligent Medicine.*
Hoffman Center
40 E. 30th St.
New York, NY 10016
(212) 779-1744
http://www.drhoffman.com
Email: drhoffman@wor710.com

Leonard Holmes, PhD, is a clinical psychologist in Virginia, with expertise in health psychology, especially treatment of chronic pain. He also runs the popular website http://mentalhealth.about.com.

Donna Hurlock, MD, is a certified menopause clinician who specializes in hormonal management for women and women's health issues.
205 S. Whiting St., #303
Alexandria, VA 22304
(703) 823-1533

Karta Purkh Singh Khalsa, known as K. P. Khalsa, is one of the world's premier herbalists. As a member of the American Herbalists Guild, with more than twenty-five years of experience with medicinal herbs and natural healing, he is co-author of the best-selling book *Herbal Defense.* His website is at http://www.kpkhalsa.com. For herbal, medical, or health care professionals interested in training, herbal consulting, or specialized herbal products and formulations, call (800) 659-2077 or email info@kpkhalsa.com.

Mary Kugler, MSN, RN, C, is an ANCC-certified pediatric nurse and health educator whose specialty is children with chronic medical problems. She has expertise in researching and educating the public on the topic of rare diseases, and runs the popular rare disease site at http://rarediseases.about.com.

Virginia T. Ladd, RT, is the founder, president, and executive director of the American Autoimmune Related Diseases Association.
American Autoimmune Related Diseases Association
National Office
22100 Gratiot Ave. E
Detroit, MI 48021
(810) 776-3900
http://www.aarda.org

Stephen Langer, MD, is author of numerous books, including *Solved: The Riddle of Illness,* co-authored with James Scheer. Dr. Langer is an expert on antiaging medicine and thyroid disease. He provides in-office and phone consultations regarding thyroiditis, hypothyroidism, fibromyalgia, chronic fatigue, orthomolecular medicine, optimal nutrition, metabolic medicine, and food allergies.

3031 Telegraph Ave., Suite 230
Berkeley, CA 94705
(510) 548-7384

Lisa Lorden is a chronic fatigue syndrome and fibromyalgia patient advocate who serves as director of communications for the National Fibromyalgia Awareness Campaign, a nonprofit organization dedicated to increasing fibromyalgia awareness and information.
National Fibromyalgia Awareness Campaign (NFAC)
2238 N. Glassell St., Suite D
Orange, CA 92865
(714) 921-0150
http://www.fmaware.org
Email: nfac@fmaware.org

John C. Lowe, DC, is a fibromyalgia, thyroid, and metabolism researcher. He is also a board-certified pain management specialist. As director of research for the Fibromyalgia Research Foundation, he has spearheaded the scientific study of two related subjects: the metabolic bases of fibromyalgia and the metabolic rehabilitation of fibromyalgia patients. He is author of the internationally acclaimed book *The Metabolic Treatment of Fibromyalgia*. **Dr. Gina Honeyman-Lowe** is an advisor to the Fibromyalgia Research Foundation and is director of the Center for Metabolic Health. She is co-author with Dr. Lowe of *Your Guide to Metabolic Health*. They practice in Colorado.
Drs. John C. Lowe and Gina Honeyman-Lowe
http://www.drlowe.com
Center of Metabolic Health
1800 30th St., Suite 217A
Boulder, CO 80301
(303) 413-9100
Fax: (303) 413-9101
Books/Publications: http://www.McDowellPublishing.com
Email: DrLowe@drlowe.com
Email: DrGHL@drlowe.com

Andrea Maloney Schara, LCSWA, is a therapist who specializes in Bowen Family Systems Theory, and individual and organizational consulting.
Georgetown Family Center
4400 MacArthur Blvd., #103
Washington, DC 20007
(202) 965-0730
http://www.ideastoaction.com

Joseph Mercola, DO, is a Chicago-area osteopathic physician and natural medicine expert who specializes in treating metabolic and immune system disorders. He also runs a popular alternative medicine website at http://www.mercola.com.
1443 W. Schaumburg Rd.
Schaumburg, IL 60194
(847) 985-1777
http://www.mercola.com

Don Michael, MD, practices holistic medicine in South Bend, Indiana. He went to Wayne State University School of Medicine, completed a neurology residency, and later completed one in psychiatry. He is board certified in psychiatry by the American Board of Psychiatry and Neurology.
328 N. Michigan St., Suite B3
South Bend, IN 46601
(219) 287-6010
Email: Dmichaelmd@aol.com

Viana Muller, PhD, is co-founder and president of Whole World Botanicals, a company that is involved in research, growing, harvesting, propagation, and distribution of certified organic and wildcrafted South American medicinal herbs. As an anthropologist, Dr. Muller has been making rainforest herb collecting/study trips to the Amazon River Basin since 1989.
Whole World Botanicals
P.O. Box 322074

Fort Washington Station
New York, NY 10032
(888) 757-6026
http://www.wholeworldbotanicals.com

Michael Phillips, PhD, is a writer, historian, professor, and a lifelong diabetes patient.

Gary Presley is a full-time freelance writer, as well as advocate for people with disabilities. Gary, who has, as he puts it, forty years of education on four wheels after a bout with polio, also runs a popular website, "Talking About Disability Issues," at http://www.aboutdisabilityissues.net.
Email: editor@aboutdisabilityissues.net

Christina Puchalski, MD, is director of the George Washington Institute for Spirituality and Health in Washington, DC.
George Washington Institute for Spirituality and Health
George Washington University Medical Center
Warwick Building, Room 336
2300 K St. NW
Washington, DC 20037
(202) 994-0971
http://www.gwish.org
Email: cpuchalski@gwish.org

Patrick Purdue, DOM, AP, is a doctor of Oriental medicine and acupuncture physician, and a graduate of the Florida Institute of Traditional Chinese Medicine. His practice focuses on women's health, gastrointestinal conditions, and autoimmune diseases.
10010 Seminole Blvd. (107th St. N)
Seminole, FL 33772
(727) 319-8819
http://www.PatrickPurdue.com
Email: PPurdue10@aol.com

Carol Roberts, MD, is a board-certified holistic physician and director of the popular Tampa Bay–area practice Wellness Works, a medical practice that specializes in integrated treatment of chronic disease and offers acupuncture, herbal medicine, nutrition therapy, and other complementary and alternative therapies. Dr. Roberts is also a frequent host on Tampa's WMNF-FM radio, talking about medicine and health.
Wellness Works
1209 Lakeside Dr.
Brandon, FL 33510
(813) 661-3662
http://www.healme.org
Email: wellnesswk@aol.com

Noel R. Rose, MD, PhD, is chairperson of the American Autoimmune Related Diseases Association's Scientific Advisory Board; professor of pathology and of molecular microbiology and immunology and director of the Autoimmune Research Center, the Johns Hopkins University. His pioneering studies on autoimmune thyroiditis ushered in the modern era of research on autoimmunity. Among his many books and publications is the definitive textbook on autoimmunity, *The Autoimmune Diseases,* edited by Dr. Rose and Ian Mackay.
720 Rutland Ave.
Baltimore, MD 21205
http://autoimmune.pathology.jhmi.edu

Marie Savard, MD, is an internationally known internist, women's health expert, and patients' rights champion. She is author of two highly acclaimed books: *How to Save Your Own Life: The Savard System for Managing—and Controlling—Your Health Care* and *The Savard Health Record.*
Savard Systems
54 Churchill Dr.
York, PA 17403
(877) SAVARDS (728-2737)
http://www.drsavard.com

Sherrill Sellman, an expert on natural hormones, psychotherapist, speaker, and health researcher, is author of *Hormone Heresy: What Women Must Know About Their Hormones.* As a women's health educator and advocate, Sherrill also provides consulting and health coaching, in addition to her educational and writing projects.
P.O. Box 690416
Tulsa, OK 74169-0416
(918) 437-1058
http://www.ssellman.com
Email: golight@earthlink.net

Richard Shames, MD, graduated from Harvard University and the University of Pennsylvania, did research at the National Institutes of Health with Nobel Prize winner Marshall Nirenberg, and has been in private practice for twenty-five years. Dr. Shames practices holistic medicine—with a focus on thyroid and autoimmune conditions—and has for twenty years been engaged in the search for answers about thyroid disease. **Karilee Halo Shames, RN, PhD,** is a clinical specialist in psychiatric nursing and a certified holistic nurse with a PhD in holistic studies. The husband-and-wife team co-authored the book *Thyroid Power: 10 Steps to Total Health.*
Richard and Karilee Shames
(561) 417-7833
http://www.shameshealth.com
Email: thyroidpower@aol.com

Melissa Stöppler, MD, is a physician, researcher, and writer with an interest in stress and its effects on the human body. Dr. Stöppler's work has focused on the role of stress in illness. She runs the popular About.com website on stress at http://stress.about.com.

Alan Tillotson, PhD, AHG, DAy, is the codirector of the Chrysalis Natural Medicine Clinic and a professional member of the American Herbalists Guild, as well as a member of its executive board. He is trained in the

Asian, Ayurvedic, and Taoist systems of medicine, healing, and meditation. He is author of *The One Earth Herbal Sourcebook*.
Chrysalis Natural Medicine Clinic
1008 Milltown Rd.
Wilmington, DE 19808
(302) 994-0565
http://www.oneearthherbs.com
Email: AlanT33@aol.com

Amber Tresca is an ulcerative colitis survivor who now works to help raise patient awareness and runs the popular website at http://ibscrohns. about.com.

APPENDIX C: REFERENCES

CHAPTER 2

American Diabetes Association website, http://www.diabetes.org.

Angier, Natalie. "Studying the Autoimmune Disease Puzzle," *New York Times,* June 19, 2001.

Arthritis Foundation website, http://www.arthritis.org.

"Autoimmune Disorder Therapies Market to Reach $18.3 Billion by 2006," Front Line Strategic Management Consulting press release, October 3, 2001.

Canaris, Gay J., et al. "The Colorado Thyroid Disease Prevalence Study," *Archives of Internal Medicine,* Vol. 160, No. 4, February 28, 2000.

Lupus Foundation of America website, http://www.lupus.org/.

Multiple Sclerosis Foundation website, http://www.msfacts.org.

National Graves' Disease Foundation website, http://www.ngdf.org.

National Vitiligo Foundation website, http://www.nvfi.org/.

Rose, Noel. "The Autoimmune Diseases," American Autoimmune Related Diseases Association website, http://www.aarda.org.

Rose, Noel. "Autoimmunity—The Common Thread," American Autoimmune Related Diseases Association website, http://www.aarda.org.

Scleroderma Foundation website, http://www.scleroderma.org/.

Sjögren's Syndrome Foundation website, http://www.sjogrens.org/.

Thyroid Foundation of America website, http://www.tsh.org.

"Understanding Autoimmune Diseases," Online brochure/National Institutes of Health/National Institute of Allergy and Infectious Diseases website, http://www.niaid.nih.gov/publications/autoimmune/.

"Understanding the Immune System," Online brochure/National Cancer Institute and the National Institute of Allergy and Infectious Diseases website, http://newscenter.cancer.gov/sciencebehind/uis/uishome.htm.

CHAPTER 3

"An Assessment of the Safety of the Anthrax Vaccine: A Letter Report," Committee on Health Effects Associated with Exposures During the Gulf War, Institute of Medicine, Washington, DC 2000.

Confavreux, Christian. "Vaccinations and the Risk of Relapse in Multiple Sclerosis," *New England Journal of Medicine,* Vol. 344, No. 5, pp. 319–326, February 1, 2001.

"Chronic Periodontal Disease Could Lead to Diabetes," American Academy of Periodontology (AAP)/National Institute of Dental and Craniofacial Research (NIDCR) press release, April 23, 2001, online, http://www.perio.org.

Elengold, Mark A. "Statement Before the Committee on Government Reform, Operations Center for Biologics Evaluation and Research, Food and Drug Administration," U.S. House of Representatives, October 3, 2000.

Faustman, Denise. "Autoimmune Diseases: What Next After Genomics?" *In Focus,* American Autoimmune Related Diseases Association newsletter, Vol. 9, No. 2., June 2001.

Guthrie, Michael. "Mycoplasmas: The Missing Link in Fatiguing Illnesses," *Alternative Medicine,* September 2001.

Hall, Carl T. "Simian Stress Lessons: When life is good, they create their own problems, researchers find," *San Francisco Chronicle,* February 26, 2001.

Hess, Evelyn V. "The Environment and Autoimmune Diseases," *In Focus,* American Autoimmune Related Diseases Association newsletter, Vol. 8, No. 4, December 2000.

Horowitz, S., et al. "Mycoplasma Fermentans in Rheumatoid Arthritis," *Journal of Rheumatology,* December 2000.

"Infections May Trigger Autoimmunity Via Rare, But Normal Process," *Science Daily Online,* December 19, 2000, Wistar Institute, http://www.wistar.upenn.edu/.

"Infectious Diseases, Chapter 162. Viral Diseases," *The Merck Manual of Diagnosis and Therapy Online Edition,* Section 13, 1995–2001.

Kenyon, Georgina. "Bacterial Protein May Help Prevent Type I Diabetes," Reuters Health Wire, December 11, 2000.

Kuman, Vijay, et. al., "Celiac Disease—Associated Autoimmune Endocrinopathies," *Clinical and Diagnostic Laboratory Immunology,* Vol. 8, No. 4., pp. 678–685, July 2001.

Lederer, Edith. "More Women Contract Disease," Associated Press Wire, March 3, 2000.

"Mechanism for Generating Autoimmunity-Suppressing Cells Identified," *Science Daily Online,* March 30, 2001, Wistar Institute, http://www.wistar.upenn.edu/.

Moran, Mark. "Autoimmune Diseases Could Share Common Genetic Etiology," *American Medical News,* October 8, 2001.

O'Shea, Tim. "Vaccination Is Not Immunization," *Alternative Medicine,* July 2001.

Perl, Andras. "Endogenous Retroviruses in Pathogenesis of Autoimmunity," *Journal of Rheumatology,* Vol. 28, No. 3, March 2000.

Reaney, Patricia. "Study Links Coffee Consumption to Arthritis Risk," Reuters Health Wire, July 25, 2000.

Rose, Noel R., and MacKay, Ian R. (editors). *The Autoimmune Diseases,* 3rd edition, Academic Press, 1998.

Siegel-Itzkovich, Judy. "Common 'Bug' May Trigger Arthritis," *Jerusalem Post,* April 1, 2001.

Kalliomäki, Marko, et al. "Probiotics in Primary Prevention of Atopic Disease: A Randomised Placebo-Controlled Trial," *The Lancet,* Vol. 357, pp. 1076–1079, April 7, 2001.

Walsh, Stephen J., and Dechello, Laurie M. "Excess Autoimmune Disease Mortality Among School Teachers," *Journal of Rheumatology*, Vol. 27, pp. 1537–1545, 2001.

CHAPTER 4

Adler, Jonathan, et al. "Reiter Syndrome," *eMedicine Journal*, May 16, 2001.

American Autoimmune Related Diseases Association website, http://www.aarda.org.

Berkow, Robert (editor). *Merck Manual of Medical Information: Home Edition*, Simon & Schuster, New York, 1999.

Doherty, Bridget. "Lupus Test May Speed Diagnosis," *Prevention*, January 2001.

Duriseti, Ram S. "Lupus," *eMedicine Journal*, June 8, 2001.

Ghaussy, N. O., et al. "Cigarette Smoking, Alcohol Consumption, and the Risk of Systemic Lupus Erythematosus: A Case-Control Study," *Journal of Rheumatology*, Vol. 28, pp. 2449–2453, November 2001.

Hoffman, Robert, et al. "Mixed Connective Tissue Disease," *eMedicine Journal*, Vol. 2, No. 6, June 21, 2001.

"Mixed Connective Tissue Disease: Section 5. Musculoskeletal and Connective Tissue Disorders, Chapter 50," *The Merck Manual of Diagnosis and Therapy*, http://www.merck.com/pubs/mmanual/section5/chapter50/50o.htm.

Phelan, Darren. "Sjögren Syndrome," *eMedicine Journal*, February 1, 2001.

"Reiter's Syndrome: Section 5. Musculoskeletal and Connective Tissue Disorders, Chapter 51. Arthritis Associated with Spondylitis," *The Merck Manual of Diagnosis and Therapy*, http://www.merck.com/pubs/mmanual/section5/chapter51/51b.htm.

Rose, Noel R., and MacKay, Ian R. (editors). *The Autoimmune Diseases*, 3rd edition, Academic Press, 1998.

"Smoking Ups Lupus Risk: Report," Reuters Health Wire, December 20, 2001.

Wallace, Daniel J. *The Lupus Book: A Guide for Patients and Their Families,* Oxford University Press, 2000.

Yakobi, M. et al. "Sarcoidosis," *eMedicine Journal,* May 16, 2001.

CHAPTER 5

"A Delicate Balance: What Changes in the Immune System Trigger Type I Diabetes?" *Diabetes News,* Joslin Diabetes Center.

Agachi, S. "The Pathology of the Thyroid Gland and Rheumatoid Arthritis in the Period of Onset," *Journal of Rheumatology,* Vol. 28, Supplement 63, 2001.

Beer, Alan E. "Thyroid Disorders and Reproductive Problems of Miscarriage, Implantation Failure and In Vitro Fertilization Failure," Finch University of Health Sciences/The Chicago Medical School.

Berkow, Robert (editor). *Merck Manual of Medical Information: Home Edition,* Simon & Schuster, New York, 1999.

Cooper, David S. "Subclinical Hypothyroidism," *New England Journal of Medicine,* Vol. 345, No. 4, July 26, 2001.

Diabetes Update, *Morbidity and Mortality Report,* October 27, 2000.

"Endocrine Autoimmunity," American Autoimmune Related Diseases Association fact sheet.

Epstein, D. et al. "Surgical Perspective in Treatment of Diabetic Foot Ulcers," *Wounds,* Vol. 13, No. 2, pp. 59–65, March/April 2001.

Holmes, G. K. "Coeliac Disease and Type I Diabetes Mellitus—The Case for Screening," *Diabetes Medicine,* Vol. 18, No. 3, pp. 169–177, March 2001.

Hypponen, E., et al. "Intake of Vitamin D and Risk of Type 1 Diabetes: A Birth-Cohort Study," *The Lancet,* Vol. 358, pp. 1476–1478, November 3, 2001.

"Insulin Injections Fail to Prevent Type I Diabetes, Separate Prevention Trial Tests Benefit of Oral Insulin," National Institute of Diabetes and Digestive and Kidney Diseases (NIDDK) press release, June 23, 2001.

Lamb, William H., and Court, Simon. "Diabetes Mellitus," *eMedicine Journal*, Vol. 2, No. 5, May 2, 2001.

Nagourney, Eric. "Exploring the Diabetes-Depression Link," *New York Times*, June 12, 2001.

"New Study Tightens the Link Between Smoking and Early Menopause," *Science Daily*, July 16, 2001.

Norris, J. M. "Can the Sunshine Vitamin Shed Light on Type 1 Diabetes?" *Journal of the American Medical Association*, Vol. 286, p. 2421, November 3, 2001.

Odeke, Sylvester, et al. "Addison Disease," *eMedicine Journal*, May 1, 2001.

"Researchers Find a Genetic Cause of Type I Diabetes and Autoimmunity," *Science Daily*, http://medinfo.wustl.edu, December 8, 2000.

Rose, Noel R., and MacKay, Ian R. (editors). *The Autoimmune Diseases*, 3rd edition, Academic Press, 1998.

Rostler, Suzanne. "Vitamin D May Cut Risk of Type I Diabetes: Study," Reuters Health Wire, November 2, 2001.

Rostler, Suzanne. "Study Links Long Menstrual Cycle to Diabetes Risk," Reuters Health Wire. November 20, 2001.

Rostler, Suzanne. "Cutting Stress Helps Diabetics Control Blood Sugar." Reuters Health Wire, December 27, 2001.

Solomon, C. G., et al. "Long or Highly Irregular Menstrual Cycles as a Marker for Risk of Type 2 Diabetes Mellitus," *Journal of the American Medical Association*, Vol. 286, p. 2421, November 21, 2001.

"The Premature Ovarian Failure Support Group Informational Booklet," online, http://www.pofsupport.org.

Votey, Scott R. "Diabetes Mellitus, Type I—A Review," *eMedicine Journal*, Vol. 2, No. 4, April 13, 2001.

Wilson, Jean D. "Prospects for Research for Disorders of the Endocrine System," *Journal of the American Medical Association,* Vol. 285, No. 5, February 7, 2001.

Weetman, Anthony P. "Autoimmune Thyroid Disease," *The Autoimmune Diseases,* 3rd edition, Edited by Noel R. Rose and Ian R. MacKay, Academic Press, 1998.

CHAPTER 6

Aarflot, T., and Bruusgaard, D. "Association Between Chronic Widespread Musculoskeletal Complaints and Thyroid Autoimmunity. Results from a Community Survey," *Scandinavian Journal of Primary Health Care,* Vol. 14, No. 2, pp. 1111–1115, 1996.

Arthritis Care Research, Vol. 45, pp. 355–361, 2001.

Cunha, Burke A., "Chronic Fatigue Syndrome," *eMedicine Journal,* Vol. 2, No. 5, May 4, 2001.

"Dealing with Anxiety, Depression and Chronic Fatigue Syndrome," *PDR Family Guide to Women's Health,* Chapter 33, http://www.healthsquare.com/fgwh/wh1ch33.htm.

Frieden, Joyce. "Stress Not a Cause of Chronic Fatigue," Reuters Health Wire, March 21, 2001.

Gilliland, Regina P. "Fibromyalgia," *eMedicine Journal,* Vol. 2, No. 6, June 8, 2001.

Lapp, Charles W. "The Treatment of Chronic Fatigue Syndrome" lecture transcript, 1997, http://www.co.cure.org/lapp.htm.

Lowe, J. C., et al. "Thyroid Status of Fibromyalgia Patients," *Clinical Bulletin of Myofascial Therapy,* Vol. 3, No. 1, pp. 69–70, 1998.

Lowe, J. C. *The Metabolic Treatment of Fibromyalgia,* McDowell Publishing Co., 2000.

Lowe, J., and Honeyman-Lowe, G. "Thyroid Disease and Fibromyalgia Syndrome," *Lyon Mediterrane Medecine du Sud-Est.,* Vol. 36, No. 1, pp. 15–17, February 2000.

Mulvihill, Keith. "Altering the Diet May Ease Fibromyalgia," Reuters Health Wire, October 25, 2001.

Reid, S., et al. "Multiple Chemical Sensitivity and Chronic Fatigue Syndrome in British Gulf War Veterans," *Americal Journal of Epidemiology*, Vol. 153, No. 6, pp. 604–609, March 15, 2001.

Rose, Noel R., and MacKay, Ian R. (editors). *The Autoimmune Diseases*, 3rd edition, Academic Press, 1998.

Rossy, I. A., et al. "A Meta-Analysis of Fibromyalgia Treatment Interventions," *Annals of Behavioral Medicine*, Vol. 21, No. 2, pp. 180–191, Spring 1999.

Schorr, Melissa. "Acupuncture May Help Relieve Fibromyalgia Symptoms," Reuters Health Wire, November 12, 2001.

Weil, Andrew. "Feeling Better with Firbomyalgia," *Self-Healing*, July 2001.

Wirrtup, Irene, et al. "Comparison of Viral Antibodies in 2 Groups of Patients with Fibromyalgia," *Journal of Rheumatology*, Vol. 28, No. 3, March 2001.

CHAPTER 7

Bolduc, Chantal, et al. "Alopecia Areata," *eMedicine Journal*, Vol. 2, No. 6, June 17, 2001.

"Genentech's Xanelim Effective for Psoriasis—Study," Genentech Inc. corporate press release, July 31, 2001, http://www.gene.com.

Hann, Seung-Kyung. "Vitiligo," *eMedicine Journal*, Vol. 2, No. 8, August 6, 2001.

Koenig, Andrew S., and Jimenez, Sergio. "Scleroderma," *eMedicine Journal*, Vol. 2, No. 5, May 17, 2001.

Macron, Doug. "Remicade Shows Promise as Psoriasis Treatment," Reuters Health Wire, March 2001.

Park, Randy. "Psoriasis," *eMedicine Journal*, Vol. 2, No. 7, July 31, 2001.

"Psoriasis/Alefacept," *New England Journal of Medicine*, Vol. 345, pp. 248–255, 284–287, July 2001.

"Reversing the Effects of Scleroderma," Interview transcript with James Dauber, M.D., *Ivanhoe Broadcast News*, November 2001.

Rose, Noel R., and MacKay, Ian R. (editors). *The Autoimmune Diseases*, 3rd edition, Academic Press, 1998.

"Study: Enbrel Effective in Psoriatic Arthritis," Reuters Health Wire, November 12, 2001.

"Targeted Immunotherapies Define Future of Psoriasis Therapeutics Markets, Says Frost & Sullivan," Business Wire press release, July 18, 2001, http://www.frost.com.

"The Case of Vitiligo," *Alternative Medicine*, online, http://www.alternativemedicine.com.

"Trials Show Positive Results for New Psoriasis Treatment; Alefacept Shows Promise for Psoriasis Relief," press release, June 22, 2001.

Wigley, Fredrick M. "When Is Scleroderma Really Scleroderma," *Journal of Rheumatology*, Vol. 28, No. 7, July 2001.

CHAPTER 8

Al-Ataie, Bashar M., et al. "Ulcerative Colitis," *eMedicine Journal*, Vol. 2, No. 6, June 29, 2001.

Anderson, Maria. "Crohn's: An Autoimmune or Bacterial-Related Disease?" *The Scientist*, August 20, 2001.

Conrad, Marcel E. "Pernicious Anemia," *eMedicine Journal*, Vol. 2, No. 6, June 19, 2001.

"FDA Approves New Treatment for Crohn's Disease," FDA press release, October 3, 2001.

Gut, Vol. 49, pp. 199–202.

Konturek, P. C., et al. "Increased Prevalence of Helicobacter Pylori Infection in Patients with Celiac Disease," *American Journal of Gastroenterology*, Vol. 95, No. 12, December 2000.

Kumar, Vijay, et al. "Celiac Disease–Associated Autoimmune Endocrin-opathies," *Clinical and Diagnostic Laboratory Immunology*, Vol. 8, No. 4, pp. 678–685, July 2001.

Rose, Noel R., and MacKay, Ian R. (editors). *The Autoimmune Diseases*, 3rd edition, Academic Press, 1998.

Rowe, William A. "Inflammatory Bowel Disease," *eMedicine Journal*, Vol. 2, No. 8, August 3, 2001.

Sherman, Neil. "Death Rate Soars with Celiac Disease," *Health Scout News*, August 6, 2001, http://www.healthscoutnews.com.

"Study Confirms Link Between Left-Handed and IBD," Reuters Health Wire, July 12, 2001.

Yang, Vincent W. "Celiac Sprue," *eMedicine Journal*, Vol. 2, No. 3, March 12, 2001.

CHAPTER 9

Agachi, S. "The Pathology of the Thyroid Gland and Rheumatoid Arthritis in the Period of Onset," *Journal of Rheumatology*, Vol. 28, Supplement 63, 2001.

Arthritis Foundation website, publications section, http://www.arthritis. org/resources.

"B Lymphocyte Depletion Therapy," Presentation to the American College of Rheumatology Annual Meeting, November 2000.

Brent, Lawrence H. "Ankylosing Spondylitis and Undifferentiated Spondy-loarthropathy," *eMedicine Journal*, Vol. 2, No. 5, May 2, 2001.

Buckingham, Thomas. "EULAR: Combination Leflunomide/Methotrexate Effective and Well Tolerated in Rheumatoid Arthritis," *PeerView Press*, June 14, 2001.

Buckingham, Thomas. "EULAR: Clinically Relevant Infections Occurring with Rheumatoid Arthritis Therapies," *PeerView Press*, June 15, 2001.

Burge, D. J. "Enbrel (Etanercept) in Addition to Methotrexate (MTX) in Rheumatoid Arthritis: Long Term Observations," Abstract W122, *Journal of Rheumatology*, Vol. 28, Supplement 63, 2001.

"Drug Helps Arthritis, But Has Side Effects: Study." Reuters Health Wire, December 31, 2001.

Genovese, Mark, and Davis IV, John S. "Current Management of Rheumatoid Arthritis," *Hospital Practice,* Vol. 36, No. 2, February 15, 2001.

King, Randall. "Rheumatoid Arthritis," *eMedicine Journal*, Vol. 2, No. 9, September 6, 2001.

Koopman, William J. "Prospects for Autoimmune Disease: Research Advances in Rheumatoid Arthritis," *Journal of the American Medical Association,* Vol. 285, No. 5, February 7, 2001.

Marzo-Ortega, Helena, et al. "Minocycline Induced Autoimmune Disease in Rheumatoid Arthritis: A Missed Diagnosis?" *Journal of Rheumatology,* Vol. 28, p. 2, 2001.

Owen, Olwen Glynn. "EULAR: Early Referral Urged for Patients Suspected of Having Rheumatoid Arthritis," *PeerView Press,* June 14, 2001.

Pincus, T., et al. "Are Long-Term Very Low Doses of Prednisone for Patients with Rheumatoid Arthritis as Helpful as High Doses Are Harmful?" *Annals of Internal Medicine,* Vol. 136, pp. 76–78, January 2002.

"Rheumatoid Arthritis May Up Risk of Gum Infection," Reuters Health Wire, July 12, 2001.

Rose, Noel R., and MacKay, Ian R. (editors). *The Autoimmune Diseases,* 3rd edition, Academic Press, 1998.

Schorr, Melissa. "Decaf Coffee Linked to Rheumatoid Arthritis Risk," Reuters Health Wire, November 13, 2001.

Siegel-Itzkovich, Judy. "Common 'Bug' May Trigger Arthritis," *Jerusalem Post,* April 4, 2001.

Spencer-Green, G., et al. "Enbrel (Etanercept) vs. Methotrexate (MTX) in Early Rheumatoid Arthritis: Two Year Follow Up," Abstract W124, *Journal of Rheumatology,* Vol. 28, Supplement 63, 2001.

"The Best Arthritis Relief," *Prevention*, January 2001.

Wolfe, Frederick, et al. "Consensus Recommendations for the Assessment and Treatment of Rheumatoid Arthritis," *Journal of Rheumatology*, Vol. 28, No. 6, 2001.

CHAPTER 10

Fanion, David. "Guillain-Barré Syndrome," *eMedicine Journal*, Vol. 2, No. 5, May 7, 2001.

Hauser, Ross A. "The Holistic Physician, Multiple Sclerosis," *Alternative Medicine* online, http://www.alternativemedicine.com.

Lisse, Jeffrey R. "Raynaud Phenomenon," *eMedicine Journal*, Vol. 2, No. 6, June 28, 2001.

Mundell, E. J. "Curry Spice May Fight Multiple Sclerosis," *Reutershealth*. April 24, 2002.

Newton, Edward. "Myasthenia Gravis," *eMedicine Journal*, Vol. 2, No. 5, May 3, 2001.

Ravicz, Simone. *Thriving with Your Autoimmune Disorder*, New Harbinger, 2000.

"Researchers Hear Human Trials of Multiple Sclerosis Drug," Reuters. March 12, 2002.

Rich, Brian C. "Multiple Sclerosis," *AAEM Emergency Medical and Family Health Guide* online, http://www.emedicine.com/aaem/contents.html.

Rose, Noel R., and MacKay, Ian R. (editors). *The Autoimmune Diseases*, 3rd edition, Academic Press, 1998.

"Study Links Multiple Sclerosis, Mono," Associated Press, December 26, 2001.

CHAPTER 11

"Diabetes and Multiple Sclerosis Patients Share Common Autoantigens," Reuters Health Wire, March 5, 2001.

"Endometriosis May Be an Autoimmune Disease," *Fertility and Sterility,* August 2001.

"MCP Hahnemann University Researcher Reports Successful Treatment of Aplastic Anemia Opens Door for Treatment of All 80 Autoimmune Diseases," MCP Hahnemann University press release, October 5, 2001.

Winer, S., et al. "Type I Diabetes and Multiple Sclerosis Patients Target Islet Plus Central Nervous System Autoantigens," *Journal of Immunology,* Vol. 166, pp. 2831–2841, February 15, 2001.

CHAPTER 12

Atkins, Robert C. *Dr. Atkins' Vita-Nutrient Solution: Nature's Answer to Drugs,* Simon & Schuster, 1999.

Edman, Joel S. *Findings of the Annual Meeting of the American College of Nutrition,* 2001.

Fuhrman, Joel. *Fasting—and Eating—for Health: A Medical Doctor's Program for Conquering Disease,* Griffin, 1998.

Groppa, Liliana. "The Effectiveness of Wobenzym as the Basic Treatment of Rheumatoid Arthritis," *Journal of Rheumatology,* Abstract W107, Vol. 28, Supplement 63, 2001.

Horstman, Judith. "More Than Medicine," *Arthritis Today* online.

Landis, Robyn, and Khalsa, Karta Purkh Singh. *Herbal Defense: Positioning Yourself to Triumph Over Illness and Aging,* Warner Books, 1997.

Smith, Lendon. *Clinical Guide to the Use of Vitamin C,* Life Sciences Press, 1991.

Tillotson, Alan Keith, et al. *The One Earth Herbal Sourcebook: Everything You Need to Know About Chinese, Western, and Ayurvedic Herbal Treatments,* Kensington Publishing, 2001.

CHAPTER 13

American Academy of Periodontology news release, *Science Daily,* April 23, 2001.

Atkins, Robert D. *Dr. Atkins' Vita-Nutrient Solution: Nature's Answer to Drugs,* Simon & Schuster, 1999.

"Changing Diet Can Help Autoimmune Disease," Reuters Health Wire, May 2001.

Chiang, B. L., et al. "Enhancing Immunity by Dietary Consumption of a Probiotic Lactic Acid Bacterium (*Bifidobacterium lactis* HN019): Optimization and Definition of Cellular Immune Responses," *European Journal of Clinical Nutrition,* Vol. 54, No. 11, pp. 849–855, November 2000.

Cohen, L., et al. "DNA Repair Capacity in Healthy Medical Students During and After Exam Stress," *Journal of Behavioral Medicine,* Vol. 23, No. 6, pp. 531–544, December 2000.

"Complementary and Alternative Therapies for Arthritis," *Intelihealth* online, April 2001, http://www.intelihealth.com.

"Consuming More Protein, Less Carbohydrates May Be Healthier," *Science Daily,* April 5, 2001.

"Diabetes Prevention," *New England Journal of Medicine,* Vol. 345, 2001.

European Journal of Clinical Nutrition, Vol. 54, pp. 849–855, 2000.

Fodor, J. G., et al. "Prevention of Type 2 Diabetes Mellitus by Changes in Lifestyle," *New England Journal of Medicine,* Vol. 345, No. 9, August 30, 2001.

Ford, Gillian. *Listening to Your Hormones,* Prima Publishing, 1997.

"Friendly Bacteria May Lend a Hand to Immune System," Reuters Health Wire, December 26, 2000.

Fruchter, O. "Prevention of Type 2 Diabetes Mellitus by Changes in Lifestyle," *New England Journal of Medicine,* Vol. 345, No. 9, August 30, 2001.

"Healing a Woman with Lupus, Seizures, and Infertility," *Alternative Medicine* online, http://www.alternativemedicine.com/digest/issue22/22036R00.shtml.

Holmes, G. K. "Coeliac Disease and Type 1 Diabetes Mellitus—The Case for Screening," *Diabetes Medicine,* Vol. 18, No. 3, pp. 169–177, March 2001.

Jibrin, Janis. "The Good Carbs Amazing New Rx for Just About Everything," *Prevention,* May 2001.

Kalliomaki, M., et al. "Probiotics in Primary Prevention of Atopic Disease: A Randomised Placebo-Controlled Trial," *The Lancet,* Vol. 357, pp. 1076–1079, April 7, 2001.

Langer, Stephen, and Scheer, James F. *Solved: The Riddle of Weight Loss,* Inner Traditions Intl. Ltd., 1989.

Mondloch, M. V., et al. "Does How You Do Depend on How You Think You'll Do? A Systematic Review of the Evidence for a Relation Between Patients' Recovery Expectations and Health Outcomes," *Canadian Medical Association Journal,* Vol. 165, pp. 174–179, July 24, 2001.

"New Study, Sponsored by Nutrition 21, Inc. Finds Chromium Picolinate and Biotin Combination Can Control Blood Sugar Levels in Type 2 Diabetics," Nutrition 21, Inc., press release, October 5, 2001.

Norton, Amy. "Stress May Be Bad for the Genes," Reuters Health Wire, January 25, 2001.

Norton, Amy. " 'Good' Bacteria May Halt Allergies in Babies," Reuters Health Wire, April 6, 2001.

Olivier, Suzannah. "Food for the Brain: A Diet Rich in Oily Fish Helps to Fight a Host of Diseases," *The Times of London,* January 16, 2001.

"Researchers Find a Genetic Cause of Type 1 Diabetes and Autoimmunity," Washington University School of Medicine, http://medinfo.wustl.edu, December 8, 2000.

Seeman, Bruce Taylor. "Sick and Tired: Life stressing you out? Planning to take a break? Get ready to become ill," *Newhouse News Service,* December 2000.

Sellman, Sherrill. *Hormone Heresy: What Women Must Know About Their Hormones,* GetWell International, 2000.

Shikany, James M., et al. "Dietary Guidelines for Chronic Disease Prevention," *Southern Medical Journal,* Vol. 93, No. 12, pp. 1157–1161, 2000.

"The Case of Vitiligo," *Alternative Medicine* online, http//www.alternative medicine.com.

The Lancet, Vol. 357, pp. 1076–1079, April 7, 2001.

Vaporean, Carole. "Selenium Research Points to Curative Powers," Reuters Health Wire, June 20, 2001.

Weil, Andrew. "Diabetes: Prevention Works," *Self Healing,* August 2001.

CHAPTER 14

Angier, Natalie. "Studying the Autoimmune Disease Puzzle," *New York Times,* June 19, 2001.

Bailey, Steve. "Happy Thoughts May Prolong Life," Associated Press, May 7, 2001.

Benson, Herbert. "Medicine and Belief," *Diane Rehm Show* interview, WAMU Radio, 88.5 AM, Washington, DC, August 9, 2001.

"Depression May Slow Wound Healing," Reuters Health Wire, April 19, 2001.

Ferguson, Elaine R. "The Self-Healing Personality," *Alternative Medicine,* May 2001.

Ferguson, Elaine R. "Cancer Recovery: Mind-Body Techniques," *Alternative Medicine,* September 2001.

Fulton, Janet. "Fast, Steady Walking Better Than Short Bouts of Exercise," *Medicine & Science in Sports & Exercise,* Vol. 33, pp. 163–170, January 2001.

Hirano, Daichi, et al. "Serum Levels of Interleukin 6 and Stress Related Substances Indicate Mental Stress Condition in Patients with

Rheumatoid Arthritis," *Journal of Rheumatology,* Vol. 28, pp. 490–495, 2001.

"Is Meditation Good Medicine?" *Harvard Women's Health Watch,* January 2001.

Kiecolt-Glaser, J. K., Marucha, P. T., Atkinson, C., and Glaser, R. "Hypnosis as a Modulator of Cellular Immune Dysregulation During Acute Stress," *Journal of Consulting and Clinical Psychology,* Vol. 69, No. 4, pp. 674–682, August 2001.

Levin, Jeff. *God, Faith, and Health: Exploring the Spirituality-Healing Connection,* John Wiley & Sons, 2001.

"Managing Stress Depends on Learning Focus and Control," Cox News Service, January 31, 2001.

"Meditation Training Lessens Symptoms of Chronic Illnesses," Harvard Medical School website, August 30, 2001, http://www.hms.harvard.edu/webweekly.

Morin, Richard. "Calling Dr. God," *Washington Post,* July 8, 2001.

Olivier, Suzannah. "It's the Gut That Suffers," *The Times of London,* January 15, 2001.

"Self-Hypnosis May Cut Stress, Boost Immune System," Reuters Health Wire, October 2, 2001.

Simonton, O. Carl, et al. *Getting Well Again,* Bantam Paperbacks, 1978, reissued 1992.

Smyth, Joshua, et al. "Effects of Writing About Stressful Experiences on Symptom Reduction in Patients with Asthma or Rheumatoid Arthritis," *Journal of the American Medical Association,* Vol. 281, pp. 1304–1309, April 14, 1999.

Weil, Andrew. "Visualization and Guided Imagery Explained," *Self Healing,* March 2001.

Yirmiya, Raz. "Depression in Medical Illness: The Role of the Immune System," *Western Journal of Medicine,* Vol. 173, No. 5, pp. 333–336, 2000.

CHAPTER 15

"Fast, Steady Walking Better Than Short Bouts of Exercise," *Med Sci Sports Exercise,* Vol. 33, pp. 163–170, January 2001.

LeShan, Lawrence. *Cancer as a Turning Point: A Handbook for People with Cancer, Their Families, and Health Professionals,* Plume, 1989, reissued 1999.

"Natural Energy Boosters," *Alternative Medicine,* January 15, 2001, http://www.alternativemedicine.com.

Reichenberg, Abraham, et al. *Archives of General Psychiatry,* Vol. 8, pp. 445–452, 2001.

Saltsman, Kirstie. "Is Bacterial Infection Carcinogenic?" *Biomednet* online, February 2, 2001, Issue 95.

"Undiagnosed Coeliac Disease and Risk of Autoimmune Disorders in Subjects with Type I Diabetes Mellitus," *Diabetologia,* Abstract Volume 44, Issue 2, pp. 151–155, 2001.

Walker, W. A., and Isselbacher, K. J. "Uptake and Transport of Macromolecular Proteins by the Intestine: Possible Role in Clinical Disorders," *Gastroenterology,* Vol. 67, p. 531, 1974.

Warshaw, A. L., et al. "Intestinal Absorption of Intake Antigenic Protein," *Surgery,* Vol. 76, No. 3, p. 567, 1974.

CHAPTER 16

"Doctors from Venus and Mars: How They Differ," *Harvard Health Letter,* Vol. 26, No. 7, May 2001.

Kristiansen, I. S., et al. "Threats from Patients and Their Effects on Medical Decision Making: A Cross-Sectional, Randomised Trial," *The Lancet,* Vol. 357, pp. 1258–1261, April 2001.

Savard, Marie. *How to Save Your Own Life: The Savard System for Managing—and Controlling—Your Health Care,* Warner Books, 2000.

Savard, Marie. *The Savard Health Record: A Six-Step System for Managing Your Healthcare,* Time Life, 2000.

Weil, Andrew. "Men's Health at Midlife," *Self Healing,* June 2001.

Weil, Andrew. "Making the Most of Your Office Visit," *Self Healing,* July 2001.

CHAPTER 17

LeShan, Lawrence. *Cancer as a Turning Point: A Handbook for People with Cancer, Their Families, and Health Professionals,* Plume, 1999.

INDEX